The Best Friends Staff

Additional titles available on Best Friends™ care practices

The Best Friends Book of Alzheimer's Activities
Volume One
Volume Two
by Virginia Bell, David Troxel,
Tonya Cox & Robin Hamon

The Best Friends Approach to Alzheimer's Care
by Virginia Bell & David Troxel

Los Mejores Amigos en el Cuidado de Alzheimer
The Best Friends Approach to Alzheimer's Care
(in Spanish)

Best Friends (DVD)
produced by the Greater Kentucky & Southern Indiana
Alzheimer's Association

For additional information on the Best Friends™ approach,
visit **www.bestfriendsapproach.com**

The Best Friends Staff

Building a Culture of Care in Alzheimer's Programs

Virginia Bell, M.S.W.
and
David Troxel, M.P.H.

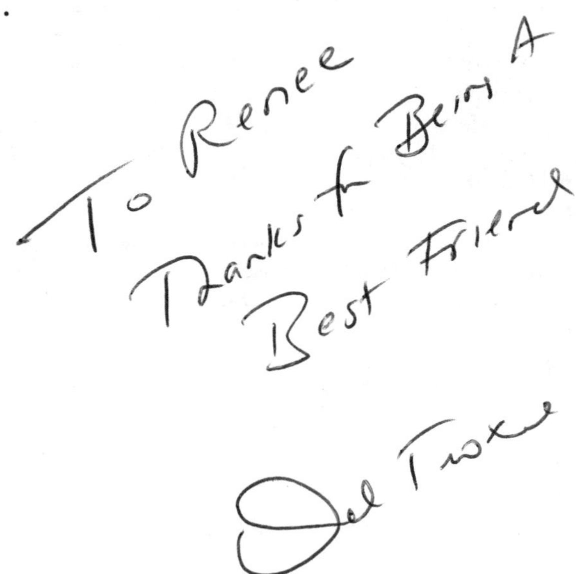

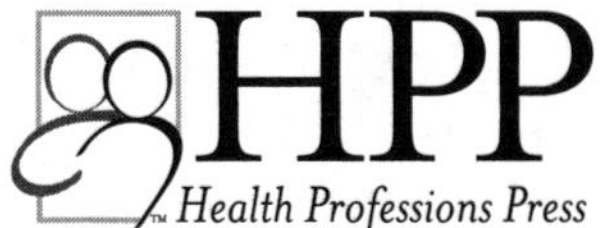

Baltimore • London • Sydney

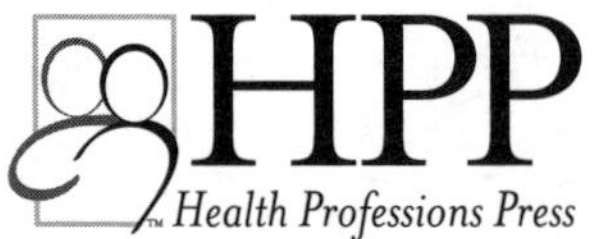

Health Professions Press, Inc.
Post Office Box 10624
Baltimore, Maryland 21285-0624

www.healthpropress.com

Second printing, October 2001
Third printing, February 2004
Fourth printing, May 2006
Fifth printing, July 2007
Sixth printing, September 2010

Typesetting by Barton, Matheson, Willse & Worthington, Baltimore, Maryland.
Manufactured in the United States of America by Versa Press, Inc., East Peoria, Illinois.
Line drawings on pages 57, 60–62, 84, and 205 were created by Robin Hamon Kern.

Names and affiliations mentioned in *The Best Friends Staff* were current as of June 2000, but may change over time. In addition, because website addresses change frequently, some of the addresses provided in this volume may not be valid. If you get a 404 or error message, try an Internet search engine or directory to search for the organization by name.

Library of Congress Cataloging-in-Publication Data

Bell, Virginia.
The best friends staff : building a culture of care in Alzheimer's programs / Virginia Bell and David Troxel.
p. cm.
Includes bibliographical references and index.
ISBN 1-878812-63-7
1. Alzheimer's disease—Patients—Long-term care. I. Troxel, David. II. Title.

RC523.B433 2000
362.1'96831—dc21 00-053954

British Cataloguing in Publication Data are available from the British Library.

Contents

Training Tool Kits

Acknowledgments

The authors thank the following programs for their contributions of stories and material for the book: ADCare, LifeSpan Services Network, Inc.: Betty Woolslayer, Barri Dymott, Pam Richards; Alzheimer's Care at Aspen Ridge: Gail Gardiner, Susan Maxwell Jones; Alzheimer's Four Seasons: Dana E. Newquist; The Breckinridge: Solomon Lee Van Meter, Marie B. Smart; Care Club of Collier County, Inc.: LuAnne Dupree Wahlstrom, Terry Elder; Carilion Adult Day Center: Carla Groff; Carinya Village Nursing Home, Churches of Christ Homes and Community Services, Inc.: Lesley Polmear, Barbara Susan Dicker; Christian Health Center, Christian Church Homes of Kentucky: Jerry Rogers; Christiana Care, Visiting Nurse Association, Evergreen Center I, Alzheimer's Day Treatment Program: Cheryl T. Weidemeyer, Carol M. Shelly; Eden Pines: Hannah Herward; Encore Senior Living, Rediscovery™ Program: Delores M. Moyer; The Fountains Continuum of Care, Inc.: Diane Will, Robin Henson; The Fountainview Center for Alzheimer's Disease: William M. Small, Jr., Linda Kimball, Kay Lloyd, Vioris Thomas, Yvonne Prosper, Mariegold Brown, Susan W. Muse, Stacy Colna, Shirley Miller, Janice Makonnen, Ann M. Helmly, Martha Shattuck, Deanna R. Pham; Friendship Adult Day Care Center: Heidi S. Holly; Haven Nursing Center: Jennifer Raeis; Helping Hand Day Center, Lexington/Bluegrass chapter, Alzheimer's Association: Tonya M. Tincher, Gwen Hutchinson, Laurie Simpson; Heritage Court, The Samarkand Retirement Community: Steven Paul Anderson, Ann Cox, Val Maxey; The Homestead, Hennis Care Center of Bolivar: David Hennis, Steven Pleili, Kari Staron; Hotel Pawnee, A Retirement Residence, the Urban Group: Bob and Alyce Parsons; Karrington Cottages, a Sunrise Assisted Living Community: Linda R. O'Connor, Barbara Lawrence; Laurel Heights Home for the Elderly: Kathey Young, Karen Wyan, Buffey Nichols, Carol Miller, Laura Stewart, Irene Brummett, Dorothy Bailey, Carol Gregory, Milton Kidd, Beulah Lincks, Jennifer Callansa, Candy Smith, Tracy Brown, Wilma McDowell; Leena's Home (Leenankoti): Leena Qvick, Paivi Voutilainen; Legacy St. Aidan's Place Daycare: Terrye Alexander; Liberty Commons Assisted Living, Liberty Healthcare Management Services, Inc.: Cindy Stancil; Margolic Psychogeriatric Center, Tel Aviv Medical Center: Debi Lahav; The Olive Branch Senior Care Center: Mary Jane Eiland; Omahanui Private Hospital: Patricia Wesley, Glennie Muir; Pinegrove Special Care, Vista Del Monte: Jeanne M. West, Rosemarie Harris; Porterville Senior Day Care: Cheri Taylor; Riverside Adult Day Program, Christiana Care Health Services: Gayle Pennington; St. Basil's Homes: Judith Montano, Sue Haroulis, Margaret Ryan; Serenity Nursing Home: Michael Livni; Sunshine Terrace Adult Day Center: Bonnie Baird Smith; Toca das Horttensias: Lilian Alicke; Villa Alamar: Bernard MacElhenny, Jr., Jackie Marston, Barbara Garman; Villa Bella Residential Alzheimer's Care Center: Ray and Faith Stazzoni, Tom Henry; The Wealshire: Carly R. Hellen; Wellington Parc of Owensboro: Holly Cecil, Susan Cecil, Stephanie K. Wilkerson; West Park Long Term Care Center: Jeanne Kaiser, Gerry Jenson, Kelli Martin, Lisa Snyder.

The authors also thank the individuals working in the field of Alzheimer's disease care and services for their contributions to this book: Joyce Beedle, Cynthia Belle, Susan D. Berry, Linda Blair, Elizabeth C. Brawley, Carole A. Bromgard, Dee Carlson, Leslie Congleton, Barbara Susan Dicker, Deborah Dunn, Mynga Futrell, Meredith Gresham, Lisa Gwyther, Carly R. Hellen, Robin Hamon Kern, Kathy Laurenhue, Cindy Lynch, Debbie McConnell, Briana Melom, Susan Peters Rachal, Joanne Rader, Carolyn Read, Lynn Ritter, Beverly Sanborn, Vicki L. Schmall, Dorothy Seman, Marie B. Smart, Beth Spencer, Virginia M. Sponsler, Tonya M. Tincher, and Jitka M. Zgola. For their assistance with Chapter 3, thanks are due to Robert Barrett, Ph.D., and Robert Harbaugh, M.D.

Thanks go to the following colleagues in the Senior and Disabled Services Division, State of Oregon, who were part of a statewide initiative to adopt the Best Friends model for providers.

From the State of Oregon Dementia Education Initiative: Megan Hornby, Kathryn Labadie, Anne Laporte, Rita Litwiller, Allison McKenzie, Linda Nickolisen, Wendy Sampels, and Gini Shaw.

Finally, a few personal acknowledgments:

From both authors—Thanks to our longtime supporters Elayne Brill, Claire Macfarlane, and Maggy Patterson and our editor at Health Professions Press, Mary Magnus, for her support and stewardship of this project. We also acknowledge our many friends and colleagues throughout the Alzheimer's Association network in the United States and Alzheimer's Disease International.

From Virginia Bell—Thanks to the Board of Directors and staff of the Lexington/Bluegrass chapter of the Alzheimer's Association, Kathy Riley, President, and staff Michael Smith, Tonya Tincher, Helen Kientz, Gwen Hutchinson, Laurie Simpson, and Ron Alpern; the volunteers in the Helping Hand Day Center; my husband, Wayne, and children, grandchildren, and great-grandchildren.

From David Troxel—Thanks to the Board of Directors and staff of the Santa Barbara chapter of the Alzheimer's Association, Lawrence Sorensen, President, and staff Marge Collins, Deborah Dunn, Debbie McConnell, Cindy Matsumura, Judy J. Miller, Cynthia Thompson, Dianne Timmerman, Anna Marie Weiner, and Donna Wick; my parents Fred and Dorothy Troxel, Harold and Joan Jorgensen, and Ronald Spingarn.

Rebecca Matheny Riley, 1925–1999

Rebecca was a devoted daughter, sister, wife, mother, grandmother, nurse, volunteer, professor, and good friend. Woven through all of her roles in life is a common thread: Rebecca was always a teacher. She probably did her best teaching after she was diagnosed with Alzheimer's disease. Rebecca was determined to make a difference. She enrolled in research studies to help find the cause of the disease, and she taught everyone who would listen what it was like to live in the world of Alzheimer's disease.

Rebecca, this book is dedicated to you, the first to teach us about this strange world. You are more than a memory. You live on in the lives of your many students all around the world.

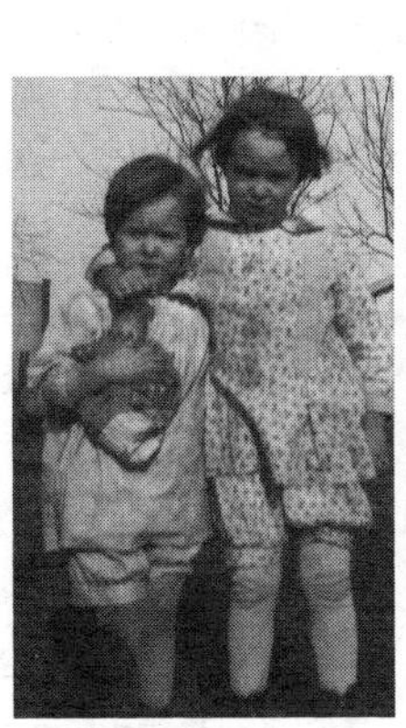
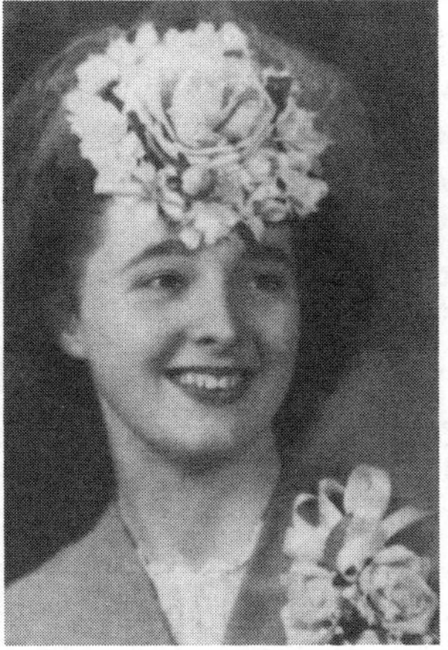
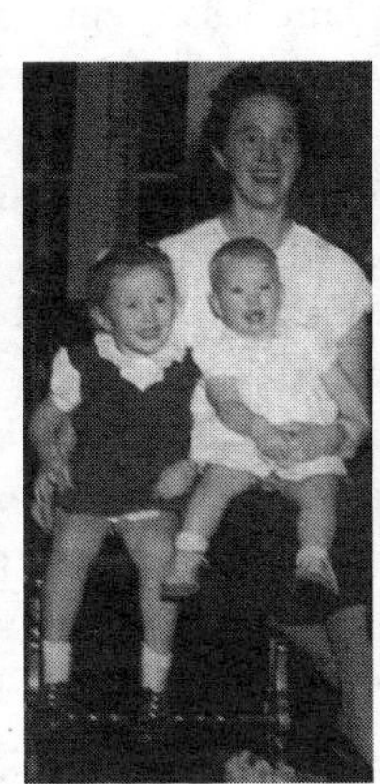
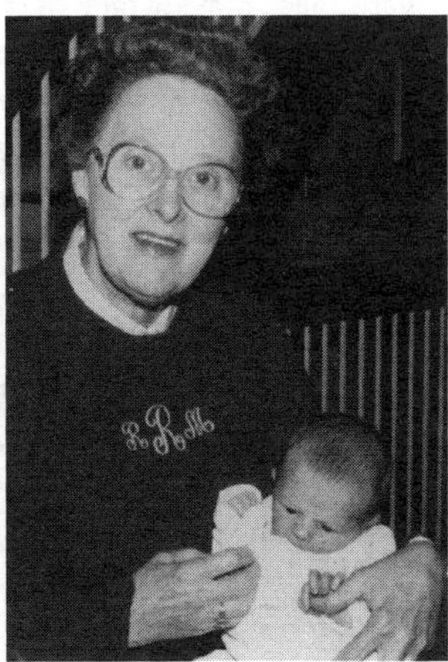
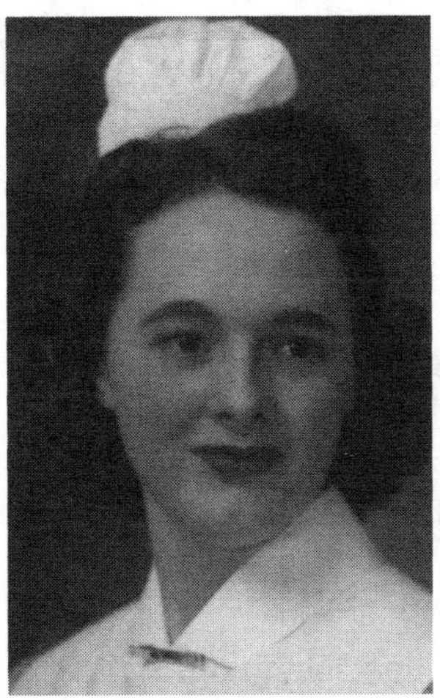
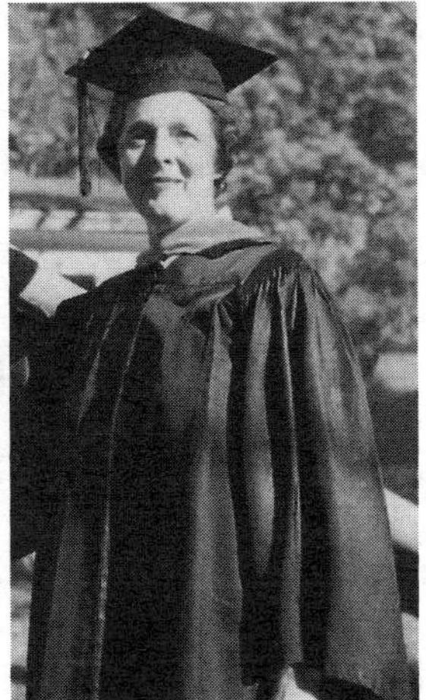
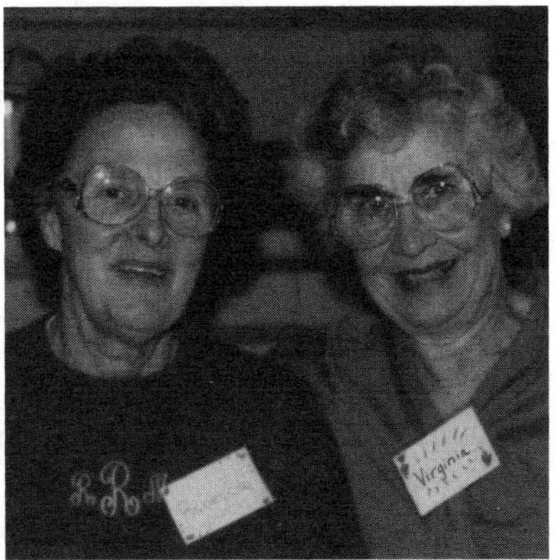

Introduction

The publication of *The Best Friends Approach to Alzheimer's Care* in 1997 introduced a model of care for *persons* with Alzheimer's disease and related disorders. Life affirming and hopeful, the Best Friends model offers new ways to solve old problems. The book argues that there is another face to Alzheimer's disease. Family and professional caregivers can learn better ways to respond to the *person* with dementia. Problem behaviors can be understood, reduced, and even prevented. Quality of life for the *person* with dementia can be improved. Caregivers can survive this illness. Long-term care communities can develop effective, outstanding programs. These improvements can be accomplished with a simple caregiving philosophy—what *persons* with Alzheimer's disease need most of all is a good friend, a Best Friend.

Families told the authors that the Best Friends approach helped them recast their relationships with loved ones. Because of the nature of Alzheimer's disease, the *person* with the disease eventually may forget a family member's name or even the exact nature of the relationship. Recasting relationships helps families accept this change; for example, they may no longer be recognized as a spouse but now can be recognized as a friend. Families also learn that the disease would not change; therefore, they had to change. They realized that they could survive the illness by learning caregiving techniques and skills, taking advantage of community services, and taking care of themselves.

Persons with early Alzheimer's disease told the authors that the Best Friends approach helped them better understand their situation. Participants in early-stage Alzheimer's support groups used the book in their sessions to talk about their feelings and share their hopes and fears about their futures. A woman with Alzheimer's disease, Ruth McReynolds, was one of the first readers of *The Best Friends Approach to Alzheimer's Care*. She took the book with her when she moved to a residential community specializing in Alzheimer's disease care, Villa Alamar, in Santa Barbara, California. She said, "This book helps me accept what I have. I even know one of the writers ... he's a friend." After a year at Villa Alamar she returned to Hawaii to be with her husband Dale as he died of cancer. Despite her diagnosis of Alzheimer's disease, Ruth was able to be a loving and helpful partner to him.

Professionals saw immediate possibilities in the Best Friends model for long-term care programs. The State of Oregon's Senior and Disabled Services Division endorsed Best Friends as its recommended statewide model for dementia care training. Maine named Best Friends as a best practice. Long-term care programs across the United States and elsewhere began to adopt the book's philosophy and to adapt the model for staff development and client programming. Here are some examples:

- Karen Wyan, assistant administrator at Laurel Heights Home for the Elderly in London, Kentucky, discovered that the Best Friends approach is "a simple approach that all staff can understand ... it really works, preventing challenging behaviors from developing out of loneliness, boredom, worry, helplessness, even loss of memory."
- After using the Best Friends philosophy for more than a year, Michael Livni, administrator, Serenity Nursing Home, Johannesburg, South Africa, reported, "The Best Friends program strengthens patient care and staff morale."
- LuAnne Walstrom, director of the Care Club of Collier County in Naples, Florida, believes that the Best Friends approach "reduces the incidence of catastrophic reactions and behav-

ioral outbursts. The philosophy has also helped develop a strong bond of trust between participants and staff."

- The Urban Group, the parent company of Hotel Pawnee, A Retirement Residence, in North Platte, Nebraska, made the book its Bible for training. New staff read and discuss each chapter of the book. Alyce Parsons, managing partner, noted, "Once they complete the book and implement the Best Friends approach into their work, we even give them a raise!"
- William M. Small, Jr., president and owner of The Fountainview Center for Alzheimer's Disease in Atlanta, Georgia, wrote, "the Best Friends concept has been most beneficial to our organization ... [It] touches on virtually every facet of our approach to Alzheimer's care."

Clearly, this model is striking a chord with many programs looking for new approaches to the challenges of Alzheimer's care. These professionals and others working in long-term settings emailed and telephoned the authors requesting more tools to help them develop Best Friends programs. This encouraged the authors to write the present book.

The Best Friends Approach to Alzheimer's Care was written for families and professionals. *The Best Friends Staff: Building a Culture of Care in Alzheimer's Programs* is directed primarily at professionals working in long-term care settings. The goal of this book is to help program leaders develop a dementia-capable staff, one that is knowledgeable about the disease, is sympathetic to the world of its residents or program participants, has a sense of fun and joy, thinks on its feet; and is dedicated to preserving dignity and enhancing quality of life for *persons* with dementia. These are the qualities of a Best Friends staff.

This book also discusses the challenge of staffing long-term care programs in the competitive and challenging job market for employers: How do you attract good line staff today, train them, and keep them? How do we retain talented leadership when news headlines frequently highlight resident neglect and million-dollar lawsuits? Although the challenges are daunting, Best Friends programs will have the greatest chance at overcoming these obstacles and changing the culture of care.

A 1997 report from a nursing facility advocates meeting in Rochester, New York, defined culture as "an organic, ongoing process that has potential for change, growth and development. There are no culprits—good guys and bad guys. Rather, there is the presence, or not, of vision, energy, and perseverance and a willingness to nurture and support one another in these change efforts." This statement reflects the philosophy of a group calling themselves "Pioneers" (see Appendix C) that have taken on the mission of changing the culture of care in long-term care. The authors embrace their definition of culture and change: Now is not the time to point fingers and assign blame; now is the time to look for new and creative ideas, to identify common goals, and to be supportive of one another as we search for enhanced job satisfaction and new models of care.

The authors have written this book for a wide audience of individuals working in long-term care settings including in-home services, adult day center care, assisted living, and skilled care. The book also may be helpful for caregivers who want to know more about issues surrounding staff training and development. Specifically:

- *Program administrators* will learn how the Best Friends model can improve client, family, and staff satisfaction. The model makes the case that training a Best Friends staff is a good investment, improving census, reducing staff turnover, and having a positive impact on "the bottom line."
- *Staff trainers or developers* will discover easy-to-use materials and programs for initial staff orientation, ongoing training, and reinforcement of lessons. Handouts, worksheets, and exercises are provided that can be copied or adapted and used in training programs and classes. The book is not a curriculum, but it does offer a framework for staff to do their work not only with skill but also with purpose and satisfaction.

- *Activities staff* will appreciate the book's philosophy that all staff who come into contact with residents or participants have a role in activities. A Best Friends program not only enriches group activities but it also encourages living between structured activities and suggests ways to make this happen. Also important, the book encourages staff to bring their own interests, hobbies, and avocations into the activity program.
- *Clinical staff* who read this book will appreciate the book's view that learning the basics of the medical and scientific aspects of dementia is important for all staff. The value of a thorough medical assessment and the importance of ongoing medical care are discussed. The book also demonstrates the value of behavioral approaches, which when combined with good medical care, promote optimal health.
- *Architects and designers,* who play such an important role in creating dementia-friendly environments, will find that this book gives them and their clients important tools for a program philosophy on which to build their designs and plans. Best Friends programs partner with these professionals to build and create a winning design.
- *Volunteer coordinators* will find that the Best Friends model helps programs expand their volunteer base. This book champions the role of volunteers in dementia care; any program can develop effective programs in this area. Notably, the book suggests that volunteers can be particularly effective when matched one-to-one with *persons* with dementia. They also can play a role in group activity programs. Because their work becomes more meaningful, volunteers are always more attracted to Best Friends programs.
- *Students* often are required to get experiential learning or to engage in community service as part of their educational programs. This book is a good resource for students, teachers, and program leaders designing hands-on learning programs. It also can be used as a textbook in gerontology and long-term care courses.
- *Family members* will discover that this book encourages them to be a partner with the long-term care community or day center serving their loved ones. Although the book is written for a professional audience, it is not technical. Families can feel comfortable mining the book for ideas that cover all aspects of Alzheimer's care, and staff should share relevant sections of the book with families.
- *Others* who work in or have an interest in long-term care, including individuals in Alzheimer's Association chapters, public policy settings, geriatric care management firms, ombudsman programs, faith communities, service and community clubs, and university or educational settings, will find that this book challenges many conventional notions about staff development and programming. New and long-established programs also will benefit. The authors hope that *The Best Friends Staff* will provide readers with inspiration and ideas to build and support better programs in this growing and dynamic sector of long-term care.

One notable concept used in *The Best Friends Approach to Alzheimer's Care* appears again in *The Best Friends Staff.* To illustrate certain concepts, the first book told true stories of almost 50 *persons* diagnosed with Alzheimer's disease. Instead of composite stories or fictitious examples, the identity and brief biography of every *person* was disclosed, and written permission was received from the *person* or a responsible party.

In *The Best Friends Staff* more than 35 long-term care programs are identified that have either adopted or embody the Best Friends approach. Also, 30 professionals and consultants in the field of dementia care from around the world have shared their experiences. They lend the material authenticity, allow the reader to benefit from the expertise of others, and give individuals interested in staff development people with whom to network. These contributors are listed in the

Acknowledgments and in Appendixes A and B. *The Best Friends Staff* was written as a companion volume to *The Best Friends Approach to Alzheimer's Care* but can stand alone. The first book is particularly helpful to family members or staff who are seeking more information about this approach to care.

Chapter 1 reviews the Best Friends model. The Alzheimer's Disease Bill of Rights is presented along with an overview of the model and introduction to one of the core concepts, the knack. Knack is the art of doing difficult things with ease, the art of using clever tricks or strategies to solve problems. Knack is what the Best Friends staff should embody. The elements of caregiving knack are listed along with examples of knack from many programs in the United States and other countries.

Chapter 2 discusses staff recruitment and development in an always-challenging labor market. One administrator at a national conference said with exasperation that the job market is so competitive in her area that she just needs "warm bodies" to show up to provide care. The need for creative recruitment and staff training and development is greater than ever before. The Best Friends approach incorporates experiential and interactive learning. It is a perfect vehicle for helping staff become empowered, to help them succeed as individuals and as employees. Just because a program starts with warm bodies does not mean that it cannot end up with warm hearts.

Chapter 3 discusses how to train staff members in the basics of the medical and research issues surrounding dementia. The chapter offers some key concepts that need to be taught to staff and suggests that the Best Friends staff must have a solid grounding in dementia care. This knowledge base should be sustained with continuing education opportunities, newsletter subscriptions, and appropriate Internet access. Still, the chapter notes that the basics of the medical and research issues surrounding dementia sometimes are taught at the expense of other topics. A balance must be struck.

Chapter 4 reveals the critical importance of teaching staff to empathize with the *person* in their care. Until staff members learn to "walk a mile in the shoes" of the *person* with Alzheimer's disease, high-quality care is not possible. Staff can also teach families this important lesson. This chapter offers a number of valuable exercises that will help staff grasp that Alzheimer's disease is as real as a broken leg or arthritis.

Chapter 5 argues that the assessment of individuals with Alzheimer's disease should be strengths-based rather than focus on disability and loss. Careful assessment allows Best Friends staff members to set appropriate expectations that can guide their overall care plan and their daily interactions. This chapter teaches staff members to think on their feet and to "stop, look, and listen" on a daily basis when caring for *persons* with dementia.

Chapter 6 goes to the heart of the Best Friends model. When staff members explore their own attitudes toward friendship, they can begin to be a Best Friend to the *person* in their care. This chapter demonstrates that the program philosophy of Best Friends is multicultural and one that speaks to staff of varying educational backgrounds. Everyone has the potential to be a Best Friend.

Chapter 7 describes how Best Friends programs can improve the social histories ("the life story") of its residents and participants. The chapter discusses techniques that encourage staff members and volunteers to learn and use these stories. The chapter concludes that good programs use facts from the person's life story regularly, including their values, traditions, and beliefs, to enhance all aspects of care.

Chapter 8 puts a new spin on one of the most critical topics of staff training—communication. *Persons* with dementia retain the desire to communicate. This chapter discusses how to teach staff effective methods of nonverbal and verbal communication. Some communication is possible with almost every *person* with dementia.

Chapter 9 helps program leaders develop strategies to greatly enrich and expand activity programming. The Best Friends model insists that every interaction be an activity and that all staff should think in these terms. For a Best Friends staff, activities can be spontaneous and inexpensive. Personal care also can be transformed into an activity rather than framed as a chore or task.

Chapter 10 discusses family issues surrounding Alzheimer's disease that can have an impact on staff. In general, families respond favorably to the improved ambiance and morale of a Best Friends program. This chapter focuses attention on how staff members learn to listen to families, understand boundaries, and help families move from denial to acceptance.

The Conclusion demonstrates the ultimate link between staff development and programming in long-term care communities or day centers, noting that the goals are surprisingly similar. The Best Friends approach creates a caring community in which staff members feel challenged, enjoy their work, and build their careers. At the same time, it benefits all aspects of care for *persons* with dementia, whatever the care setting.

A number of quotations appear in the margins of most of the chapters and provide commentary or complementary examples of the concepts being discussed in that chapter. The authors hope that these quotations from staff members, *persons* with dementia and family members, and famous writers will speak to the reader and provide another tool for relating the material in the book to the reader's own work situation.

At the end of Chapters 2 through 10, a Training Tool Kit is presented to help readers learn and teach concepts from the specific chapter. These sections contain a variety of materials that can be copied or adapted for quick-and-easy training programs. The tools were developed by the authors and long-term care professionals from around the world. The elements of each Tool Kit include the following:

Warm-ups—These suggested exercises can be used to begin each training class to focus staff attention on the task at hand, work as a team, and even have a few laughs. Sometimes just taking several minutes for a funny story, joke, or a group exercise can build a sense of togetherness in staff. These activities are often called "icebreakers," but the authors prefer the more friendly image of "warm-ups."

Program Pointers—These handouts, checklists, originals for transparencies, articles for bulletin boards or newsletters, and other items can build a Best Friends program. Program leaders can use them as they are or adapt them for their own facilities.

Games for Learning—These group activities or games reinforce the material covered in the chapter. They also help staff work with the concepts being taught and make them their own. This is active learning at its best.

Knack and No-Knack Exercises—These exercises feature a series of statements/myths about Alzheimer's care that the group leader can discuss with staff. They also can serve as the basis of fun role-play skits that can be acted out for staff discussion and learning.

In reading the book, note the following:

1. Although this book addresses Alzheimer's disease, the concepts apply to the care of any individual with an irreversible dementing disorder. Thus, individuals with multi-infarct dementia (multiple strokes), Parkinson's disease, frontotemporal dementia, Lewy body disease, or other irreversible dementias can benefit from the Best Friends model.
2. The authors use the term *long-term care* to discuss support programs across the continuum of care, from in-home services to residential skilled nursing care.
3. The authors have adopted the terms *long-term care communities, residential care communities,* or *communities* to describe any independent living, assisted living, board and care home, or residential or skilled facility caring for *persons* with dementia. The term *adult day centers*

describes adult day care programs. Sometimes the word *program* is used to describe situations that apply to any long-term care setting.

4. Family members are called *caregivers* in this book. Professionals provide caring support, but this term is more commonly applied to family members.
5. The authors use the word *staff* to describe all members of the team who work in long-term care programs or settings. The terms *line staff, staff member,* or *certified nursing assistants (CNAs)* are used to describe the hands-on, direct care workers who perform much of the personal care in residential communities. The term *activities staff* is used to describe staff members who organize activities as their primary job function. Other titles commonly used in this book include Administrator, Director of Nursing, Licensed Practical Nurse (LPN), Director of Activities, and Director of Staff Development. When discussing these supervisory and management positions, the authors use the term *program leader.*
6. Individuals in long-term care communities are called *residents,* and people in adult day centers are referred to as *participants.*
7. Writers often struggle with the question of how to describe the man or woman with dementia. The authors reject labels such as "Alzheimer's victim," "memory-affected individual," and "Alzheimer's person" because these terms collapse the *person* into the pathology of the disease. The word *patient* should be applied only in settings in which an individual is being attended to by a medical professional. Labels such as "the person with Alzheimer's disease," "those with dementia," and "the person with memory loss" are bulky and laborious for readers. This book uses the italicized *person* to describe an individual with Alzheimer's disease or a related dementia. The authors hope that this designation will be more economical for readers. At the same time, the term gently reminds us that there is a person beneath the cloak of dementia—one who has feelings, one who has led a life full of rich experiences, and one who deserves dignified care.

I

The Best Friends Model

The authors began developing the Best Friends model as they visited adult day centers throughout the United States in the 1980s. These centers provided some of the first specific programs for *persons* with dementia and largely preceded the national movement for dementia special care units in residential care communities. These programs have been the laboratories for learning about dementia care.

The authors worked in the 1980s with the University of Kentucky Alzheimer's Disease Research Center and the Lexington/Bluegrass chapter of the Alzheimer's Association to develop an adult day center, the Helping Hand Day Center. The program was an immediate success when it opened in 1984, and 4 years later it received one of the first Robert Wood Johnson Foundation grants supporting adult day center care. This nationally recognized model program operates 6 days a week, with more than 150 volunteers who provide one-to-one care under professional supervision.

The authors' experience in adult day center settings led to a number of conclusions. First, these programs care successfully for many *persons* with Alzheimer's disease whose own families label them "difficult," even "impossible." It seems that the ambiance and programming of most centers evoke the amazingly intact social graces of the *person* with dementia. Manners and customs learned in childhood seem to remain intact; thus, *persons* work harder, try harder, and, in general, exhibit better behavior in front of "friends" and "company."

In outstanding programs there was a sense of give and take, equality, and fun. It was as if a group of friends had gathered to spend the day together. There was no "us" and "them." In fact, on more than one occasion, the authors mistook some staff members and volunteers for participants and some participants for staff members and volunteers. The authors learned that a strong relationship exists between good friendship and the best Alzheimer's care.

This work in adult day centers helped the authors develop a philosophy of care that forms the foundation for the Best Friends model that is described later in this chapter.

In good dementia care:

Language matters—The language of the past, when *persons* with Alzheimer's disease were described as *victims* or *ghosts,* has been replaced with more positive and life-affirming words such as *person.* When language is employed that objectifies or victimizes the *person* (and caregivers), it negatively affects staff attitudes. If he or she is indeed "gone," then why bother with efforts to provide good care? The Best Friends staff are deliberate about language and employ a positive vocabulary.

Care should be person *centered*—The individual with Alzheimer's disease should be treated as individuals without Alzheimer's disease would want to be treated if this had happened to them. *Persons* have all of the same feelings and emotions as do individuals without Alzheimer's disease. Good care stems from a philosophy that the *person* has value, has feelings that need recognition, and has a spirit that needs nourishing.

When you've met one person *with Alzheimer's disease, you've met just one* person *with Alzheimer's disease*—Each *person* with Alzheimer's disease seems to follow his or her own path when it comes to the course of the illness. Some individuals lose language skills early and others remain reasonably articulate for years. Some *persons* become very demented over a short course of time; others have a decades-long experience with the disease. Ultimately, the authors believe that each *person* has his or her own individual remaining strengths and that Alzheimer's disease should be looked at as more of a continuum than a series of proscribed stages.

With good Alzheimer's care, it is not necessarily what you do, it is in the doing—Dementia care cannot be taught strictly through laundry lists of "do's and don'ts"; staff cannot memorize the best way to respond to every situation. Staff members need to develop empathy for their participants or residents while they learn ways of dealing naturally with situations as they arise. Problem-solving skills used morning, noon, and night also are essential. For example, a well-trained Best Friends staff member might spend some time with an anxious day center participant, empathize with his or her feelings, determine the problem, and then make things better by telling a story from the *person's* past and starting a favorite activity to provide an appropriate distraction.

The following summarizes the Best Friends model as seen in Figure 1.1. The model describes a way of thinking about Alzheimer's disease that redefines dementia care. Each chapter that follows expands on this basic summary, to give program leaders ideas and tools for helping employees and volunteers learn and embrace the Best Friends model.

To be a Best Friend to a *person* with dementia, one must:

Empathize with and understand the experience of Alzheimer's disease—Best Friends staff members always "walk a mile in the *person's* shoes." Good care is possible only when staff members imagine what it would be like to have dementia. This means taking thoughtful time to understand the losses that are experienced by those for whom they care. The Best Friends staff recognize that many behaviors that at first seem strange and unsettling can be understood. Often, the behaviors are the result of the *person's* trying to make sense of and cope with his or her world.

Know the basics of the medical and scientific aspects of Alzheimer's disease—Best Friends staff members do not need expertise in all medical and scientific aspects of the disease. They do need to understand the basics. For example, knowing that Alzheimer's disease typically unfolds over an extended period of time can cue an alert certified nursing assistant (CNA) that a sudden change in behavior might be the result of a treatable medical condition, such as an infection or dehydration. The basics of the medical and scientific aspects are the building blocks for the development of caregiving skills—what line staff most need.

Invest time in an initial and ongoing strengths-based assessment—Best Friends staff members engage in the assessment process to complete a comprehensive evaluation of the resident or participant. It should always be strengths based, focusing on what the *person* can still do rather than the losses that he or she has experienced. A Best Friends staff member continually "checks the daily traffic," by observing the *person's* moods, actions, words, and expressions. A good evaluation coupled with keen observation help staff to avoid setting expectations too high (inviting failure) or too low (reducing self-esteem and function).

Support basic rights for the person *with dementia*—Best Friends staff members support the goals that are outlined in the Alzheimer's Disease Bill of Rights (see Figure 1.2). Written by the authors in 1994, this document has been translated into more than a dozen languages; many long-term care programs and even some national and local Alzheimer's Associations have adopted it. It provides programs with a simple and clear set of goals for providing high-quality care while preserving resident or participant rights.

Know the person's *life story very well*—Best Friends staff members thoroughly study and learn the life history, values, attitudes, and traditions of the *persons* for whom they care. Well-informed staff can use this biographical information in every area of care, including understanding behaviors, providing clues and cues for conversation, designing appropriate activities, and avoiding catastrophic reactions.

Apply the qualities and lessons of friendship—Best Friends staff members understand that the elements of friendship, when put into play, evoke intact social graces and allow staff to relate better to *persons* with dementia. The use of these elements of friendship can have a positive impact on almost any dementia care program. They also are something that all staff members can understand, whatever their background. Traditions may be different from culture to culture, but the basic tenets of friendship remain the same. Thus, the Best Friends model is multicultural and easy to adapt for today's diverse long-term care staff. This adaptability is demonstrated throughout this book by the stories and examples of the use of Best Friends concepts from around the world.

Recast relationships—Best Friends staff members recast their relationships with participants or residents to become less task oriented and more person oriented, to treat *persons* as they would a friend. When a problem arises, staff can simply ask themselves, "How can I be a Best Friend to this *person?*" The answer might call for being more patient or understanding, forgiving or forgetting an incident, discovering a common interest in an activity, or even just giving the *person* a hug.

Learn the knack—Best Friends staff members have a magic touch in their work with or care of *persons* with Alzheimer's disease, what the authors call the "knack." Staff with knack can do difficult things with ease and use clever tricks or strategies in daily care. Some people are born with this natural ability. The Best Friends model suggests that everyone can learn some elements of knack, as outlined in the next section. It is the desired outcome of a staff training and development program. It is the Best Friends way.

STAFF WITH KNACK

Every long-term care program should aspire to having a staff that has knack. The elements of knack are outlined in Figure 1.3 and discussed in the following sections.

Being Well Informed

Staff members with knack learn as much as they can about the nature of Alzheimer's disease, techniques for caregiving, family issues, and community resources. They are encouraged to attend workshops. They recognize that the more that they know about Alzheimer's disease, the less stressful and difficult the job of caregiving is.

A well-informed staff member at the Serenity Nursing Home in Johannesburg, South Africa, reacted with calm when a resident tried to hit her. The staff member's insight about the disease allowed her to put the incident aside and continue working with the resident in a positive way.

This staff member equated the resident's anger with the losses caused by Alzheimer's disease and immediately looked for the causes that might have triggered the anger. At the same time, the staff member learned to be cautious to protect herself from future incidents. More basic medical information about Alzheimer's disease is presented in Chapter 3.

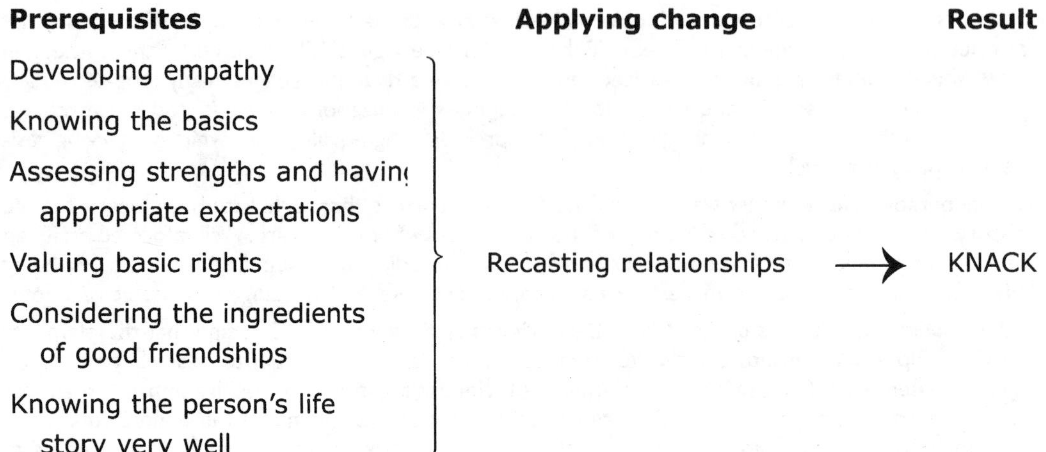

Figure 1.1. The Best Friends model of Alzheimer's care: A road map to success. (From Bell, V., & Troxel, D. [1997]. The best friends approach to Alzheimer's care *[p. 101]. Baltimore: Health Professions Press; reprinted by permission.)*

Having Empathy

Staff members with knack have taken the time to imagine what it would be like to have Alzheimer's disease. This knowledge helps them understand that the world of Alzheimer's disease can be difficult and frightening. In the following example, having empathy helped staff members reach out to a *person* who needed their support:

A very young male participant was enrolled in the Carilion Adult Day Center in Bedford, Virginia. When he started to show symptoms of dementia, many of his friends abandoned him, which often left him feeling lonely, frustrated, and helpless. The staff understood his feelings and stood by him "every step of the way, with a best friends touch."

Carilion's staff realized that this participant would have moments of loneliness and sadness and that it would be awkward to be a younger individual in a program of predominantly older participants. Staff worked to compensate for this; close bonds formed, particularly between the resident and staff members who were close to his age. When he died, a staff member delivered his eulogy, which is reprinted in the margin on pages 12–13. More discussion of the experience of having Alzheimer's disease can be found in Chapter 4.

Respecting the Basic Rights of the *Person*

Staff members with knack are dedicated to basic rights and high-quality care for *persons* with Alzheimer's disease. Staff operate in an ethical fashion. They embrace the Alzheimer's disease bill of rights (see Figure 1.2), as in the following example:

One day, a participant in the Care Club of Collier County, Inc., Naples, Florida, was angry with a staff member. Another staff member intervened. While the participant told his story, the staff member actively listened and then assured him that he would "look into the matter at once!"

Every person diagnosed with Alzheimer's disease or a related disorder deserves the following rights:

To be informed of one's diagnosis

To have appropriate, ongoing medical care

To be productive in work and play for as long as possible

To be treated like an adult, not like a child

To have expressed feelings taken seriously

To be free from psychotropic medications, if possible

To live in a safe, structured, and predictable environment

To enjoy meaningful activities that fill each day

To be outdoors on a regular basis

To have physical contact, including hugging, caressing, and hand-holding

To be with individuals who know one's life story, including cultural and religious traditions

To be cared for by individuals who are well trained in dementia care

Figure 1.2. The Alzheimer's disease bill of rights. (From Bell, V., & Troxel, D. [1997]. The best friends approach to Alzheimer's care *[p. 38]. Baltimore: Health Professions Press; reprinted by permission.* Note: *Copies of the bill of rights are available in other languages. For a copy, email the authors at* VBellKY@aol.com *or* SBDavidT@aol.com.*)*

Elements of Knack

Being well informed

Having empathy

Respecting the basic rights of the *person*

Maintaining caregiver integrity

Employing finesse

Knowing it is easier to get forgiveness than to get permission

Using common sense

Communicating skillfully

Maintaining optimism

Setting realistic expectations

Using humor

Employing spontaneity

Practicing patience

Developing flexibility

Staying focused

Remaining nonjudgmental

Valuing the moment

Maintaining self-confidence

Using cues that are tied to the life story

Taking care of oneself

Figure 1.3. Elements of knack. (Adapted from Bell, V., & Troxel, D. [1997]. The best friends approach to Alzheimer's care *[p. 94]. Baltimore: Health Professions Press.)*

The staff member respected the basic right of the *person* to have expressed feelings taken seriously. The participant felt listened to, and his anger was diffused.

Maintaining Caregiver Integrity

Staff members with knack approach problems and decision making with an attitude of good will toward the *person*. Staff should always start from a position of truth. The following example reveals how caregiving integrity can be maintained in a potentially trying situation:

At Villa Alamar, in Santa Barbara, California, a resident became very upset because his shaver was not working. He showed staff that when he moved it across his face, it did not work and asked if it could be fixed. In fact, he was trying to shave with his small tape recorder. A staff member said, "This old shaver doesn't work anymore. I'll get you a better one." She handed him his cordless shaver and he thanked her profusely.

The staff member's artful reply preserved the resident's dignity, for if she had pointed out his mistake, it could have caused him embarrassment and frustration, or worse. By giving him a real shaver, he was able to finish shaving, making him feel capable and in control instead of helpless. Here, actions and words were applied with integrity even though they did not represent the literal truth.

Employing Finesse

Staff members with knack use the art of finesse to respond to difficult situations. They employ skillful, subtle, tactful, diplomatic, and well-timed maneuvers to handle problems. When a *person* attending day center care says, "I want to go home," and staff respond, "Soon," finesse is being employed to give the *person* a reassuring answer. Perhaps he or she will accept the statement and move on to another topic, later forgetting that he or she wanted to go home. Skillful finesse is part of the knack of good Alzheimer's care, as seen in this second example involving shaving.

A nursing assistant at The Fountainview Center in Atlanta, Georgia, tried to give a resident a much-needed bath, but he continually refused. She was, however, successful in getting him to say yes to a shave. Using finesse, she talked about his day and hers and moved him to the sink near the shower. Just as she was finishing the shave, she "accidentally" got some shaving cream on his shirt. Of course, he had to take the shirt off. She apologized profusely and confessed that she was not having a good day. She continued to be "clumsy" with the shaving cream and more and more clothing came off. Before the resident knew it, he was in and out of the shower and "feeling pretty sorry for the staff member and the horrible day she was having." Humorously, he chided the staff member after the fact: "You know, next time, you need to be more careful!"

Here, a confident—even gutsy—CNA showed finesse with a can of shaving cream. Her willingness to make fun of herself allowed her to accomplish this task and give the resident a long-overdue shower. The approach might fail if tried by a CNA without knack.

Knowing It Is Easier to Get Forgiveness than to Get Permission

Staff members with knack know that dignified care calls for asking permission whenever possible, but asking permission often is unsuccessful with a *person* who has dementia. Because problem solving and judgment are diminished, a *person's* response to questions calling for decisions often is, "no." This is the safest answer for the *person* to give when he or she may not fully comprehend the question. (See Chapter 8 for more information on this topic.)

A participant in the Helping Hand Day Center in Lexington, Kentucky, wanted to wear his overcoat all day long, becoming overly warm. When he slid the coat off behind his chair, a volunteer took away his coat and hung it out of sight. When he missed his coat, she said, "I'm sorry I didn't ask you, but I checked your overcoat to keep it in a safe place."

If asked, he never would have given permission to take his coat. When the volunteer acted without permission, the participant accepted the results and did not think about the coat any longer. Usually, "out of sight, out of mind" works well, but, when the coat was asked for, it was returned to him.

The Alzheimer's Society of Finland has embraced the Alzheimer's Disease Bill of Rights, and Leena's Home has found that the document touches on all aspects of its work with residents and families: The Alzheimer's Disease Bill of Rights forms the ideological basis of care in our facility.

—Paivi Voutilainen and Leena Qvick, Administrators, Leena's Home (Leenankoti), Alzheimer's Society of Finland, Helsinki, Finland

Using Common Sense

Staff members with knack use common sense, finding simple solutions to sometimes-complex problems. For example, a staff member's noticing a resident's agitation might look for some commonsense answer. Perhaps the program is serving too many sweets and too much caffeinated coffee. Perhaps the group activities are in a cold room or are lasting too long. Problems also can come up unexpectedly, as in the following example:

The new window blinds purchased for Porterville Senior Day Care in Porterville, California, did not fit. The vice president of the board of directors said, "No problem! I'll take them back immediately." As he turned around to gather them up, a participant said, "No! You are not *leaving with this one. This one is mine!" She continued to hold on to the blind until she was called for lunch sometime later.*

The board member returned later to pick up the window blind and make the exchange. His well-timed retreat delayed the exchange of the window blinds, but his commonsense approach prevented what could have been a major disruption. By the time he returned to pick up the blinds, the participant had forgotten about them.

Communicating Skillfully

Staff members with knack communicate skillfully, cueing the *person* with appropriate words from his or her life story, using positive body language, and knowing the right and wrong ways to give directions and ask and answer questions.

Staff at the Alzheimer's Four Seasons in Santa Barbara, California, use what they called "care"-ful statements and questions for effective communications. These are defined as caring statements that are full of descriptive detail. For example, to get someone to sit down, a "care"-ful statement might be, "It's so good to be with you, Pablo. Come sit with me, here, in this comfortable green chair [patting the chair]."

Staff members at the Alzheimer's Four Seasons call the resident by his or her preferred name and communicate in a caring, descriptive way. Effective communication also involves skilled listening. More information about communication is presented in Chapter 8.

I believe the Best Friends model can be summed up by the qualities of total acceptance of each individual and just being there whatever the situation may be.
—Gayle Pennington, Director, Riverside Adult Day Program, Christiana Care Health Services, Wilmington, Delaware

Maintaining Optimism

Staff members with knack do not dwell on the losses caused by the *person's* disease. They project an upbeat, positive attitude in their work and look for small successes. Because *persons* with dementia are sensitive to their environment, their behaviors are influenced positively by staff members' attitudes. The glass is always half-full for a Best Friends staff member.

While a student at Madonna University in Livonia, Michigan, Rachel Everett was working on a service/learning project at a local assisted living facility. She was told that it was difficult to relate to one resident of German descent who had reverted to her native language. The student created a poster with key words and phrases in German and English to hang in the resident's room. Staff use these phrases to encourage the resident to complete her activities of daily living (ADLs) and become more involved in all activities.

This student was certain that *something* could be done to improve this situation. Thanks to her optimism, staff can communicate better with this resident, vastly improving the quality of care.

Setting Realistic Expectations

Staff members with knack focus on what *persons* with Alzheimer's disease can still do. They have a good sense of these individuals' remaining cognitive strengths, the state of their physical health, and their personal interests and values. Staff also know that setting expectations too high can lead to failure and frustration. Setting expectations too low leads to diminished self-esteem and a lessened ability to function. In the following story, staff set appropriate expectations that were fulfilled:

A physically frail participant in the Helping Hand Day Center was struggling to walk the short distance from the bathroom to the program room. The volunteers and staff encouraged her to finish the walk and get to her chair because they knew that the doctor wanted her to walk as much as possible. "Just a bit farther," they encouraged. "We don't want you to lose your front-row seat," they said, teasingly. She made it to her chair safely.

Every day at the program is special to me—everyone goes out of their way to help one another.

—Audrey Taylor, participant, Riverside Adult Day Program, Wilmington, Delaware

If staff had not been so in tune with her situation, then they might have either given up (and she would have missed much of the program sitting in the hallway) or pushed her inappropriately, causing her physical pain or distress. Instead, their patient encouragement supported the goals of the care plan and allowed her to sit down, smile, and feel good that she had made it to her chair. More about setting expectations and assessment is featured in Chapter 5.

Using Humor

Staff members with knack enjoy telling funny stories and jokes, and they laugh when humorous things happen. They understand that even when the *person* does not "get" a funny story or joke, laughter and good feelings are contagious, as in the following story:

A volunteer at Heritage Court, The Samarkand Retirement Community, Santa Barbara, California, remarked one day that he was wearing one brown shoe and one black shoe. Residents roared with laughter as he showed them the shoes and admitted his embarrassing gaffe.

As demonstrated in this example, volunteers and staff with knack should not be afraid to make fun of themselves now and then. Self-deprecation levels the playing field. It can preserve the dignity of *persons* by helping them feel that they are not the only ones with problems.

Employing Spontaneity

Staff members with knack know how to be spontaneous. A horticultural therapy class in a facility's garden might take a half-hour of unplanned bird watching when colorful cardinals are spotted in the trees. *Persons* with Alzheimer's disease live in a world full of spontaneous events; they can teach us to appreciate this quality, too.

The Gourmet Club of The Fountains Continuum of Care, Inc., in Tucson, Arizona, planned a cookie-making project. The plan was to bake cookies in the morning, frost them in the afternoon, and then enjoy them for an evening snack. At 11:00 A.M., the cookies came out of the oven. The smell of freshly baked cookies filled the room, proving too good to pass up. Despite the careful planning, all of the cookies were eaten before lunch. Fruit was substituted for the evening snack.

The group leader was able to enjoy the moment, be flexible and spontaneous, and capture the enthusiasm of the residents.

Our facility has adopted the Best Friends model with great success. It has inspired us to move from task oriented care to people care. There is an atmosphere of excitement and joy as we see residents and staff responding.

—Karen Wyan, Assistant Administrator, Laurel Heights Home for the Elderly, London, Kentucky

Practicing Patience

Staff members with knack realize that it takes the *person* with dementia longer to complete tasks and to respond to words and events. They also know that losing patience, getting frustrated, or becoming angry almost always makes matters worse. Taking time with someone is an activity, a valuable gift for a resident or participant. It builds relationships that ultimately help staff members be more effective in all aspects of daily care and programming.

A participant in ADCare adult day service centers in San Luis Obispo County, California, operated by LifeSpan Services Network, Inc., has a great uncle who was a famous writer. She loves to talk about him, often repeating the same stories. The program director, Pam Richards, said, "Even though we have heard the story many times, we listen since she gets so much pleasure from talking about him."

It would be easy to become impatient or disinterested. In this case, staff members with knack respond to the participant's smiles and excitement about telling the story, and so are patient about listening to it once again.

I would like to say a few words about Bryan on behalf of his friends at the Carilion Adult Day Center—Nancy, Vicki, Dinah, Jeff, and I. We didn't know Bryan as many of you did. We met Bryan after he became ill and his parents came to us for help. From the first time we met Bryan, he had an effect on us that no other participant has ever had. His warmth and vulnerability drew us to him. We shared with him and his family in the feelings of frustration, helplessness, and hope. We protected him from those who judged. We laughed with him. We cried with him. But most of all, we simply loved him. Bryan, although he couldn't speak to us, communicated his love of life, family, nature, and friendship. He brought treasures to show us—pictures of his boat, his artwork, his poetry, his pocketknife.

Developing Flexibility

Staff members with knack recognize that schedules cannot be set in stone. Residents or participants may have their own ideas about how their day will transpire. Some residential programs have taken this philosophy a step further and have built in flexible bathing, dressing, waking, and eating times.

Mealtime at Omahanui Private Hospital in New Plymouth, New Zealand, had become noisy and difficult, with some residents constantly getting up and sitting down and bothering others during the meal. The staff decided to change the routine from one seating to three. They removed one table to make the dining room less crowded and even invited some residents to help themselves from silver serving dishes. Now, according to the administrator, Patricia Wesley, "No one wanders from the dining room, and meals have become pleasurable, social occasions."

Sometimes a program will rush residents through a meal to get to an activity. These programs are missing the point: Staff should make the most of every part of every day. By reorganizing, the staff of Omahanui changed mealtimes from a task to a warm and social activity.

Jitka M. Zgola, a writer and dementia care consultant, made a similar point when she described a CNA's rushing a resident through a bath: "Don't worry Mrs. L., you'll be done in time for your two o'clock sensory stimulation group."

This example draws attention to the common practice of not making the most of every situation for the benefit of the resident and to forgetting that life is about living between structured activities.

Staying Focused

Staff members with knack overcome the distractions that are present in most long-term care settings. They learn the value of being present for the *person.* Being present involves really listening to *persons* when they speak, making eye contact, and getting the most out of every encounter. It also involves putting a staff member's concerns or problems on hold. When a staff member is thinking about what to cook for dinner that night, care suffers.

In the following example, a CNA demonstrated the knack of being focused when she spent good-quality time with a resident at mealtime every day.

A resident at The Fountainview Center for Alzheimer's Disease seemed very sad and refused to eat most of her meals. A caring CNA, Vioris Thomas, began to sit with her at mealtime. They talked together about her interest in history, exchanged hugs, and discussed what foods she liked best and what she did not like at all. They joked and kidded with each other. Thomas confessed, "Sometimes I had to use everything in the book, but I kept trying."

Soon the resident was eating again, improving her health and quality of life.

Remaining Nonjudgmental

Staff members with knack are nonjudgmental. With Alzheimer's disease, it is important for everyone to remain sensitive to, accepting of, and nonjudgmental about others' feelings.

A resident at West Park Long Term Care Center in Cody, Wyoming, was crying and said, "I wish I was dead." Some staff members may have judged the resident's statement, labeling it "wrong" or measuring it against their own religious beliefs and values. Instead, a staff member did not dismiss these feelings or try to argue the point. She offered a hug and a back rub and just sat with the resident, offering her comfort and companionship.

This staff member recognized that, like everyone else, *persons* with dementia have feelings that need to be expressed. She did not judge the resident's statement, but instead offered unconditional support.

Bryan continued to communicate this need for friendship when Nancy, Vicki, and I visited him in the hospital. He reached out to me in the only way he still could. He placed his foot on my chest, and the twinkle in his eyes told me he was saying, "I'm glad to see you, friends," and we were glad to be there. We are thankful to have known Bryan and feel honored that we were entrusted with his care. Bryan and his parents have taught us so much and have caused us to reflect on the true meaning of love, compassion, commitment, and the sanctity of life, no matter how fragile. The family, as well as Bryan's dear friends, Linda and Doug, have been an inspiration to us all. Now is the time to end the long battle, and begin to rejoice in the fact that our friend, Bryan, has enriched our lives.

—Carla Groff, Manager, Carilion Adult Day Center

Valuing the Moment

Staff members with knack know the importance of living in the moment and finding joy in it. Activities including a pleasant lunch, time spent arranging flowers, or a joyful game may soon be forgotten, but it can be pleasurable in the moment. When staff members string together these positive moments, good Alzheimer's care can be achieved.

A housekeeper at Wellington Parc of Owensboro, in Owensboro, Kentucky, befriended a restless resident who wandered aimlessly in a hallway. The housekeeper knew that the resident had been a carpenter and handyman, so she took his hand and asked him to be in charge of pushing her cart from room to room.

At the moment the staff member with knack took his hand, this resident felt connected to life. Their work became a regular activity for him, making him feel appreciated and productive. The housekeeper took pride in the fact that her involvement with this resident was making such a difference in his daily life and happiness. All it took was for this housekeeper to look beyond the strict requirements of her job and to include a resident in her routine.

Maintaining Self-Confidence

Staff members with knack exhibit self-confidence in their daily interactions with participants and residents. Confidence evokes trust and feelings of security for the *person.* Confident staff members are willing to take chances as in the following example.

When Milo was admitted to the Sunshine Terrace Adult Day Center, in Logan, Utah, his children mentioned that he had cleaned and repaired furnaces all of his life. They did not think that he would want to play in the center's bell choir or participate in any musical activities because they thought that he would not be interested and would be shy and embarrassed. Sunshine's music therapist sensed, however, that he was interested, and one day encouraged him to try to play the Autoharp. He hesitated and then said, "I don't think I can, but if you think I can, I'll try." Months later at the center's talent show, his family, sitting in the front row, was pleasantly surprised when he accompanied the center's choir on the Autoharp.

The confidence of the program staff proved to be inviting, even irresistible, to the participant. This is a good example of ambitious activity programming. Some things one might think never would work do, in fact, work. More material on activity programming is presented in Chapter 9.

Using Cues that Are Tied to the Life Story

Staff members with knack incorporate the *person's* life story into all aspects of care. Examples include cueing the *person* to recall certain names, places, and things; telling familiar stories; and reminding him or her of achievements.

From one resident's life story, staff at Laurel Heights Home for the Elderly, London, Kentucky, knew that she always insisted that her children and husband get cleaned up as soon as they came in from working on the farm. Whenever it was time for a bath and to get dressed, staff evoked this tradition, saying, "It's time to clean up, just like you did on the farm."

The life story helps staff establish a successful personal care routine for this resident. Even better, it gives staff members much to talk about with her; they can tell stories about farming, joke about cleaning up, and talk about their own lives in the rural community where this facility is based. Further information on using the life story can be found in Chapter 7.

Taking Care of Oneself

Staff members with knack take time out for themselves to let go of the stress and strain that can accompany their work. They learn that humor is important. They learn techniques for stress and anger management, conflict resolution, assertiveness training, and other life skills.

At Liberty Commons Assisted Living, Liberty Healthcare Management Services, Inc., in Wilmington, North Carolina, staff are offered stress management and nutrition information workshops. Also, an exercise program is held three times a week for staff who are interested in getting into shape. The director of operations, Cindy Stancil, said, "The programs help keep mind and body strong."

This wellness program helps staff members operate at their best. It is difficult to take care of someone else when staff members are not feeling well themselves.

Overall wellness is never more important than in situations in which staff members confront death and dying. Dementia programs sometimes overlook the real feelings that staff have when a *person* becomes worse, leaves a program, or dies.

Linda Blair, a grief and bereavement counselor in Frankfort, Kentucky, teaches staff members how to cope with issues surrounding grief and loss. She acknowledges, "It is very tough for staff to see a favorite resident or participant decline or die. For many, grief issues resonate in their personal lives; the death of a favorite resident may evoke memories of the death of a beloved grandmother."

Linda's class helps staff to address these issues. It is important to build this support for staff because many feel these losses deeply.

West Park Long Term Care Center conducts a balloon liftoff each spring for staff to celebrate the lives of residents who have died. Celebration lifts and renews the spirit. This tradition gives staff a sense of closure, allows them to support one another, and, ultimately, helps staff take care of themselves emotionally and spiritually.

Conclusion

When the authors were attending an international Alzheimer's disease conference in 1991 in Amsterdam, the Netherlands, they met a woman who ran an adult day center who had a unique approach to staffing challenges. To staff her program, she said that she looked for former barmaids and beauticians. These individuals share many of the qualities of knack: They are good listeners, good conversationalists, upbeat, funloving, and people who love people. They have knack.

Programs cannot hire only "barmaids and beauticians" in today's complex long-term care environment, but a staff with these qualities can be developed (see Chapter 2). Cheri Taylor, executive director of Porterville Senior Day Care, agreed, saying, "Knack doesn't always come naturally, but it can be shared and learned." New staff members come to a job with differing strengths and weaknesses; variations in education, reading, and language skills; and different personality types, but it is the authors' belief that everyone is *capable* of friendship. This insight may be why the Best Friends model has been such a success in long-term care settings.

The model provides programs with a framework for resident care and staff development. It is easy to implement, life affirming, and inexpensive. It will not solve a long-term care community's or program's problems overnight, nor will it remove the very real challenges of providing good-quality dementia care. Yet when implemented in the ways suggested in this book, the Best Friends model always enhances staff skills, improves morale, energizes activities, and has a positive impact on the quality of care.

2

Staff Recruiting, Training, & Development

Who works in long-term care and why? The authors spoke with certified nursing assistants (CNAs) in various residential care settings. Many come from diverse backgrounds and challenging circumstances. Many are recent immigrants, are single parents, have incomes at or below poverty levels, or live in inadequate housing. Many speak English as a second or even third language. Many work more than one job.

Arguably, many of these individuals could find work in easier jobs with fewer responsibilities. Many could possibly earn higher wages in other, less demanding settings. The authors asked them why they worked in long-term care. Here are some of the answers:

I feel good about helping others.
It was the first job I found when I moved here.
I like the older people. They are nice to me.
It's the one place where I get love. They [the residents] like me and I feel like a success because of that.
It feels like home. I like it there.

The authors particularly appreciated one young man's answer that his job was a place for him to find love and success. This is possible because *persons* with Alzheimer's disease can be amazingly accepting of people from differing social, economic, and ethnic backgrounds. Sometimes the disease helps them let go of prejudices. They have great capacity to give love.

It seems clear that many line staff members are finding satisfaction in their jobs. It is a place to help others, feel successful, and even receive love from the residents. It is a place to find a community. This may be why they work in a long-term care environment. The Best Friends program supports its staff's hopes and aspirations. It builds on this quest for community, fulfillment, and success.

The following sections discuss staffing issues in greater detail. Let's start with one fictional facility with some staff openings to fill.

A Day in the Life of a Skilled Nursing Facility Administrator

It is going to be a good week, the administrator thought, until she arrived at work. Before she even had finished lunch, two of the best CNAs gave notice. One was moving to a different city to be closer to her family; the other had been scooped up by a competitor. Fortunately, it was not too late to make the deadline for the weekend newspaper, and an advertisement was placed.

Several days passed, and, as the administrator was driving to work, she wondered if she would ever fill the positions. As she walked into the building, she noticed a group of about 15 people milling about the lobby. Who could they be?

The receptionist spoke up immediately: "This is your lucky day!" The administrator seemed puzzled until the receptionist added, "All these people are here for our job openings." Surprised, the administrator jumped right into the interviews. She thought, "If I'm lucky I'll fill these positions soon."

Candidate 1 was well dressed and had a nice smile and a firm handshake. Asked to talk about himself, he quickly replied, "I just felt my career in teaching wasn't satisfying. In between my volunteer work with the local theatre company and my Ph.D. studies, I decided to do some hands-on work with elders." After a pleasant interview, the administrator thanked him and went on to the next candidate. The next candidate had worked as a CNA for 5 years, liked to play the piano for the residents, and had a friendly laugh. Candidate 3 was not available for her interview because she had already walked down the hall and was helping several residents get to their rooms. Candidate 4 said that she could start working that day, and asked, "If the dietary staff okay it, do you mind if I bring in a batch of cookies every few days? I enjoy doing extra things."

The administrator was ecstatic. She smiled and thought, "My problems are over. What a great group of candidates! I'm going to hire them all." Just then, she felt something cold and wet on her nose; she opened her eyes to see her Golden Retriever licking her face to remind her that it was time for his morning walk. "Oh, no!" she exclaimed. "It was all a dream."

If "dream staff" walked into every long-term care program every day, then there would be little need for extensive staff training. Yet few staff members arrive with outstanding skills and the knack in place. It is up to effective program

We honor the ongoing living of life, enjoying dignity and well-being in a shared, caring relationship with residents, family and staff.

—Mission statement, The Wealshire, Lincolnshire, Illinois

The CNAs love to tell stories about what they do well.

—Joanne Rader, dementia consultant and Associate Professor, Oregon Health Sciences, University, School of Nursing, Portland, Oregon

I believe that in order for a staff to really learn, the training should be experiential. The training that I conduct has the participant actively involved.

—Susan D. Berry, Alzheimer's disease consultant and trainer, Warsaw, Indiana

Focus on the problem, not whose fault it is . . . this increases the confidence and ultimately the enthusiasm of the staff in the quality process.

—Margaret Ryan, Quality Manager, St. Basil's Homes, New South Wales, Australia

leaders to provide new staff members with the training that they need to succeed.

Even more disturbing is that the question of "How do I get *good* staff?" is being replaced by "How do I get *enough* staff?" Some residential facilities in certain parts of the United States, for example, are leaving rooms vacant that could be filled with paying residents. The reason? They do not have enough line staff to take care of these residents.

The problem exists not just at this level of staffing; developers, owners, and nonprofit boards of directors have told the authors that there also is a shortage of talented program leaders and administrators in long-term care settings.

Alyce and Bob Parsons, managing partners of Hotel Pawnee, Santa Barbara, California, told the authors that one of their greatest challenges as long-term care managers and developers is finding skilled managers. Alyce noted, "We will not go forward with a project until we know that we can attract the right staff, those who have ability mixed with compassion."

Strong leadership is an essential ingredient of an excellent dementia care program.

These trends create major challenges for dementia care programs, which are so dependent on good staff. How can these problems be solved?

The answers are complex and overlapping. Ideally, every dementia care program will offer competitive wages and benefits. An attractive physical environment can be an incentive for new employees. Strong leadership that employees can respect is always important. Flexible hours and an opportunity for growth and advancement come into play. Good working conditions, including high staff morale, also attract potential employees. What makes the most difference is a comprehensive and effective program philosophy that pulls all of these factors together. The Best Friends model can give program leaders something positive to dream about. Even better, it can help them develop a staff with knack and a long-term care program that is a good place to work and live.

Let's turn to the issues surrounding the recruitment, hiring, training, and retention of staff.

Recruitment and Hiring

During the interview process, the Best Friends program looks first for individuals with knack or the potential to de-

Part of the emphasis of training is on putting as much if not more emphasis on meeting the spiritual, emotional, and social needs of residents rather than focusing solely on their physical and personal care needs. We work on prioritizing so that residents' quality of life and contentment is more important than the number of baths they receive each week. We work on recognizing that I cannot possibly help Rachel with her bath if I don't recognize how worried she is about her ill daughter and take time to assure her that her family is safe and well.

—Briana Melom, Director of Education and Family Services, Alzheimer's Disease Center, Mayo Clinic, Rochester, Minnesota

No one is useless in this world who lightens the burden of it to anyone else.

–Charles Dickens

velop it. (See Tool 2.7 for some tips on hiring staff with knack.)

Carly R. Hellen, director of Alzheimer's care, The Wealshire, Lincolnshire, Illinois, measures knack by asking nontraditional questions such as, "Tell me about an older person you know," and, "Who is your personal mentor or hero?" During the interview, potential employees also can be given an object such as a funny hat, a button, a brochure on new cars, or an apple. They are asked to come up with as many ideas as they can for ways to use the object in an activity. If the individual comes up with a dozen or more inventive answers, then they already have knack.

Prospective employees who perform poorly in these initial tests may, surprisingly, still be excellent candidates for jobs in dementia care programs. Sometimes a staff member who has faced tough times or has a shy personality blossoms when exposed to a caring Best Friends community.

I find that staff respond well to a multisensory teaching style which includes visual, auditory and kinesthetic modes.

—Leslie Congleton, Program Coordinator, Legacy Health Systems Trinity Place Alzheimer's Day Respite Program, Portland, Oregon

I believe more is caught than taught.

—Kay Lloyd, Director of Staff Education, The Fountainview Center for Alzheimer's Disease, Atlanta, Georgia

At the opening of the training session, staff members enter a room with a television set blaring and a rock radio station turned on high. Their purses and other personal items are taken from them, and they are asked to sit in the brown chairs

Potential Employees

To expand the pool of potential staff members, the authors encourage programs to look for nontraditional sources of staffing, including students, retirees, and even individuals with no previous background in long-term care.

The Friendship Adult Day Care Center in Santa Barbara, California, prides itself on its staff with knack. The director enjoys line dancing, the associate director drives a hand-painted multicolor Honda, and staff members have included a professional musician who played music for the participants and a surfer who enjoyed sharing his exploits on the ocean, which is located just a few blocks from the center.

The administrators believe that if staff members with an adventurous spirit and a sense of humor are hired, then these individuals have great potential to develop knack. Good training can later fill in any educational gaps. In addition to frequent staff in-service programs, the Friendship Adult Day Care Center sends new staff members to local educational events that are sponsored by the Alzheimer's Association.

Former caregivers also can provide valuable volunteer support to long-term care programs or sometimes become paid staff members. Some family members find it rewarding to use the caregiving skills they have learned at home by working in a dementia program after they are no longer involved in direct care. This is one way to turn the tough and challenging experience of being a caregiver into something more meaningful—of "turning lemons into lemonade."

When Staff Fail

One of the toughest aspects of any administrator's job is to dismiss employees who are not succeeding. The view of Beverly Sanborn, director of Alzheimer's field services, Marriott Corporation Senior Living Services, Washington, D.C., and former long-term care administrator, is particularly interesting. She does not believe in writing people up for minor infractions. "When programs manage by shame, it flows from top to bottom, owners to administrators to staff and then to residents." This negative style can work against the goals of a Best Friends program.

She recommends dismissing staff members who "don't get it." Her opinion is that some people are not cut out to work in dementia care programs. When staff members cannot make a connection with residents or participants, prove to be rigid, or are unable to grow and thrive, they should be encouraged to seek different employment sooner rather than later. They may thrive in other jobs but do not belong in a Best Friends program. When a dismissal must be made, it should reflect the caring philosophy of the program: "I tell them that their passions and talents lie elsewhere."

(no such chairs were in the room). They are asked to discuss how it feels to be misunderstood, oversupervised, overstimulated, frustrated, and scared—the world of Alzheimer's disease.

—Briana Melom, Director of Education and Family Services, Alzheimer's Disease Center, Mayo Clinic, Rochester, Minnesota

I try to catch them at a success rather than a failure.

—Beverly Sanborn, Director of Alzheimer's Field Services, Marriott Corporation Senior Living Services, Washington, D.C., redefined the role of an administrator as first and foremost a teacher and trainer. This helps staff understand and welcome her on-the-floor feedback about their work.

Students can play a valuable role in a nursing home. I involve them in creating life stories, developing communication strategies, and other simple, meaningful activities.

—Beth Spencer, Assistant Professor of Gerontology, Madonna University, Livonia, Michigan

Training and Retention

Training Programs that Do Not Work—The Old Idea Care Center

> It is payday at the Old Idea Care Center, and everyone is ready to get his or her check and make a run for the bank. An in-service on communication is about to begin. A few staff members who have been up late the night before look pretty drowsy. The administrator will give today's talk. She comes in, says hello, and introduces a new 40-minute-long video. The lights are dimmed. She says that she has seen the video before, so she is going to sneak out for a few minutes to do some paperwork. The film starts, and around the room, eyes begin to close. At the end of the video, the lights come back on and the

administrator asks whether anyone has questions. Hearing none, she dismisses the class. Many staff members go to work or leave the building to cash their paychecks.

After the in-service, one staff member goes straight to the Alzheimer's care unit, and the administrator happens to wander by. She could not help noticing that the staff member who had just sat in on the training was still making the same mistakes. "What's wrong with my staff?" the administrator wondered. "Why can't they learn this stuff?" Meanwhile, the staff training coordinator crosses the topic off her list: "Good! We've got communication covered. We don't need to do this topic again until next year."

The next in-service is scheduled in 4 weeks. A physician will talk to the staff. His topic is the neurobiology of aging. He comes to the facility with his carousel of slides. He notices that the staff do not seem too welcoming or enthused. He does his best to get them involved. Fortunately, he is a good speaker, but his handouts are hard to read and understand.

A few staff members notice that something has come up, and the director of nursing and the administrator leave the room. One staff member whispers to another, "If they don't need to hear this, why do we?" The other asks, "Do you know what all these words mean?"

The Wealshire involves our line staff, called Resident Living Assistants (RLAs), in interviewing potential employees and giving facility tours to prospective families.

—Carly R. Hellen, Director of Alzheimer's Care, The Wealshire, Lincolnshire, Illinois

Making learning fun is different from being entertained.

—Vicki L. Schmall, Executive Director, Aging Concerns, West Linn, Oregon

Traditionally we have sent administrators and leaders to conferences. More CNAs should have this opportunity. I also like to have programs for CNAs only. It makes them feel special.

—Cynthia Belle, dementia care consultant and trainer, Chicago, Illinois

These rather depressing examples of poor training happen every day in long-term care settings throughout the United States. The wrong things often are taught to the staff (teaching line staff more about neurobiology than bathing). There is no follow-up (the lessons on communication were not reinforced in the dementia care unit once the staff member left the class). Administration does not have a true commitment to training (key staff members left during the in-service). Teaching is too passive (lectures and videos are presented instead of interactive learning). The environment does not lend itself to learning (darkened rooms). Materials may not be culturally appropriate (English language only). Materials may be educationally inappropriate (the reading level is too advanced). Finally, training does not include all staff members who need it (training sessions did not include housekeeping, kitchen, marketing, and other support staff members).

Training Programs that Work—The New Idea Care Center

It is payday at the New Idea Care Center, and everyone is ready to get his or her check and make a run for the bank. An in-service on communication is about to begin. The staff file into the room and notice that the lighting is bright, and there are balloons and flowers on the front desk. There are a few new people at the in-service—the administrator's secretary and the community's gardener are there.

The guest speaker comes in and immediately greets everyone, shaking hands and introducing herself to the staff. She quickly asks everyone to stand, and a fun group game is played in which everyone has to guess some things about one another. One staff member later comments, "It was a little dumb, but, hey, we all laughed. It woke me up, too." The talk continues, with three main points being made.

The speaker asks numerous questions of the audience, but they are easy to answer. Everyone present says at least something. The staff laughs at the cartoons that the speaker presents, and likes the skits that the director of nursing and guest speaker role-play. "I didn't think that she had a sense of humor," one staff member says about the head nurse.

Then an interesting thing happens. The speaker asks everyone to leave the room and talk with a resident for 5 minutes, to practice what they have just learned, and then return to discuss what happened. When all of the participants come back, she asks them to describe their interactions with the residents. At the end of the training program, the guest speaker hands out a colorful one-page flyer with the main points of her presentation highlighted and says that a larger version will be posted on the bulletin board. Then she announces a competition. A big sheet of butcher paper will be posted in the staff lunchroom. "Everyone who writes down an idea about how to improve communication will be entered into a drawing for a large pizza at Taffy's Pizza. It doesn't have to be the best idea, just anything that works for you during the next week." On the way out, many staff members still rush to the bank, but they leave smiling. "I'm going to win that pizza, I hope," says one housekeeper. "I already have a few good ideas to post on the sheet."

Best Friends staff members are trained using some or all of the concepts presented in the description of the fictional New Idea Care Center. This training program is interactive and fun. Some core concepts are taught and reinforced. The staff pay attention and are treated with respect. (See Figure 2.1 for a summary of differences between "Old Idea Care Centers" and "New Idea Care Centers.")

Old Idea Care Center	**New Idea Care Center**
Hires "warm bodies"/anyone	Innovative recruitment
Little or no training	Investment in training
Minimal wages	Competitive wages
Only activity staff do activities	Everyone does activities, bringing in their own interests and skills
Training by lecture and video only	Interactive, innovative training
Little or no follow-through	Knowledge is reinforced by modeling, practicum, role play, or other method
No feedback from staff	Evaluation of training
Quick staff entry onto job	Staff orientation about program history, philosophy, and mission
Work is task oriented	Work is person oriented
Staff do only assigned tasks	Staff are self-starters, take initiative, team oriented
Staff struggle in interactions with residents	Staff experience successes
Staff feel put upon, under seige	Staff feel appreciated
High turnover	Good staff stay
Low morale	High morale
Staff resist change	New ideas welcomed by staff
Shame-based management "looking for mistakes"	Reward-based management "looking for successes"
Many residents exhibit challenging behaviors, restlessness	More residents seem happy, enjoying and feeling secure in the community

Figure 2.1. *A comparison of the "Old Idea Care Center" and the "New Idea Care Center."*

Ideas for Training Programs that Work*

Training that works should have the following qualities.

Be Taken Seriously, Be Consistent, and Be Part of a Well-Defined Set of Expectations

A Best Friends program makes a commitment to training and expects the staff to do the same. More important, training must be consistent; if a 12-week class is established, then it is important that it be offered and supported by management. If staff members get the message that something is not important, then they will not be invested in the process.

The staff educator at The Fountainview Center supports the importance of training by ensuring that no one who has been at work the night before attends a mid-morning class if this class time interferes with his or her normal sleep pattern. This type of scheduling increases the likelihood that each staff member will be alert, be able to learn the material, and be able to participate in the training. Affected staff can either request the night off before the training (if possible) or be trained at another time.

Approaching training in this way may cause some scheduling headaches, but it demonstrates the organization's commitment to the training program. It also lays out an expectation that staff members be active participants in training.

Teach the Organization's Mission, Values, and Philosophy

All staff members should be oriented to the organization's purpose and mission. Staff members are program ambassadors to the community; they should be able to deliver a consistent message about the program's services when asked by family members or prospective clients.

Staff members at The Fountains Continuum of Care begin their training by studying the materials, brochures, and handouts that are used to publicize their community. They provide the staff with a basic understanding and overview of what potential residents and families have read about the community and what they expect to see when they walk in the door. (See Tool 2.4, the ENTHUSIASTIC sheet.)

Such training clearly benefits staff members as they interact with existing and potential residents and their families.

Include Program Leaders

It makes a good impression on the staff when they see administrators attending training programs. Good training programs include all staff.

Administrative staff at The Wealshire are encouraged to attend training sessions and spend a day "walking in the shoes" of their nursing assistants, the RLAs (resident living assistants). The managers experience first hand the many aspects of the RLA's job. They call this the "RLA for the Day" program.

---

*The authors thank Debbie McConnell, director of education, Alzheimer's Association, Santa Barbara (California) chapter, for her contributions to this section.

This example not only teaches administrative staff to empathize better with the difficult job of being a RLA but it also makes staff feel more appreciated. In addition, it helps program leaders become more knowledgeable about the program that they manage—to know what is working and what is not working.

Best Friends programs also provide these program leaders with training in the areas of supervision, time management, strategic planning, and interpersonal skills. Leadership coaches can be hired to help these program leaders excel at meeting goals and building a successful team. Without an effective leader, most dementia programs flounder.

Meredith Gresham, a coordinator and developer of dementia training programs in Avon, Connecticut, offered another view of effective leadership: "As a manager, it is too easy to forget just how much of a relationship develops between your staff and the person with dementia. Like any relationship, it has its ups and downs. Managers need to be there to celebrate the ups and cushion the downs."

Meredith recognizes that staff need to feel that program leaders support them in both good times and bad times.

Involve Non-Direct Care Staff

Training should include staff who traditionally have been overlooked or not included. Best Friends programs include gardeners, cooks, administrative support staff, marketing staff, housekeepers, and others in the training sessions.

A broad array of staff at The Samarkand Retirement Community are involved in an intensive Alzheimer's disease training program, including some who are not directly working in its Heritage Court Alzheimer's program. The campus administrator, Steven Anderson, noted, "Their enthusiasm was equal to or greater than the direct care staff, in part because it was their first exposure to this type of training program."

In a residential community or day center, all employees inevitably have contact with *persons* with dementia. Why not give them the training they need to be Best Friends, too?

Teach the Right Content

Be certain that the content is appropriate for the jobs that the workers are doing. Hands-on staff members need to acquire practical skills. Other staff members may benefit from learning more about diagnosis and treatment. One faculty member defines appropriate content this way:

Beth Spencer, assistant professor of gerontology, Madonna University, Livonia, Michigan, wrote to the authors that "over the years as I have done training in the field of dementia, I have increasingly become convinced that the most important part of training is helping staff think about what it feels like to have dementia."

For Beth and her students, this is the right content or core concept to teach. Everything else flows from this point.

All staff members who have achieved the needed competency in their areas should have the opportunity to attend training programs on topic areas that are outside their normal work activity. This allows them to grow and develop as individuals and allows a facility to cross-train staff in important areas.

Teach in the Right Way

The average individual's attention span for traditional learning (reading and lecture) has fallen, while his or her attention span for other types of learning has increased. Today's staff learn best through active learning, games, short videos, group exercises, storytelling, and discussions with family members telling their stories (see Tool 2.8).

Dee Carlson, president of Alzheimer's Care: Consultation, Education & Training, Inc. (ACCET), Lexington, Kentucky, wrote that in general, adult learners are cautious about change, have their own beliefs and experiences, and have other distractions and responsibilities. They profit most from training that is enjoyable, interactive, exceedingly person centered, and applicable to care.

Effective trainers walk out in the audience, make eye contact, and, when appropriate, even touch the shoulders of or shake hands with staff in the class. Moving away from a podium or away from the "front of the class" can dramatically change the mood of the room and get staff more involved in training. It also makes it harder for some staff members to hide in the back row.

Having staff teach one another can be an effective tool for learning. Carly R. Hellen developed a mentoring system for new staff at The Wealshire. She asks each staff member to sign up to demonstrate a skill that reflects his or her identified personal strength. For example, if Mary is especially capable of helping a particular resident to bathe, then Mary will demonstrate this skill to a new staff member. Staff can be excellent teachers on the job and also in class training sessions.

Staff also should be engaged by the print materials that are handed out. Sometimes handouts and materials look as if they have been copied and recopied dozens of times. Staff are attracted to nice-looking materials reproduced on colored paper or created with colorful art and backgrounds.

Kathy Laurenhue, a writer and dementia trainer and president of Better Directions in San Diego, California, says, "If you want to make a splash with training materials be certain to make your handouts colorful and inviting."

Presentations like these not only capture the interest of staff but also show that the trainer has put some time and effort into them (see Tool 2.9 for some examples).

Do Not Teach Too Much Material in Any One Class

Many training programs try to teach too much material in a given session.

Joyce Beedle, president of Alzheimer's Consulting Service, Portland, Oregon, said, "It is dangerously easy to provide so much information that key concepts are lost in the detail. The learner returns to work wondering how to put the information to use and ends up not using the information at all. A few key points well defined, with time to practice and apply information, is best. The practice and application time fosters confidence in the use of the new tool, and confidence increases the likelihood of the tool actually being used. Ultimately, the goal is that the learner will go back to the worksite with new tools ready to use."

Limiting an in-service program to two or three points and then giving staff time to practice them is the key to successful training.

Be Culturally Appropriate and Sensitive

Good staff development programs recognize and respect diversity. Staff training should take into account the cultural norms, values, and traditions of staff. For example, a staff member told the authors that he found it disrespectful that his facility celebrated Groundhog Day and Valentine's Day but not Cinco de Mayo or Martin Luther King Day.

The authors also believe that in cases in which a preponderance of staff speak English as a second language, some training programs and materials should be offered in the primary language of staff. This provides these staff members with a greater opportunity to understand and learn the material being taught. One example is a list of medical terms in various languages. Peer-to-peer learning also can be helpful with a multicultural staff.

Deborah Dunn, director of patient and family services for the Santa Barbara, California, chapter of the Alzheimer's Association, often leads staff in-services completely in Spanish for the Latino staff of local programs. "While most, if not all, of the staff speak English, it's often a second language for them. When I do the program in Spanish, the staff lights up and participates more enthusiastically. My Spanish isn't perfect, but they appreciate my efforts and help me through the talk."

When staff members feel respected, they make a greater investment in the training program. One program in Australia serves many residents of Greek descent and has staff whose first language also is Greek:

"We are unique in that we offer care and services to a population primarily of Greek origin, while still catering to elderly mainstream Australians who, as a population, are from a diverse range of cultural backgrounds," wrote Judith Montano, director of care services, St. Basil's Homes, New South Wales, Australia. Senior bilingual staff at the homes have translated and typed forms and information into Greek. Doing so allows multicultural staff to examine issues in Greek, English, or both.

The predominantly Greek staff at St. Basil's Homes benefit from materials that have been translated into their native language. Nothing in the content is designed to discourage them from learning English. Yet having material in their primary language can help staff make a better transition into Australian life and be more effective in their jobs.

Get Staff to Talk

Successful training programs encourage staff members to talk about themselves, the problems they have that are related to resident care, and their response to the material being taught. Techniques include asking staff to present material themselves or breaking the class into smaller groups for discussion. A skilled instructor also can ask questions that are nonthreatening and invite staff to join the discussion.

At Wellington Parc of Owensboro, staff first discuss their own actions and reactions when working with persons *with Alzheimer's disease. Questions are posed such as how does it feel when one is try-*

ing to help a person sit down who has forgotten how? Staff list these feelings and then discuss how the person *might have felt while trying to sit. This exercise allows staff to recognize that they may at times share similar feelings, such as frustration and fear.*

When staff are encouraged to talk openly about their work, they are able to vent built-up pressure, to laugh, and to learn new ideas. Many of the games for learning and warm-ups in this chapter and subsequent chapters fulfill a similar purpose.

"Getting to Know Me" is a favorite activity at The Fountainview Center in which new staff fill out a form that is distributed widely. The biographies can then be discussed at staff meetings.

There are many approaches that work. The Fountainview Center's activity is one approach that encourages staff to voluntarily share their lives, express themselves, and talk with one another during an in-service for the most effective learning to take place. Use of warm-up exercises, as suggested in the Training Tool Kit section of each chapter, also can be an effective way to encourage staff to talk and become involved.

Use Games and Role Plays

The beauty of using games and role plays is that they break down the barriers between staff and get everyone on their feet actively learning. For role-play situations, it is best not to call on staff at random but instead to preplan with specific staff members who enjoy being in front of a crowd (see Tool 2.11). This and the remaining chapters include Games for Learning in each Tool Kit.

The following are some examples of games and role-play exercises being used in long-term care programs:

Kay Lloyd, the staff educator at The Fountainview Center plays a game called "Who Am I?," in which key facts about residents are shared in a question-and-answer format. The first staff member who guesses correctly wins a prize. For example, a series of questions may be read, such as "I was born in Providence, Rhode Island. Who am I?" "I enjoy gardening and crafts. Who am I?" and "My cat, 'Miss Kitty,' kept me company. Who am I?"

Dee Carlson, president of ACCET, Inc., uses a number of games in her training sessions not only to break the ice with staff but to get them to think about new ways to solve problems, stretch their thinking, and challenge their attitudes.

There are many ways you can learn. Susan D. Berry, Alzheimer's disease consultant and trainer in Warsaw, Indiana, likes to teach by "Putting the Pieces Together" (see, e.g., Tools 3.8 and 5.7). At each session the group puts together a puzzle around a theme. This allows staff to have a visual experience seeing the pieces of the lesson come together.

Debi Lahav, the coordinator of activities at Margolic Psychogeriatric Center, Tel Aviv, Israel, uses collage as a teaching tool. The idea of staff working together, even over a period of time, to create a collage is very appealing. It evokes good discussion and can be displayed as a gentle reminder and reinforcement of the concepts being taught. It also allows staff to jump into a creative art activity, something that they may not have done since childhood.

Examples of these games are shown in the Tool Kits.

Training classes at Laurel Heights Home for the Elderly feature role plays—"Knack and No-Knack"—in which situations are created and then discussed. How would a staff member react if he or she had "no knack"? How would he or she react with knack?

This concept was first suggested in *The Best Friends Approach to Alzheimer's Care* and has proved successful in many settings. If a scene is created in which a staff member with shoulders slumped, a frown, and a downcast expression says to a group of residents, "Let's do a fun activity!", then staff witnessing this during training can laugh and name that behavior as "no knack." Staff respond very well to concrete examples of "the wrong way" and "the right way," particularly when these are demonstrated with humor. Examples of this technique are given in the Tool Kits.

Involve Storytelling

Many teachers use anecdotes or stories to make their points. In this book, both real anecdotes and fictional stories (the imaginary long-term care programs at the beginning of some chapters) are used to highlight the points that the book makes. Program leaders should develop their own collection of these stories to engage their students and enhance learning. Families also have stories to tell:

Marie B. Smart, Alzheimer's care specialist at The Breckinridge, Lexington, Kentucky, noted, "Families who are living with Alzheimer's disease have many stories to tell staff about their experiences. In their own ways, they become care experts. Their stories can help staff members better understand the disease and the person *and give staff helpful tips and pointers."*

When programs ask families to "teach" staff about their loved ones, it is never an admission of defeat or failure. Instead, it recognizes the expertise and experience of caregivers.

Take Place in an Environment that Facilitates Learning

The environment for learning is important. Is the room free from distractions? Are the lighting and sound good? Are the chairs comfortable? Is the temperature too hot or too cold? Trainers with knack also create a festive, positive atmosphere for learning that is inviting and welcoming.

During The Fountainview Center's staff education series, the director of community relations, Anne M. Helmly, enters the classroom with a bouquet of balloons and a greeting card for all the new staff scheduled to be in the class. She wrote, "By giving new staff members a warm welcome and a sense of importance, they will in turn experience how a wonderful welcome makes the resident and their family feel on the first day at the center."

A special effort was made to welcome new staff to the in-service and to their new positions.

Involve Follow-Through and Modeling

Good training features follow-through and modeling by the teacher or senior staff. The "New Idea Care Center" example given previously in this chapter demonstrates a number of these techniques, including asking staff to practice during the in-service and report on successes during the week.

At The Wealshire, staff are asked to complete a miniature case study on a resident of their choice following the completion of their training program. This challenging exercise has proven successful because it helps staff apply knowledge they have learned to a resident they know.

One reason that this exercise is so successful is that staff can choose the resident and work with one another to complete the assignment. Administrative staff members are also always available to help.

The Santa Barbara Alzheimer's Association conducts a 32-hour training program for long-term care staff at The Samarkand Retirement Community in a jointly sponsored Teaching Learning Center Program. After each class segment, students immediately go to the dementia program, Heritage Court, to work hands-on with residents to practice what they have learned. Faculty members observe, help when needed, and offer feedback and evaluation.

Staff at this innovative project, which has trained staff from programs throughout central California, plan to develop a similar program for family caregivers.

Teach Life Skills

A successful training program teaches life skills to staff, such as assertiveness training, problem solving, and stress management. These training sessions can include talks by community experts or knowledgeable staff members telling their own stories about what has worked well for them in certain settings. Other topics can include anger management or conflict resolution, both skills that can be valuable in a long-term care setting and in life.

Beverly Sanborn teaches life skills to long-term care employees. She believes that problem solving and assertiveness training classes are particularly effective. "Younger people also seem to have had little training in redirecting anger or frustration; training in this area can pay dividends," she noted.

Life skills can include English classes for staff members who are not fluent in English. This is yet another way a program can support staff members to learn skills that will help them not only on the jobs but also in their lives.

Another area of growth and development is community involvement:

Riverside Adult Day Program in Wilmington, Delaware, encourages staff to sit on various committees for the local chapter of the Alzheimer's Association and attend support groups. This allows staff to feel the self-esteem acquired through community involvement while learning new skills such as public speaking, teamwork, and planning of events.

Such community service allows staff to try new skills they may never have used before and to reinforce skills learned in staff training programs.

Involve *Persons* with Alzheimer's Disease

The growing number of *persons* diagnosed early in the disease process presents staff developers with an opportunity to involve them in training programs. When a *person* tells staff members how he or she wants to be treated in a long-term care setting, it sends a powerful message.

Friendship Adult Day Care Center created a video called My Challenge with Alzheimer's Disease. *It has become a successful tool for learning about early Alzheimer's disease through an interview with Beverly Wheeler, a woman diagnosed in her late 50s, who speaks movingly about her experiences.*

Tool 4.7 offers ideas for incorporating *persons* with Alzheimer's disease in training programs. When inclusion is not possible, staff can turn to a number of videotapes that feature interviews with or portrayals of people with Alzheimer's disease (see Appendix C).

Provide Incentives for Learning and Growing

Concerned about creating undue competition or compromising professionalism, some program leaders oppose offering prizes to staff, but all programs should offer some form of recognition or incentives for success. Incentives can include days off with pay, bonuses, raises, and even scholarships for further education. Prizes can motivate staff, but it often seems best to put each staff member who participates in a particular activity in a "prize pool" to win a gift certificate or other award.

Wellington Parc of Owensboro has implemented buttons for the staff that say, "I've got it!" "It" means the knack. Whenever someone sees a staff member using good techniques and interventions that are respectful of the residents, or simply doing something "right," that staff member gets points. A certain amount of points entitles the staff member to a button proclaiming, "I've got it!"

The Fountainview Center conducts a "graduation ceremony" after staff complete the center's dementia curriculum. Much fanfare is made during the ceremony, and a certificate of accomplishment and a graduation pin are presented.

Many staff members may never have received an award or recognition before. These activities can build a staff member's self-esteem and pride.

Encore Senior Living Rediscovery™ in Portland, Oregon, publishes newsletters that recognize volunteers and staff members. "We have developed incentives and recognition programs that have reduced turnover 20%–30% per year. When staff are acknowledged, they feel valued and part of the team. Incentives include extra pay, T-shirts, sweatshirts, and, of course, verbal acknowledgment when staff reach measurable, achievable goals," comments Delores M. Moyer, senior vice president.

One form of recognition should never be overlooked: It is important for program leaders to thank staff for the work that they do. Cynthia Belle, a dementia care consultant and trainer in Chicago, does this well in her training of CNAs. When staff have finished her course, she praises them with the following words: "You now know more than most people in the country about Alzheimer's disease. Your expertise can be valuable not only in your work but to your friends and family. Congratulations and thank you for the job you do." This elevates staff and motivates them to learn more.

Be Evaluated by Staff on a Regular Basis

The Best Friends program evaluates its training efforts by asking staff for feedback and comments. The authors recommend Kathy Laurenhue's simple list of evaluation questions for any long-term care training program:

1. *Did staff learn something new?* Effective training keeps the staff's interest by providing new information to help them be their best.
2. *Did staff like the process?* Do staff appreciate the teaching methods used in the program? Was training interesting, even fun? Even when the information is good, staff should be asked to comment on whether the material was presented well.
3. *Did staff like how they were treated during the process?* Did the class start on time? Were the instructors respectful to staff, or did staff feel talked down to?

Asking these hard questions may sometimes be painful for program leaders, but the answers will help build better staff training programs.

Conclusion

The Best Friends program acknowledges that how staff members are trained is as important as what staff members are taught. This is true because the best curriculum will fail if taught in a series of lectures with little or no opportunity for the learning to be experiential. An effective training program must teach the basics, but it also should be a staff development program, building a staff member's knowledge base while giving him or her enhanced work and life skills and hope for the future.

For example, many programs employ activity assistants. A Best Friends training program might target these individuals with good information, well-conceived and interactive training, follow-up, and reinforcement. The program also might provide coaching in communication, time management, and problem solving, and perhaps offer incentives for further education. Maybe a CNA who receives this help will someday become the facility administrator.

The benefits of involving staff in an effective Best Friends training program are great. Consider this example from Briana Melom, director of education and family services at the Alzheimer's Disease Center, Mayo Clinic, Rochester, Minnesota. She trained one staff member in residential care, Carol, in the Best Friends approach. Here are Carol's remarks after she embraced the Best Friends concepts:

"I used to come to work thinking my job was to cook, clean, and give baths. Residents who were resistive were just in the way of getting my job done. Now I realize I'm here for the people. I've always thought Meg, in particular was difficult but listening to her story I thought I should be bowing down and kissing her feet. She has done so much in her life; I've had such little experience in comparison. I feel like now I can enjoy my job and enjoy the people I work with."

The authors are particularly struck by the statement, "Residents who were resistive were just in the way of getting my job done." Being exposed to the Best Friends model and being trained in a creative, respectful, and effective way helped this staff member fundamentally change her approach and attitude. Briana tells us that this staff member now gives love (and good personal care) freely. "What a gift for the staff member and Meg to have the opportunity to become Best Friends." It is this shift away from being task oriented to being *person-*oriented that will change the culture of long-term care.

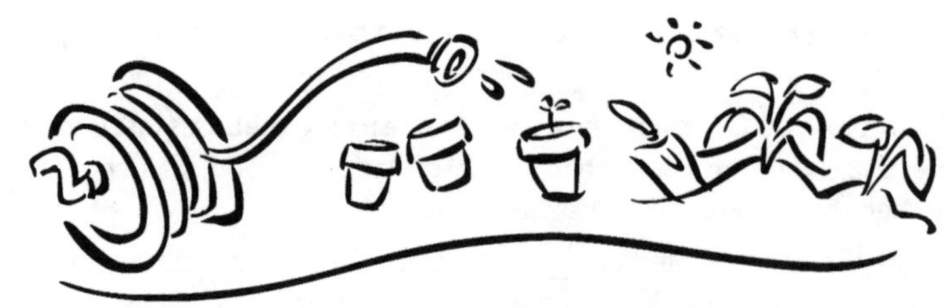

Training Tool Kit

Tool 2.0 / Warm-Up
Here Comes the Sun

Use this exercise to show that most situations have an up side and a down side, a "sunny" and a "dark" side, depending on how you look at them. In good Alzheimer's care, the idea is to find as many positives in the situation as you can, to look for the "sunny side of life."

Draw a large picture of the sun on a flipchart or board. Ask staff to take a few moments to think about the sun and sunshine. Then ask the questions below. Write the staff's answers underneath the picture you have drawn of the sun.

What happy feelings or positive experiences do we have when we think about the sun or sunshine?

What distressing feelings or negative experiences do we have when we think about the sun or sunshine?

This exercise helps the class come up with positive examples such as warmth, brightness, happiness, and the beach. Negative examples might include sunburn, sweat, glare, or humidity. The group leader can then make the point that we can look at the same situation in many ways.

Suggested by Cheryl T. Weidemeyer, program director, Christiana Care/Visiting Nurse Association, Evergreen Center I, Alzheimer's Day Treatment Program, Wilmington, Delaware.

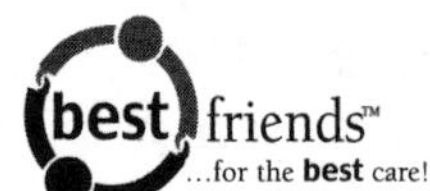

Tool 2.1 / Games for Learning

Numbers Game

This game demonstrates that things get easier with practice; the same is true in Alzheimer's care.

Distribute three copies of the game to the class and have them put the copies face down. Ask them to turn the first page over and connect as many numbers as they can in 1 minute, beginning with the number 1. After 1 minute, ask everyone to stop. How much progress did each staff member make? After the discussion, ask them to turn the next page over and repeat the exercise. Note how the staff got much further this time around. Repeat the exercise a third and final time.

18

23 21

27

24 11

36

15 10 38

3

22 13 28

35

9 16

12 7

5 37

25 2

8

6 34 31 14

20 4

19 33

17

32

26 39

29 1

40

30

Adapted from Newstrom, J.W., & Scannell, E.E. (1989). Games trainers play *(p. 156). New York: McGraw-Hill; reprinted by permission. (Suggested by Dee Carlson.)*

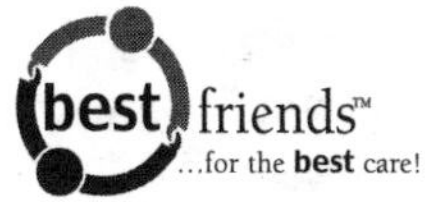

Tool 2.2 / Games for Learning
Word Game

This game teaches that tasks work out better when simplified. Relate the results of this game to Alzheimer's disease care, including dressing and communication.

Divide the class into two teams. Give one group List A and another group List B. They should look at their list for 1 minute, then turn the page over and write down as many words as they remember from their list. Begin the class discussion and find out how many words each group was able to retain (write them on a flipchart or board).

List A

Animals	*Cloths*	*Fuels*
Dog	Cotton	Oil
Cat	Wool	Gas
Horse	Silk	Coal
Cow	Rayon	Wood
Fruits	*Colors*	*Professions*
Apple	Blue	Doctor
Orange	Red	Lawyer
Pear	Green	Teacher
Banana	Yellow	Dentist
Furniture	*Utensils*	*Sports*
Chair	Knife	Football
Table	Spoon	Baseball
Bed	Fork	Basketball
Sofa	Pan	Tennis
Weapons	*Tools*	*Clothing*
Dagger	Hammer	Shirts
Gun	Saw	Socks
Rifle	Nails	Pants
Bomb	Screwdriver	Shoes

List B

Dog	Gas	Pants
Animals	Silk	Coal
Oil	Cotton	Cat
Table	Cloths	Fuels
Wool	Baseball	Hammer
Cow	Knife	Basketball
Fruit	Tennis	Bomb
Pan	Chair	Yellow
Green	Colors	Professions
Sofa	Screwdriver	Dentist
Doctor	Shoes	Football
Furniture	Teacher	Rifle
Horse	Blue	Apple
Rayon	Utensils	Sports
Saw	Orange	Weapons
Wood	Tools	Clothing
Nails	Spoon	Lawyer
Gun	Shirt	Pear
Socks	Fork	Banana
Red	Bed	Dagger

The members of Group A typically will remember more words because things are easier to remember when categorized or simplified.

Original source unknown. (Suggested by Dee Carlson.)

Tool 2.3 / Games for Learning
Making a Collage

Collage is often used in activity programming. Debi Lahav suggests how it can be used in training:

A collage is an artistic composition of materials and objects pasted on a surface. It was first used by Picasso and Braque and then used by Matisse for his famous paper cuts. He used the technique when he became disabled, confined to a rocking chair or bed.

> Collage is one of the easiest, most nonthreatening techniques in the creative arts. Anyone can succeed in creating a collage with little or no artistic talent or expertise. Old magazines, newspapers, scraps of paper, material, or assorted objects can be used. The materials are recycled; something new is created from the old. New connections and combinations are found and new meanings are conveyed.
>
> It is a valuable technique when training because the final product can be a metaphor for a staff member's feelings, thoughts, dreams, and hopes.
>
> Making a collage can be compared to using the Best Friends approach to Alzheimer's disease care. The Best Friend connects to the *person* and helps give new meaning in life by activating his or her remaining strengths.

Collage can be used as both a training tool and an activity. For training purposes, it can be used to celebrate the diversity of families and staff, symbolize the experience of Alzheimer's disease, or be a representation of feelings. It can depict friendship, portray life stories, or show that activities are everywhere.

Submitted by Debi Lahav, occupational and art therapist, Margolic Psychogeriatric Center, Tel Aviv Medical Center, Tel Aviv, Israel; reprinted by permission. (See examples in Tool 4.4.)

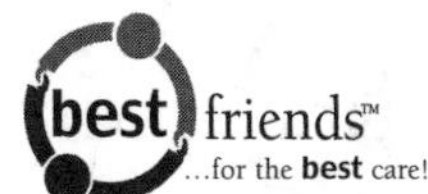

Tool 2.4 / Program Pointer
ENTHUSIASTIC

Use this list for bulletin boards and newsletters or to hand out and discuss with staff. These traits help to build enthusiastic staff and encourage high-quality care.

Enjoy	Enjoy working with older adults.
Natural	Be authentic and genuine. Families and residents can tell when you truly care. Treat your residents as you would your friends.
Thoughtful	Be considerate and attentive. Show real concern as you would with your friends.
Honest	Be honest with your other associates (staff members).
Understand	Picture in your mind what the resident is feeling. Be a friend.
Sincere	Be sincere and caring. Let your words and actions show "I Care."
Initiative	Be self-directed. Don't wait for things to happen; you must make things happen.
Attitude	Employ positive thinking. Staff who feel good about themselves produce good results.
Spirited	Be energetic. You are in a profession in which everyone can win, so enjoy and have fun.
Trustworthy	Be dependable. Families and residents trust you to provide the best care possible.
Involved	Be attentive. Involve the resident by listening.
Change	Employ flexibility. Adjust to changing circumstances every day.

Adapted from a list created by Diane Will, national community life director, The Fountains Continuum of Care, Inc., Tucson, Arizona.

Tool 2.5 / Program Pointer

Knack for Best Friends Newsletter

Create your own newsletter and include statements from staff and residents that are similar to these examples from the newsletter of Laurel Heights Home for the Elderly:

When I told my Best Friend that I wanted to be his Best Friend, you should have seen the look on his face! You could tell that he was touched and pleased. It means a lot, he said, to have a special visit each day from someone who cares.

—*Irene Brummett, Laundry*

I could not pick just one Best Friend, so I chose two. I look forward to visiting with them each day. I feel like we are really getting to know each other in a way I have never thought about. I look forward to it as much or more than they do.

—*Carol Gregory, Business*

My day is not complete unless my Best Friend and I visit. I just cannot go by her door without going in and seeing how she is doing and if she has slept well or needs something. She is so kind. Being her Best Friend is my favorite part of the day.

—*Laura Stewart, Billing*

Look at my life story that the student wrote for me. I've got to show it to Mrs. Young. She is my Best Friend. She will be very interested in all these facts about me.

—*Milton Kidd, Resident*

I look forward so much to see Ruth come in that door or when she sits down with me when I smoke—even though she doesn't smoke. She really cares for me. I can tell because she always comes if she is here. And she will smile, we visit, and I feel better.

—*Beulah Lincks, Resident*

From Knack for Best Friends, *Laurel Heights Home for the Elderly, London, Kentucky, January 1999; reprinted by permission.*

Tool 2.6 / Program Pointer
Elements of Successful Staff Training

Hang this list on bulletin boards, include it in a newsletter, or use it as a handout to discuss with staff.

Successful training programs should

- Be taken seriously, be consistent, and be part of a well-defined set of expectations
- Teach the organization's mission, values, and philosophy
- Include program leaders
- Involve staff who are not involved in direct care
- Teach the right content
- Teach in the right way
- Not teach too much material in any one class
- Be culturally appropriate and sensitive
- Get staff to talk
- Use games and role plays
- Involve storytelling
- Take place in an environment that facilitates learning
- Involve follow-through and modeling
- Teach life skills
- Involve *persons* with Alzheimer's disease
- Provide incentives for learning and growing
- Be evaluated by the staff on a regular basis

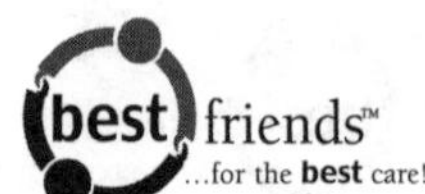

Tool 2.7 / Program Pointer
Tips for Hiring Staff with Knack

Share this list with the individuals who are in charge of hiring and recruitment.

Look for nontraditional candidates who can be trained (e.g., individuals from other service-related fields, older adults, students).

Walk them around the program during the interview and see how they relate to *persons* and other staff.

Have other line staff meet with them one-to-one and ask their future peers for their assessment of the candidate.

During the interview, hand them an object (e.g., stuffed animal, apple, scarf) and see whether the potential employee is willing to be creative and have some fun.

Ask them questions about their personal "best friends." See how they describe those friends. Is it done in a caring and loving way?

Tell them about your program's Best Friends philosophy. Notice how they react.

Talk to them about activities. Do they have any special interests or hobbies that they could contribute to the program, if hired?

Tell them that staff are encouraged to have fun in the program. Can they think of something funny that has happened to them in recent weeks or an embarrassing moment that they had? Observe whether they have a sense of humor.

Ask candidates how they would handle the following situations:

- A resident is pacing and seems upset.
- A resident will not eat his or her dinner no matter how hard the CNA tries. Should the CNA continue trying to feed the resident?
- A resident gets up during the night and wants to talk.
- A participant arrives at the day center with his wife, and he will not get out of the car.

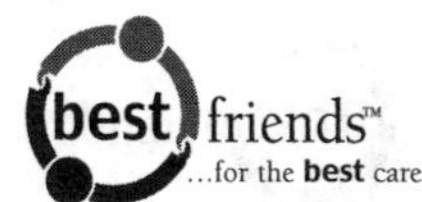

Tool 2.8 / Program Pointer

20 Progressive Ways to Teach a Concept

Share this list with all staff educators. Send it out ahead of time to guest speakers.

Games
Puzzles
Collage
Role play and drama
Debate
Small-group discussion
Peer-to-peer teaching
Poetry
Warm-ups
Charades/pantomime
Guessing games/trivia
Skits
Newsletter
Trainers modeling and reinforcing in the dementia program
Making an acrostic or a list
Short lecture with ample time for discussion
Practice
Observation
Writing songs or special song lyrics
Short video clips with discussion

Tool 2.9 / Program Pointer
Making a Splash with Handouts for Training

Here are some examples of innovative ways to create handouts. Many similar originals or templates can be found at art and office supply stores or copy stores. Have fun!

Making the Communication Connection

Do speak clearly and slowly

Use positive body language

Smile often

Use the life story

Practice good body language

Use 30 second activities

Do this and you will
Meet your Caregiving

GOAL!

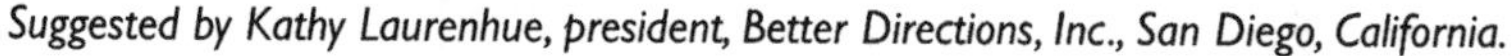

Suggested by Kathy Laurenhue, president, Better Directions, Inc., San Diego, California.

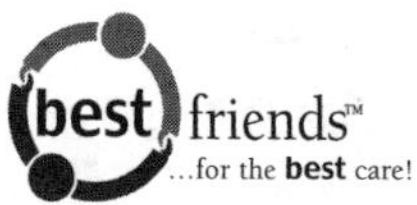

Tool 2.10 / Program Pointer
Developing a Theme for Your Handouts

Creating a theme for lessons is one creative way to teach them. For example:

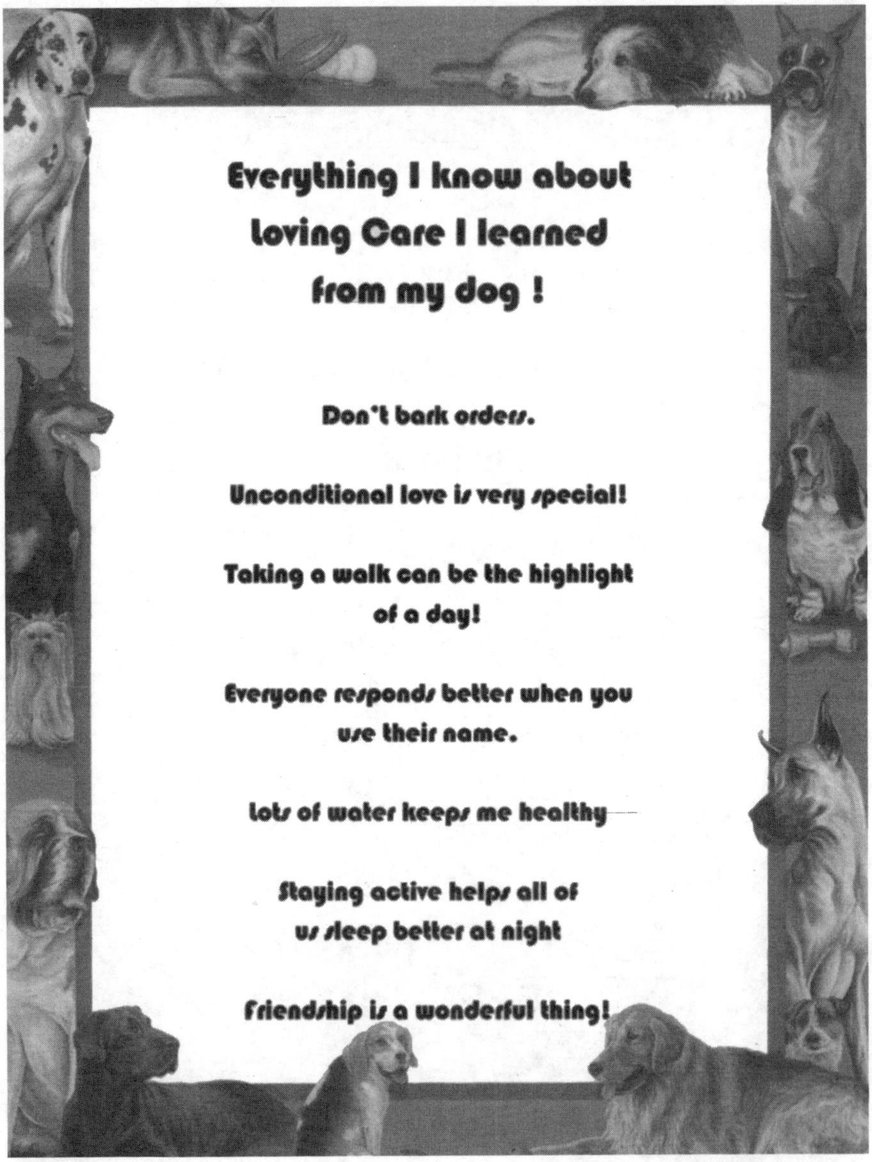

**Everything I know about
Loving Care I learned
from my dog !**

Don't bark orders.

Unconditional love is very special!

**Taking a walk can be the highlight
of a day!**

**Everyone responds better when you
use their name.**

Lots of water keeps me healthy

**Staying active helps all of
us sleep better at night**

Friendship is a wonderful thing!

Suggested by Kathy Laurenhue, president, Better Directions, San Diego, California

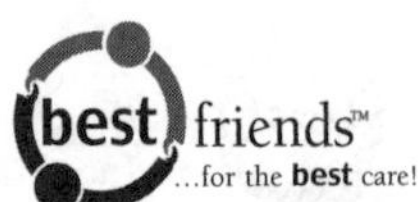

Tool 2.11 / Games for Learning
How to Create a Successful Role Play

Role-play concepts that are built around a "wrong way" and a "right way" are some of the best ways to learn while having fun. Here are some suggestions to help you develop successful role plays, as well as a sample role play from which you can model your own.

- Line up the "actors" first. When possible, choose a "cast" from a variety of staff positions. Meet with the actors ahead of time to explain the concept or lesson being taught.
- In general, it is not a good idea to select actors on the spot. Sometimes a staff member will feel uncomfortable or not really understand the point of the skit.
- Employ humor or exaggeration in the skit or dialogue. When supervisors, for example, are willing to poke fun at themselves, it helps the line staff have even more fun and pay more attention to what is being taught.
- Role-play the wrong way first, then stop and discuss the situation. Write the mistakes on the board.
- Do the skit all over again the right way. Try to incorporate or address some of the concerns that are raised. Now discuss the second scenario and list on the board all of the right ways to address a problem.

Here is a short example of the situation. The actual role plays can be much richer.

Role Play: The Argument
Purpose: To show that you cannot argue with residents with dementia.
Set up: Have the director of nursing play a resident, "Mrs. T."
Have the activities director play a staff member, "CNA."
Scene: Mrs. T is certain that she is late for work.
Staff member tries to explain her situation and ends up arguing with her about it.

MRS. T: I'm late for work. I need to run and catch the bus.
CNA: [*not making eye contact, talking fast, being abrupt*] No, you're retired now.
MRS. T: I'm sorry, you're wrong. I just got promoted.
CNA: No, you haven't worked in 10 years.
MRS. T: What's the matter with you? I was there yesterday.
CNA: You were *here* yesterday, I saw you myself.
MRS. T: [*getting anxious, angry, worried*]. Why are you . . . What are you saying? I don't like you. I want to leave now!
CNA: Don't you remember anything? You *do not* work!

The class can be asked to discuss what went wrong with this approach and should be able to come up with many problems (lack of eye contact, not caring, being argumentative, not providing a distraction, not using the life story, and more). The following is an example of the right way to approach the situation.

(continued)

MRS. T: I'm late for work. I need to run and catch the bus.
CNA: [Smiling, making eye contact] How are you today, Marge?
MRS. T: Fine, but I'm late for the office.
CNA: May I walk with you while you tell me about your work?
MRS. T: Oh, how nice you are. I'm a writer.
CNA: And a very good one I hear! You look terrific today. How is your son, Michael, and your two darling grandchildren, Toby and Annette?
MRS. T: They are wonderful, but I'm late.
CNA: You are so talented. I hear you are one of the most successful graduates of your school. Berkeley, isn't it?
MRS. T: Yes, Berkeley, I went there.
CNA: I think the bus is running late today, let's just sit for a while. Tell me about your days at college.

The class can then be asked why this approach might work (employing empathy, using the life story, providing a gentle distraction, reminiscing, not arguing). Maybe by the time they are finished chatting, Mrs. T will have forgotten about getting to the office.

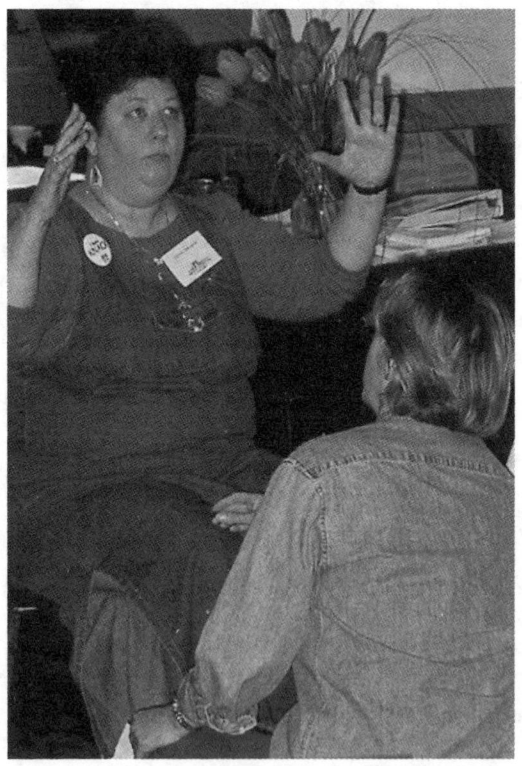

Wendy Sampels (left) and Joanne Rader role playing the "right way" to communicate with a person with dementia.

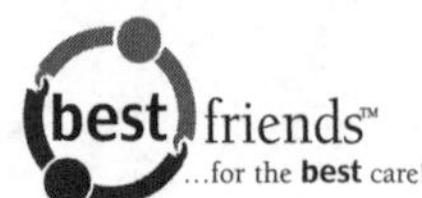

3

Medical & Scientific Basics

Learning the basics about the medical and scientific aspects of Alzheimer's disease is an important part of staff training and development. This knowledge helps staff understand that the disease is real, and it gives them the tools they need to implement the best plan of care for the *person* with Alzheimer's disease. Staff members do not need to become experts on the disease, but they should acquire the skills that are necessary to do their jobs with confidence and care.

This chapter reviews the basics of what should be taught to a Best Friends staff member about Alzheimer's disease. Suggestions on how the following key concepts can be taught are offered in the Training Tool Kit at the end of the chapter.

What Does the Word *Dementia* Mean? Is It the Same as *Senility*?

Senility is an outdated word that is often used to refer to the physical and mental deterioration of old age. It should not be used because it reinforces many stereotypes about aging, particularly the notion that every individual who gets old loses his or her mind. The preferred term is *dementia*. With its Latin roots (*de* means "away from," and *mens* means "mind"), dementia actually means "away from the mind." It is the universally accepted phrase to describe losses in intellectual functioning, including one or more of the following: memory loss, language deficits, diminished judgment, decline in problem-solving ability, and lack of initiative. Dementia implies a chronic (months or years) malady, in contrast to the term *organic mental syndrome,* which is transient (hours or days). Young people can have dementia, but it is usually related to a situational event such as high fever or drug or alcohol use/abuse. In elderly individuals, symptoms of dementia usually (but not always) reveal an irreversible health problem.

Dementia is a global term describing a neurological condition that has many potential causes. By itself, dementia is not a complete or an appropriate diagnosis. It is as if a physician were to diagnose cancer without providing any further details. Someone who sees a doctor should expect to receive a diagnosis that describes a specific type of dementia, or at least a working diagnosis, and should be confident that other potentially treatable causes of loss of cognition, such as multiple strokes or a tumor, have been excluded.

To help explain this concept, staff members can be asked to imagine that the word "dementia" is painted on a large umbrella. Underneath that umbrella, the disorders that can cause reversible and irreversible dementias are listed. This simple visualization exercise can help teach the idea that Alzheimer's disease is a form of dementia and that there are related disorders that also cause dementia (see Tool 3.2).

What Is Alzheimer's Disease?

The disease was described initially in 1907 by a German doctor, Alois Alzheimer, for whom it was named. It has probably always been present, but it has gotten more attention as the world population has grown larger and older. Although younger individuals do develop Alzheimer's disease, the disease is primarily one that affects people 65 years of age and older.

The national Alzheimer's Association has said, "Alzheimer's disease usually begins gradually, causing a person to forget recent events and to have difficulty performing familiar tasks. How rapidly the disease advances varies from person to person with the disease, causing confusion, personality and behavior change, and impaired judgment. Communication becomes difficult as the person with Alzheimer's disease struggles to find words, finish thoughts, or follow directions." A description of the impact of Alzheimer's disease on language is seen in Figure 3.1. Over a number of years, *persons* with Alzheimer's disease become totally unable to care for themselves. This creates enormous demands on family and professional caregivers.

Agnosia—The inability to interpret sensations and recognize familiar objects. The person has trouble knowing the meaning of what is seen, heard, smelled, touched, and tasted. He or she may not recognize familiar faces, may not recognize where he or she is, and may not recognize what belongs to him or her or others.

Anomia—The inability to find the right word, to name an object, or express an idea.

Aphasia—Difficulty understanding and/or expressing language. Affects an individual's ability to follow instructions, participate in conversations, and express needs.

Apraxia—Difficulty translating thought into action. Someone with apraxia may agree to brush her teeth, but will be unable to organize and carry out the process.

Paraphrasia—Syllables, words, and phrases become jumbled and mixed up. Speech can become meaningless sounds, although it may retain the tone and expression of normal language.

Perseveration—A persistent repetition of an activity, word, phrase, or movement such as tapping, wiping, or picking. People with dementia can "get stuck" on certain words or actions.

Word salad—The use of words that are mixed up or used together without meaningful content.

Figure 3.1. Impact of dementia on language. (From Alzheimer's Association. [1995]. Terms & tips: An Alzheimer care handbook *[Publication PF 303Z]. Chicago: Author; reprinted by permission.)*

The disease is very real, causing physiological changes to the brain that take a devastating toll on the *person,* who eventually may be unable to swallow and eat, unable to walk, and unable to manage most or all activities of daily living (ADLs). Alzheimer's disease ultimately takes the life of the affected *person.* On death certificates, Alzheimer's disease often is listed as a secondary cause of death, with the more immediate cause (e.g., heart attack, stroke, pneumonia) listed first.

What Is the Difference Between Alzheimer's Disease and Normal Age-Associated Memory Loss?

Many individuals become more forgetful under stress because of medication or simply because of the normal aging process. One way to determine whether a problem exists is by using the following tongue twister: *If you remember forgetting, that's OK. If you forget you forgot, that's not.* Thus, an individual who forgets a business appointment but later remembers, calls his or her colleague, and apologizes may have nothing to fear. If he or she does not remember the appointment or makes an implausible excuse for the mistake ("We never had an appointment," "I showed up and someone said you canceled"), then an assessment for Alzheimer's disease or another form of dementia may be in order.

Forgetfulness is not the only sign of a potential problem. Sometimes apathy or personality changes can mark the beginning of a dementing illness. The 10 warning signs of Alzheimer's disease are described in Figure 3.2. These warning signs can be a useful tool for families who are concerned about dementia. Be certain to present them with an appropriate medical referral because it is always possible that a reversible dementia is present.

1. Recent memory loss that affects job skills.
2. Difficulty performing familiar tasks.
3. Problems with language.
4. Disorientation of time and place.
5. Poor or decreased judgment.
6. Problems with abstract thinking.
7. Misplacing things.
8. Changes in mood or behavior.
9. Changes in personality.
10. Loss of initiative.

Figure 3.2. The 10 warning signs of Alzheimer's disease. (From Alzheimer's Association. [1996]. Is it Alzheimer's? Warning signs you need to know. *[Publication PR/301/Z]. Chicago: Author; reprinted by permission.)*

What Are the Related Irreversible Dementias?

Alzheimer's disease is the most common irreversible dementia in older adults. Other forms of irreversible dementia include:

- Vascular dementia—brain damage caused by multiple strokes; also called multi-infarct dementia
- Parkinson's disease—can include some symptoms of dementia
- Frontotemporal dementia—includes Pick's disease and a variety of other disorders; a leading cause of dementia in younger *persons*
- Lewy body disease—*persons* often have muscular symptoms that are similar to those of Parkinson's disease, and they sometimes have visual hallucinations and significant sensitivity to psychotropic medications

A more comprehensive list and description of these disorders is included in Figure 3.3.

What Are the Most Common Irreversible Dementias in Older Adults?

Alzheimer's disease is by far the most common dementing illness. The next most common form of dementia is vascular or multi-infarct dementia, or multiple strokes. Together these disorders account for the majority of irreversible dementias in elderly people.

What Are the Related Reversible Dementias?

Some dementing disorders are reversible or partially treatable. For example, if an older person mixes prescription drugs with over-the-counter drugs inappropriately, then an adverse drug interaction can cause symptoms of dementia. Other reversible problems include vitamin B_{12} deficiency and thyroid disorders. Depression also can mimic the symptoms of dementia; with medication, counseling, or both, an elderly individual often can bounce back to good health. A number of causes of reversible dementias are described in Figure 3.4.

Should Everyone Who Has Symptoms Get a Thorough Diagnosis?

Best Friends staff members recognize that whatever someone's age, if he or she is exhibiting symptoms of dementia, then a complete medical evaluation is mandatory. There is always hope that an evaluation will reveal a reversible or treatable disorder. A good evaluation also will help identify problems that, if left untreated, could make the *person's* dementia worse. Getting a thorough diagnosis can help *persons* and their families plan for the future.

This evaluation should include a thorough medical history, a neuropsychological or mental status examination, a neurological examination, laboratory tests, and other tests as ordered. Testing may also include a computerized tomography (CT) scan or magnetic resonance imaging (MRI), which look for problems such as stroke, hydrocephalus, or tumors.

Alzheimer's disease (AD)—Discovered in 1907 by a German doctor for which the disease is named, AD is a progressive, degenerative disease of the brain that gradually causes declines in intellectual ability, including memory, problem solving, and judgment. Eventually the disease leaves *persons* unable to care for themselves. Medications are available and under development that may improve thinking or slow the advance of the disease, but no cure is yet available.

Creutzfeldt-Jakob disease (CJD)—CJD is a rare, fatal brain disease caused by infection. Symptoms are failing memory, changes in behavior and lack of muscular coordination. CJD progresses rapidly, usually causing death within a year. No treatment is currently available.

Multi-infarct dementia (MID)—Also known as vascular dementia, MID results from brain damage caused by multiple strokes (infarcts) within the brain. Symptoms can include disorientation, confusion, and behavioral changes. MID is neither reversible nor curable, but treatment of underlying conditions (e.g., high blood pressure) may halt progression.

Frontotemporal dementia—Personality changes and disorientation may precede memory loss in this dementia. Visual hallucinations and sensitivity to medications may occur. Pick's disease is one example.

Parkinson's disease (PD)—PD is a disease affecting control of muscle activity, resulting in tremors, stiffness, and speech impediment. In late stages, dementia can occur, including AD. Antiparkinsonian drugs can improve steadiness and control, but they have no effect on mental deterioration.

Lewy body disease—Recognized only since the 1980s, this is a disease in which the symptoms are a combination of AD and Pick's disease. Usually dementia symptoms are initially present followed by the abnormal movements associated with Pick's disease. Other symptoms include hallucinations and delusions, falls, and varying consciousness. People with Lewy body disease also can be very sensitive to psychotropic medications. There is no treatment currently available.

Huntington's disease—Huntington's disease is a hereditary disorder characterized by irregular movements of the limbs and facial muscles, a decline in thinking ability, and personality changes. It can be positively diagnosed and symptoms controlled with drugs. The progressive nature of the disease, however, cannot be stopped.

Figure 3.3. Selected irreversible dementias. (Adapted from Alzheimer's Association. [1997]. An overview of Alzheimer's disease and related dementias *[Publication ED205Z]. Chicago: Author.)*

Are All *Persons* with Alzheimer's Disease Alike?

As the saying goes, when you've met one *person* with Alzheimer's disease, you've met just one *person* with Alzheimer's disease. Best Friends staff members understand that there can be tremendous variations in the manifestation of dementia; the impact on visual/spatial abilities, judgment, and even short- and long-term memory can vary. Also, symptoms and behaviors

Depression—Depression is a psychiatric condition marked by sadness, inactivity, difficulty with thinking and concentration, feelings of hopelessness, and, in some cases, suicidal tendencies. Many severely depressed people also display symptoms of memory loss. Often, depression can be reversed with medical treatment and counseling.

Medication interactions—Many older people take a variety of prescription and nonprescription "over-the-counter" medications. Misuse of these medications or use of medications that are not compatible can cause symptoms of dementia.

Normal-pressure hydrocephalus (NPH)—NPH is a rare disease caused by an obstruction in the flow of spinal fluid. Symptoms include difficulty in walking, memory loss, and incontinence. NPH may be related to a history of meningitis, encephalitis, or brain injury and is often correctable with surgery.

Vitamin B_{12} deficiency—Low levels of vitamin B_{12} and folic acid can cause symptoms of dementia. Treatment can often improve or reverse the dementia.

Infections—Left unchecked, infections can cause symptoms of dementia. Fortunately, this problem usually responds to medical attention.

Hormonal—Very low or very high levels of thyroid hormone can cause symptoms of dementia. Correcting the problem will usually reverse these symptoms.

Malnutrition—When someone does not eat well, he or she can actually become malnourished. This is particularly a problem when an individual lives alone. At its worst, malnutrition can contribute to dementia.

Figure 3.4. Selected reversible causes of dementia. (Adapted from Alzheimer's Association. [1997]. An overview of Alzheimer's disease and related dementias *[Publication ED205Z]. Chicago: Author.)*

change over time. This is a good news/bad news situation for staff. The good news is that problems that seem daunting sometimes diminish or end. The bad news is that care would be easier if the future could be predicted.

Can Alzheimer's Disease Be Inherited?

Best Friends staff members know that Alzheimer's disease does run in some families (i.e., it can be familial) but that a *person's* children, siblings, or other relatives may never develop it (i.e., it may not be inheritable). The consensus among researchers seems to be that an individual's chances of developing Alzheimer's disease are higher if a parent had the disease, particularly if the parent's onset came at a younger age (e.g., ages 40–70).

It is important to stress that even if someone is at genetic risk for developing Alzheimer's disease, it may not manifest itself. There also is optimism that the enormous strides being made in research will lead to preventive methods, treatments, or even a cure.

Can Alzheimer's Disease Be Prevented?

Best Friends staff members understand that although there is no known way to prevent Alzheimer's disease, some researchers feel that this is an area of great hope. Alzheimer's disease may actually develop years before symptoms appear; it may be that medication or lifestyle changes will be discovered that will delay onset or prevent it.

Some physicians and studies have suggested that antioxidant vitamins (notably vitamin E) and anti-inflammatory medications (e.g., ibuprofen), taken over long periods of time, can have preventive qualities. More research studies on this subject are forthcoming. A physician's advice should be sought before starting any new medication or vitamin regimen.

There also have been studies suggesting that the adage "use it or lose it" may in fact have some validity. These researchers believe that staying intellectually active probably will not prevent Alzheimer's disease altogether, but it might delay its onset.

How Can Excess Disabilities Be Prevented?

The Best Friends staff maximizes a *person's* physical health and well-being to prevent excess disabilities. Excess disabilities are any treatable medical or health-related condition that, left untreated, will increase a *person's* dementia. An example of this is the *person* with a treatable vision problem that has not been dealt with, thus increasing his or her disorientation and confusion. Getting this *person* new glasses and asking a thoughtful CNA to encourage their use could eliminate one excess disability. Other examples of treatable problems include bladder infections, bowel impaction, pneumonia, and dehydration.

Depression often accompanies Alzheimer's disease. It can be treated effectively and should be regarded as an important excess disability to detect and treat. See Tool 3.6 for more on excess disabilities.

Do Sudden Changes Suggest Problems Other than Alzheimer's Disease?

Best Friends staff members recognize that sudden changes in mood, energy, or behavior can be indicative of physical problems that are unrelated to Alzheimer's disease. If a woman with Alzheimer's disease who usually is alert and happy-go-lucky suddenly becomes angry and acts out, then it is possible that she is in pain and cannot say so. She also may have a serious medical problem that requires immediate attention. Well-trained staff always will be sensitive to the fact that a "behavioral problem" might be an excess disability, which, once treated, will allow the *person* to function at his or her full potential.

What Is the Role of Psychotropic and Other Drugs?

Best Friends staff members work hard to create an environment in which psychotropic, or mood-altering drugs, are used with care. These medications have their place and can often make an enormous difference when problems such as sleeplessness or anxiety occur. A competent physician can devise an effective treatment plan, but finding the right medication and right dosage for older, frail individuals with dementia can be challenging. The challenge and paradox of these drugs are that some of the drugs effectively treat problems such as anxiety, hallucinations and delusions, sleeplessness, or aggression, but they also may have unacceptable side effects or increase the underlying confusion that they are designed to combat.

New medications that may improve cognition and slow the ongoing disease process continue to be developed. Many people believe that these drugs also will have a positive impact on behavior, without the disadvantages of many psychotropic drugs.

In the near future hugs *and* drugs may both make the lives of *persons* with dementia better.

Resources for the Best Friends Staff

The pace of change in Alzheimer's disease research has been fast and furious. A more hopeful time has arrived when effective treatments and preventive measures are on the horizon. A Best Friends staff member keeps abreast of these changes. To do this, long-term care programs should subscribe to local and national Alzheimer's Association publications, check out reputable websites, and affiliate whenever possible with local or regional university research centers. There also are a number of professional journals and publications that can help program leaders keep up with developments. See Appendix C for a list of resources for program staff.

Conclusion

Staff who are well versed in dementia care have more confidence in their daily work and are better able to empathize with *persons* with dementia. This basic knowledge about Alzheimer's disease also helps staff recognize that the disease is real and that the symptoms are part of a disease process. They also will have more skills to do their job well. When a *person* says something mean or hateful, well-educated staff members recognize that it is probably the disease talking, not the *person*.

The authors believe that when training programs are conducted in the Best Friends way, staff members will embrace lifelong learning and will want to learn more about their chosen field. Whether it be through university-sponsored or Alzheimer's Association courses, a physician guest speaker, a guest speaker with early Alzheimer's disease, one of the growing numbers of excellent videotapes, role plays, or a presentation, education is a gift that programs can give staff.

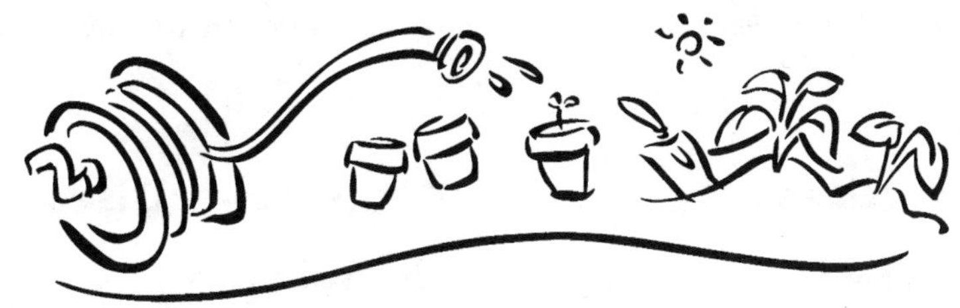

Training Tool Kit

Tool 3.0 / Warm-Up
The Leadership Lineup

Ask everyone to line up according to the length of time they have worked in the field of aging or Alzheimer's disease. The newest staff member should be first in line. Give the group about 5 minutes to sort this out. Then, when everyone is in line, ask each staff member to name the number of days, months, or years that they have worked in this field.

Give a round of applause to the newest and oldest members of the field.

Variation: Some programs may choose to have those present line up on the basis of how long they have worked at that particular program.

Variation: Add up the number of years of work experience in the room.

Make the point that staff members have varying levels of expertise and experience. New staff members can look to senior members for ideas and help. New staff can sometimes offer different approaches to senior staff. The group also should celebrate the combined wealth of experience in the room.

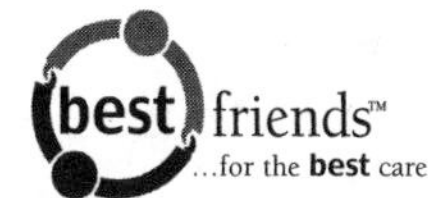

Tool 3.1 / Program Pointer
Alzheimer's Disease Is/Is Not

This list can be tacked on bulletin boards and included in newsletters or used to hand out and discuss with staff.

Alzheimer's Disease Is

Real

A disease that has an impact on a *person's* memory, judgment, language, problem-solving ability, initiative, and personality

A disease that attacks selected areas of the brain

A disease (or diseases)

One form of dementia

Progressive

Irreversible

Age related

Worldwide

The fourth leading cause of death among adults in the U.S.

Alzheimer's Disease Is Not

Normal aging

Inevitable

Faked symptoms, stubbornness

A disease of only older *persons*

Senility

Sudden

The same as dementia caused by stroke, Parkinson's disease, depression, etc.

A disease of any one culture, socioeconomic group, or gender

Imagined

A mental condition

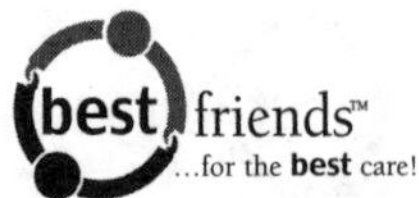

Tool 3.2 / Program Pointer
The Dementia Umbrella

Use the drawing of the dementia umbrella for bulletin boards and newsletters or to hand out and discuss with staff. Dementia is a global, or umbrella, term that is applied when an individual presents with memory loss, confusion, declining problem-solving and judgment skills, and language deficits. Under the umbrella at left are examples of the irreversible causes of dementia; at right are examples of reversible causes.

*Variation:** Write the conditions on index cards. Use a real umbrella and hang the cards from it to allow staff to comprehend how they all are part of the world of dementia.

Variation: Create a bulletin board to teach the concept.

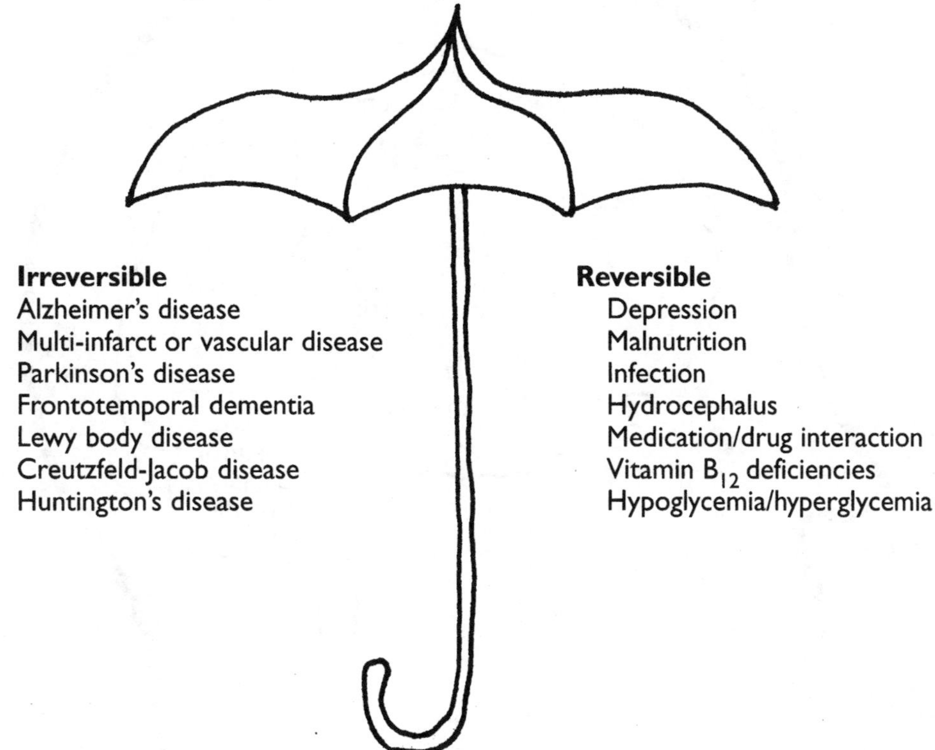

**Variation suggested by Debbie McConnell, Director of Education, Alzheimer's Association, Santa Barbara, California.*

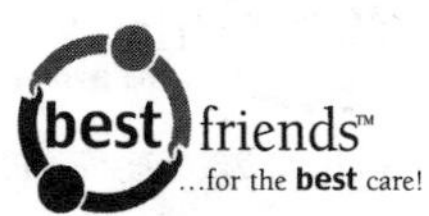

Tool 3.3 / Program Pointer
A Map of the Brain

Use this tool as a handout to remind staff how Alzheimer's disease has an impact on different parts of the brain. The disease affects some people differently than others. Alzheimer's disease affects the brain selectively, leaving some skills and functions intact and damaging others. The areas that are most typically affected are those that control memory and language. Some people may have damage to areas of the brain that affect language, whereas others may have damage in areas of the brain that affect memory.

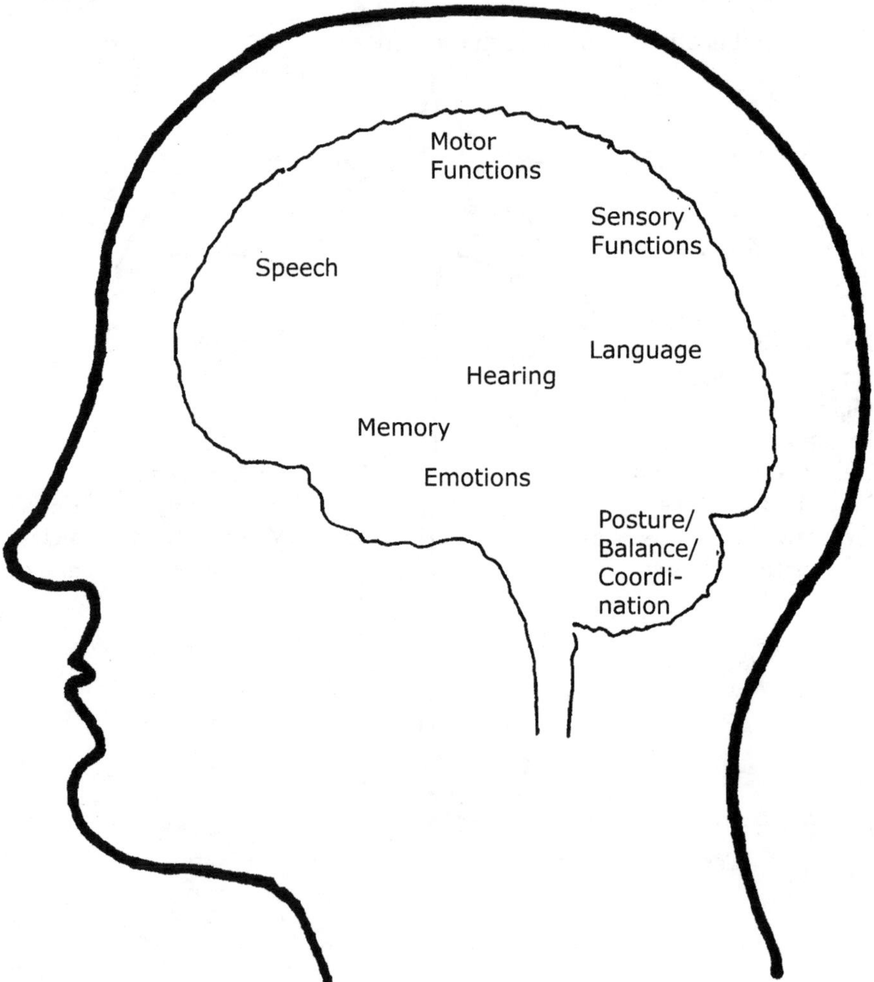

best friends™ ...for the best care!

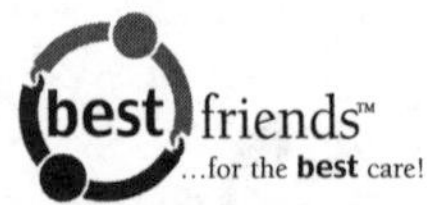

Tool 3.4 / Program Pointer
The Impact of Alzheimer's Disease

Use this tool as a handout or an overhead to remind staff that Alzheimer's disease is real. Alzheimer's disease takes a physical toll on the brain. These photographs show how the disease attacks the brain. The top photograph is a healthy cross-sectional view; the one at bottom shows atrophy (shrinkage) and gaps where there should be tissue.

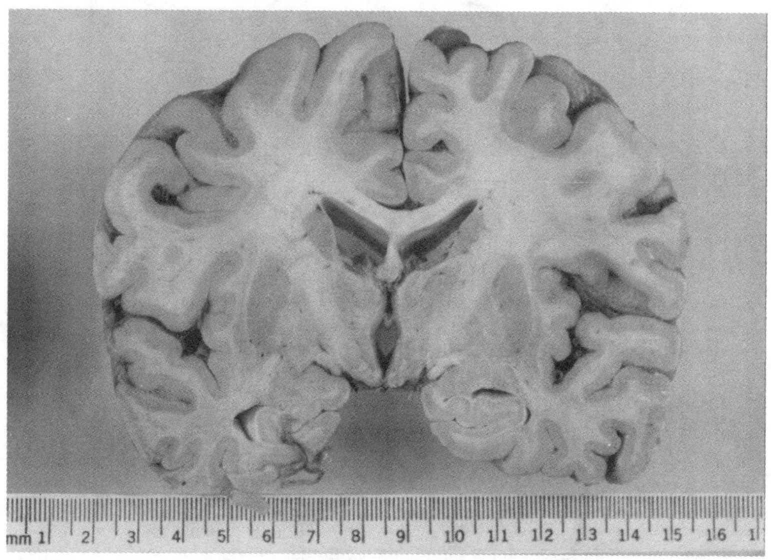

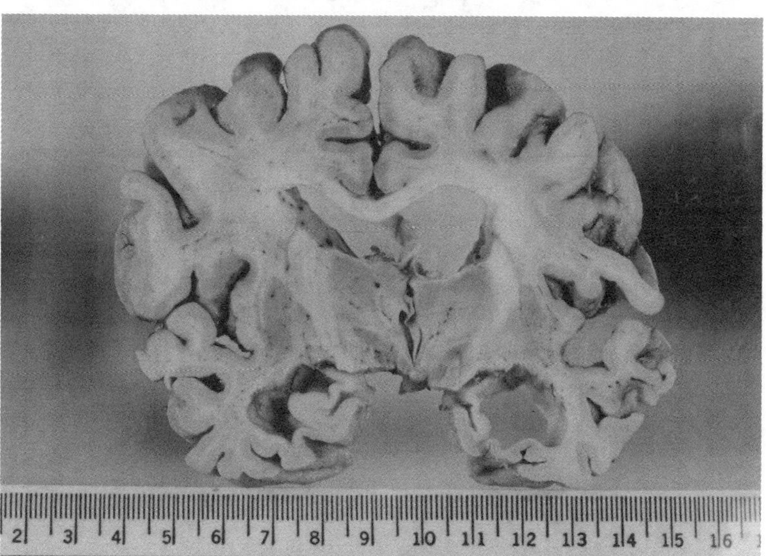

Photographs courtesy of Alzheimer's Disease Research Center, Sanders-Brown Center on Aging, University of Kentucky, Lexington.

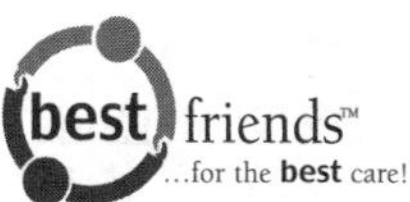

Tool 3.5 / Program Pointer
The World of Alzheimer's Disease

Draw on and around the illustration of the face the problems listed below as typical symptoms/problems of the person *with dementia. Use for group discussion or as an individual exercise. (This activity is particularly effective for new or inexperienced staff.)*

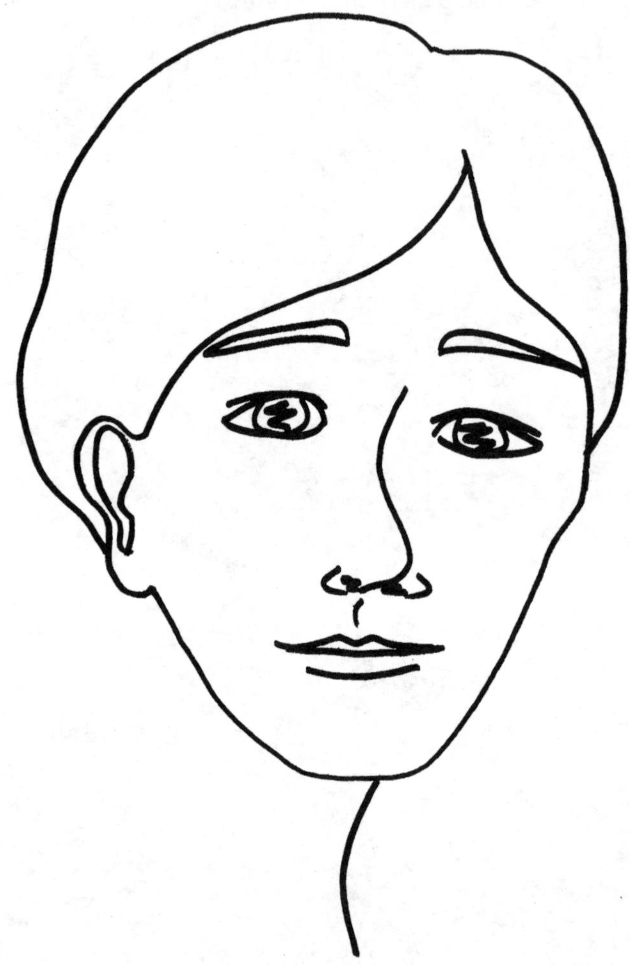

The *person* with dementia faces losses in the following areas:

Memory loss (notably short-term memory)
Language
Judgment
Initiative
Problem solving
Sequencing
Visual/spatial

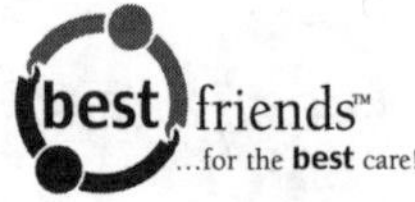

Tool 3.6 / Program Pointer
The Excess Baggage of Alzheimer's Disease

Use this tool for group discussion. Compare excess disabilities to being weighed down with too much baggage. Contrast with Tool 3.7.

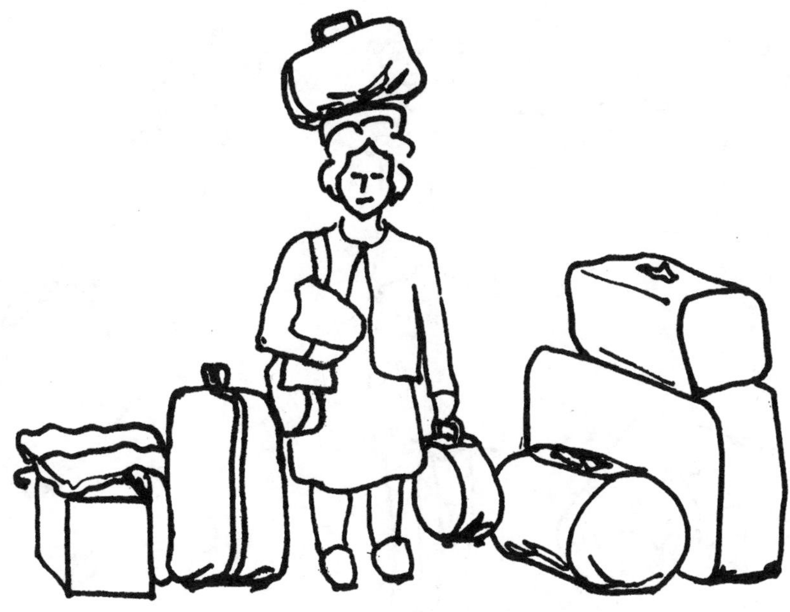

Excess disabilities that can occur:

- Infection
- Nutritional problems
- Pain
- Vision loss
- Hearing loss
- Toothaches/mouth problems
- Heart problems
- Foot problems
- Uncontrolled diabetes
- High/low blood pressure
- Dehydration
- Hypothermia
- Depression
- Bowel/bladder problems

Variation: Tennis balls. Use this activity as an analogy of how excess disabilities can build up and overwhelm a *person.* Ask a volunteer staff member to stand in front of the class. Class members should gently toss tennis balls to the staff member. See how many balls the staff member can hold without dropping one or more.

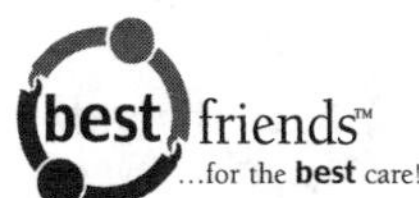

Tool 3.7 / Program Pointer
Let's Get Rid of Excess Baggage!

Use this as a handout or an overhead for discussion, showing the benefits of treating excess disabilities.

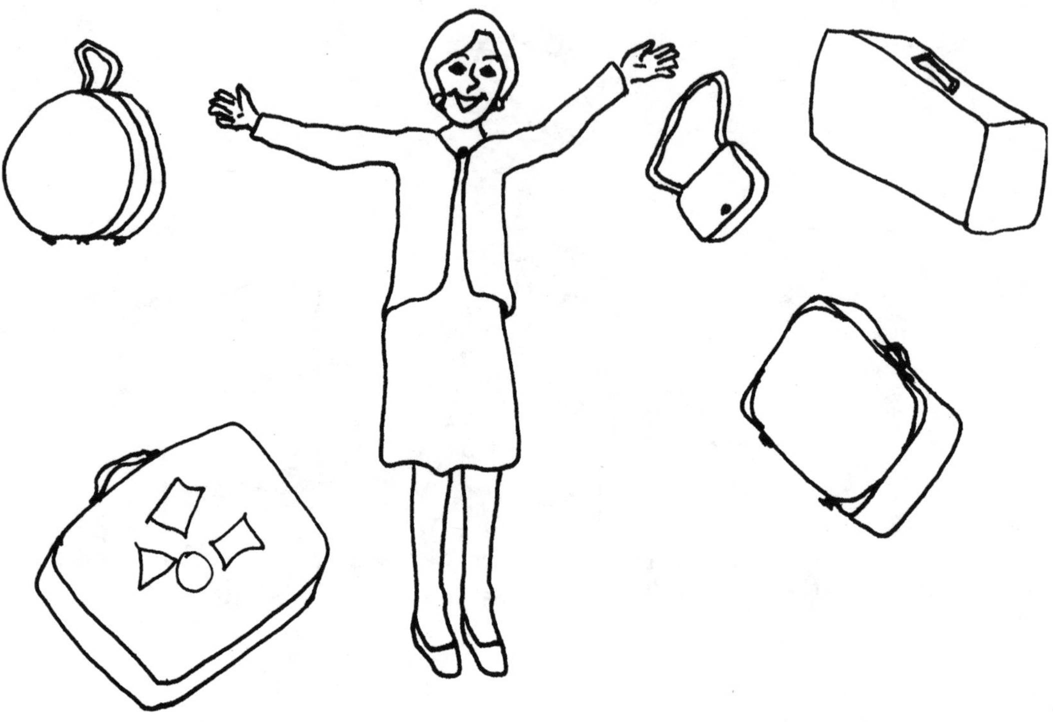

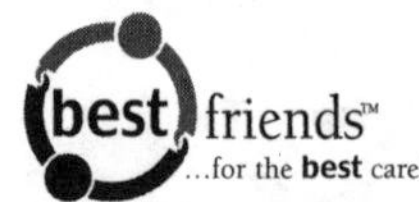

Tool 3.8 / Games for Learning
Putting the Pieces Together

The purpose of this exercise is to help staff understand the symptoms of Alzheimer's disease.

Prior to the training session, cut foam board from an art supply store into puzzle pieces and place a piece of Velcro on the back of each piece. On a piece of paper, write the terms from the possibilities listed below that you have decided to use. Cut out each term and stick one on each puzzle piece.

Divide the class into small groups and give each group one or more puzzle pieces. Ask the group to discuss the content of its puzzle piece and how it relates to Alzheimer's disease. At the end, ask a volunteer from each group to come to the front of the class and put its piece back into the puzzle. (You can create a master outline for the tabletop.)

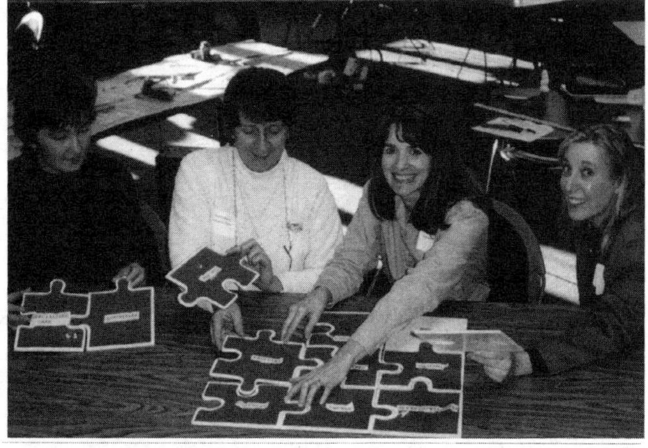

From left: Lila Turner Chandler, Beverly Zahl, Debbie Wayner, and Beverly Walker put the pieces together during an in-service.

Repeats old stories
Makes bad decisions
Loses car keys
Loses car
Leaves the stove on
Has trouble getting dressed
Cannot follow a favorite recipe
Makes false accusations
Thinks strangers are in the house
Gets angry for no apparent reason
Has trouble walking on a patterned floor
Gets lost in a familiar neighborhood

Variation: Use the 10 warning signs of Alzheimer's disease from Figure 3.2 as puzzle pieces.

Make the point that, in and of themselves, these symptoms or behaviors cannot lead to a definitive diagnosis of Alzheimer's disease, but that when you put them together, you get a good picture of Alzheimer's disease. All of the above-listed symptoms can be symptoms of a dementia. It is always important to get a good medical evaluation to uncover any treatable problems.

Exercise courtesy of Susan D. Berry, Alzheimer's consultant and trainer, Warsaw, Indiana.

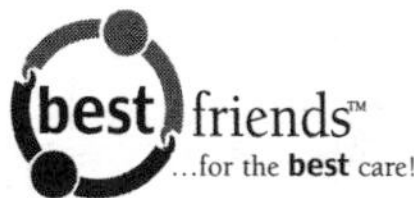

Tool 3.9

Turning No Knack into Knack

The purpose of this exercise is to show, with a dash of humor, the wrong way to do something. This is active learning that really sinks in, particularly when class members themselves volunteer to take part in the role plays.

The following statements represent stereotypes or falsehoods about dementia. These examples of "no knack" can be used in a number of ways to explore staff attitudes and reinforce the lessons that are presented in this chapter. Draw the examples from a hat to discuss as a group or incorporate them in role plays. Invite staff to comment on the mistakes in the statements below. Then role-play or discuss the right way. The authors discuss the art of role plays in Tool 2.11. Use your creativity to have fun turning these examples of "no knack" into "knack."

That old guy is just senile. They all get that way.

All of them become violent.

She could do more things, but she's just being stubborn.

If you take care of yourself you won't get Alzheimer's. I eat a lot of carrots and I think that will do it.

Alzheimer's can be cured by the latest drugs.

Why bother taking Mom to the doctor? There's no need for regular checkups now.

I just picked up the new *National Star* at the grocery store. Madonna is having triplets, and now they have a cure for Alzheimer's.

I lost my car keys. I must have Alzheimer's.

When you've seen one *person* with Alzheimer's, you've seen them all. They're all the same.

Why get a diagnosis if nothing can be done?

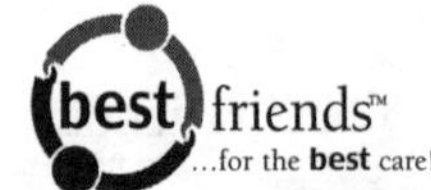

4

The Experience of Alzheimer's Disease

Teaching staff to understand what it would be like to have Alzheimer's disease is a vital component of any comprehensive and effective staff training program. This understanding, what the authors have described as "walking a mile in the *person's* shoes," helps staff in all aspects of care. When staff are able to imagine the feelings, losses, and challenges of having dementia, many puzzling behaviors can be explained and thus prevented. Having this understanding also can help staff be more patient with *persons* and solve problems as they arise. It builds empathy that allows staff members to give care in a more loving and compassionate manner.

This chapter discusses the experience of Alzheimer's disease and ways in which to build the quality of empathy in a Best Friends staff. The following story demonstrates what can happen when staff do not have empathy or understanding.

When Staff Don't Get It

The evening was off to another rocky start at Unhappy Valley Alzheimer's Home. It was already 7:00 P.M. when Richard wondered, "Why aren't they in bed yet?" Richard rolled his eyes as he talked to the other staff member on duty that evening. "I don't understand it, Maria. Why does Mr. Smathers keep getting up and wanting to walk into the other rooms?" Maria responded, "I've told him over and over again not to do it. I'm so frustrated that he won't listen." Richard agreed and approached the resident, saying, "Hi, Mr. Smathers. Why don't you go to bed. You look really tired."

Mr. Smathers pointed down at the floor. There were some small strips of paper on the floor that must have landed there during the afternoon craft activity. "That's kind of dirty," Mr. Smathers said. "It needs cleaning up." Maria chimed in, "I'm sure that the day shift cleaners will take care of it like they do every morning at 9. Now, you go back to your room. Room 8, it's around the corner and the third from the left, next to the green couch." Mr. Smathers looked worried, even agitated; it was clear that he was becoming angry. Richard thought to himself, Now what? I hope we don't get another combative, angry resident on our hands. Maybe Mr. Smathers is entering that stage tonight.

This example demonstrates what can happen when staff in a dementia care program do not understand the experience of Alzheimer's disease. Clearly, there is no connection between staff and Mr. Smathers; they do not try to understand his feelings or actions. Because they did not have a basic understanding of the impact of dementia on a *person,* staff members gave overly complex instructions to Mr. Smathers. They did not pick up his verbal clues—that he could be upset by a dirty floor. Many other mistakes were made, but fundamentally the staff demonstrated no empathy for this resident.

Here is what can happen with the same cast of characters but in a Best Friends program.

I am now teaching a long-term care class that is for future administrators. I am introducing them to the Best Friends model and have taken some of the students to long-term care residences to see firsthand the model in action.

—Susan Peters Rachal, faculty member in gerontology education, University of Louisiana, Monroe

I often talk about what I call the 3 H's of training—heart (empathy), head (knowledge), and hands-on (skills). All three are important. However, all too often the focus of training programs is primarily (and sometimes solely) on imparting information to staff, that is, providing knowledge. The most successful training programs also instill empathy (the heart). The knowledge and hands-on skills will be applied more meaningfully by staff when "building the heart" is also a part of the training program.

—Vicki L. Schmall, Executive Director, Aging Concerns, West Linn, Oregon

The Best Friends Way

The evening was going well at Sunny Mountain Alzheimer's Home. It was 7:00 P.M. and the after-dinner music hour had been a success. The two residents who did not usually participate in the music program had returned safely from their walks (thank goodness for those great volunteers, Richard thought), and he and Maria began to help a few residents who would be going to bed soon to reach their rooms. For the others, staff would serve some milk and cookies and wind the evening down.

Richard suddenly noticed that Mr. Smathers seemed a bit agitated and was walking in the hallway, looking down at something on the floor. There were some small strips of paper on the floor that must have landed there during the afternoon craft activity. "That's kind of dirty," Mr. Smathers said. "It needs cleaning up."

Maria chimed in, "The cleaners must have missed that. What do you think, should we clean up this mess?" Mr. Smathers nodded, and Maria went to get a broom and dustpan. She handed Mr. Smathers the broom and leaned down, holding the dustpan against the paper scraps. "Here, right here. Sweep the broom toward me and let's get this cleaned up." They worked together for about 5 minutes and finished the job. Maria looked into Mr. Smathers's eyes and asked, "Mr. Smathers, what would I do without you? We really make a great team." Mr. Smathers smiled broadly and walked to his room.

Richard complimented Maria on doing just the right thing. "Oh, it was an easy call," Maria noted. Maria then reminded Richard that Mr. Smathers had worked hard his whole life as a custodian. "His family told us that he always liked things very clean and neat." Richard then said, "That's right! It was probably stressful for him to see things any other way!"

Here, an empathetic staff responded to a situation with knack, connected to Mr. Smathers's feelings, and supported his need to be helpful.

What follows are key concepts that help staff learn to understand better the experience of Alzheimer's disease. Once gained, empathy can help staff cope with the ups and downs of Alzheimer's disease. It can turn "unhappy valley" programs into ones full of "sunny mountain tops."

When I told him that I wanted to be his Best Friend, you should have seen the look on his face. You could tell that he was touched and pleased. He tells me that it means a lot to have a special visit from someone who cares each day.

—Irene Brummett, Laundry, Laurel Heights Home for the Elderly, London, Kentucky

No soul is desolate as long as there is a human being for whom it can feel trust and reverence.

—George Eliot

To Know Someone, You Must Walk a Mile in His or Her Shoes

Best Friends staff members understand what it might be like to have Alzheimer's disease. They have learned the symptoms of dementia, and they have thought about and internalized the meaning of and impact on a *person* of poor memory, diminished judgment, lack of initiative, and the other manifestations of dementia.

One way of explaining this concept is through analogy: Having Alzheimer's disease is like arriving at a strange airport for the first time and not knowing your way around. There is a lot of noise and conversation in the terminal. Instructions are confusing or complex (go to the lower level, get on Shuttle Bus A, get off on Concourse B, then look for the red sign that leads to the escalator). It can be hard at an airport to keep track of your belongings ("Do I have all of my luggage or have I left something behind?"). This example can help staff realize that any of us would have feelings of frustration, fear, and even anger when put in certain situations. It can be true even in "imaginary" situations:

As staff, we have to constantly monitor ourselves to remain sensitive to those in our care and to avoid imposing our own values or choices on them. The person inside must always be honored. It is very easy for busy caregivers to take over all decision making in the best interests of those they are caring for. I strongly encourage staff to avoid this practice.

—Gayle Pennington, Director, Riverside Adult Day Program, Wilmington, Delaware

One resident at West Park Long Term Care Center was frantic after breakfast because she imagined that company was coming. She was upset that the dishes had not been washed. The staff did not argue the point. Instead, they got a few dishes, a basin, and a dishcloth and helped her do the dishes. She was so relieved to get the place cleaned up and was no longer anxious about guests seeing a messy house.

Here, staff empathized with the resident's feelings even though no company was coming. They jumped in and engaged her in a work-related activity. She forgot that she was ever expecting guests. A sensitive staff member later explained, "It's important to 'be' where they are at that moment."

I have become very close to a resident that no one else wanted. She kicked and scratched other staff, but she likes me. I have become her Best Friend.

—Janice Makonnen, CNA, The Fountainview Center for Alzheimer's Disease, Atlanta, Georgia

Person-Centered Care Is Central

Best Friends staff members treat *persons* the way any of us would want to be treated if we had dementia. They recognize that a *person* has value even when he or she has diminished memory or thought processes. They also recognize that focusing on the positive—the *person's* remaining skills and talents—can create a new paradigm for care within their program. Whether it be success or failure, you get what you look for.

Cheri Taylor, executive director at Porterville Senior Day Care, wrote to the authors, "We work very hard to separate the disease from the person, and use every possible avenue to learn about the person behind the disease. We remind each other constantly to treat our participants like we would want to be treated."

This caring approach reminds staff of the program's mission to provide the best person-centered care.

Having Alzheimer's Disease

Depression

Can't say what I want.

Afraid I can't express my thoughts and words—thus I remain silent and become depressed.

I need conversation to be slowly.

It is difficult to follow conversations with so much noise.

I feel that people turn me off because I cannot express myself.

I dislike social workers, nurses, and friends who do not treat me as a real person.

It is difficult to live one day at a time.

My philosophy, adopted July 30, 1984

—Rebecca Riley, diagnosed with Alzheimer's disease at age 59

Losses Caused by Dementia Can Evoke a Wide Range of Distressing Feelings and Emotions

Best Friends staff members understand that Alzheimer's disease dramatically affects *persons'* lives and restricts their ability to do the things that they have always enjoyed. Thus, they are at great risk for experiencing a variety of distressing feelings such as loss, loneliness, sadness, confusion, worry, frustration, fear, paranoia, anger, and embarrassment. Left unchecked, any one of these feelings can magnify and fuel depression, anxiety, or angry and distressing behaviors.

A resident at The Fountains often cried out that she wanted to go home. At first, a staff member tried to explain where she was in a futile effort to convince her to stay. Later, an empathetic staff member asked, "How can I help you?" He learned that she wanted to go home to her mother, and engaged her in conversation: "You sound like you really love your mother. Would you tell me more about her?"

A staff member with knack allowed the resident to express herself and share her feelings. This action ultimately diffused her desire to leave. Her attention became focused on her mother and her early childhood. For that moment and afterward she was more "at home" because she no longer felt alone.

PERSONS WITH DEMENTIA CAN EXPERIENCE JOY, LOVE, AND HAPPINESS

Best Friends staff members are aware that although the journey of Alzheimer's disease can be a very rough one, it is not totally full of despair for *persons*. Many become happy-go-lucky or let go of past worries and fears. Even when *persons* are having a tough time emotionally, they can still experience positive moments, as described in the following story:

A participant in the Helping Hand Day Center arrives each day in a great mood. She greets each person warmly, although she cannot remember names. She enjoys funny stories and playful conversation and teasing. In her own way, she participates in various activities throughout the day. When her husband comes to pick her up at the end of the day, he always asks, "How was it today?" She responds, "The best one yet!"

Some people with dementia maintain a very positive, upbeat spirit.

THE FEELINGS OF *PERSONS* WITH DEMENTIA ARE AS REAL AS YOURS AND MINE

Best Friends staff members realize that *persons* share the same range of emotions and feelings as an individual without cognitive impairment. This means that anyone can, and will, experience moments of happiness and sadness and contentment and anger, and good and bad times.

A nurse at Villa Alamar remembers a male resident who became very frightened. "Please hurry, we must close the drapes. They are coming!" he cried. They went from room to room, closing the

The Experience of Alzheimer's Disease

We had a gentleman who was in the early stages of Alzheimer's and he tried to explain to me what it was like to have Alzheimer's. He sometimes knew that things he said were wrong, but he couldn't make them come out of his mouth right. This was very upsetting to him and he asked for forgiveness for anything that he might say in the future that I would think inappropriate.

He said that in his head, things just became very confused and it was sometimes hard to express his feelings. He would also forget his response and ask me to repeat the question, saying that he wasn't sure if he had heard me right. On occasion, I would tell him things that he had just said and ask if that was what he meant.

He told me that if I had not repeated things back to him, he would never have believed that these were his words. It was disturbing to him that he could not remember things that had just happened that day and that *drapes. When he was satisfied that he was safe, he threw his arms around the nurse and wept with relief, saying, "Thank you, thank you." The nurse was speechless.*

Even though this behavior surprised a normally unflappable nurse, she remembered that he was of Jewish descent and had been in hiding during World War II. She went with his feelings, rather than seek to change them or explain his actual situation. She realized that his fear was very real, and she worked with him to solve the imagined safety issue.

Behaviors that Seem Out of Place Are Not

Best Friends staff members realize that behaviors that at first seem strange or inappropriate or that are disruptive may result from the logical efforts of *persons* to cope with the world in which they find themselves. If a resident of a special care unit takes another resident's coat, he or she is not necessarily a thief. The *person* may actually believe it is his or her coat. *Persons* who disrobe may be doing so not because they are exhibitionists but because they are hot. However distressing or shocking, a man who makes a sexually suggestive comment to his daughter may be mistaking her for his wife. He is not a "dirty old man," as the authors once heard an angry staff member respond.

A resident of West Park Long Term Care Center had been a ranch owner and outfitter (someone who readies groups for trail expeditions). Often, his behavior was disruptive and disturbing, especially to other residents. Sometimes at night he would make rounds, opening every closed door at the center and asking, "Got enough blankets?" The staff learned that he was responsible for providing blankets to his guests so that they could be warm enough during the cool Wyoming nights. Once staff realized this, his behavior became much easier to understand. Nurse Kelli Martin said, "One must simply step into his reality to help him through his days. To do this, we became ranch hands, cowgirls, and dudes!"

Knowing that behaviors often can be explained is an important concept because it can help staff enter into the *person's* world and offer him or her comfort, reassurance, or redirection. It also can help staff moderate their responses when surprising behavior occurs. In such cases, staff might

thoughts could get so mixed up in his head. Once he told me that he wished that his head could be cleaned out and it was like having cobwebs in there all the time. His long-term memory was still very good and he repeated his life history to me several times, always the same.

Being a religious man, he could tell Bible stories and interpret them with a message he felt was important. In the early stages, he told me that he had concerns about the future, seeing the other residents very confused and behaving in ways that he felt very inappropriate and knowing that he would be like that someday. Being part of a very close knit family, he was afraid of not remembering those he loved.

—*Martha Shattuck, Program Coordinator, The Fountainview Center for Alzheimer's Disease, Atlanta, Georgia*

Modeling a Best Friends approach is what teaches it.

—*Beth Spencer, Assistant Professor of Gerontology, Madonna University, Livonia, Michigan*

The person *with Alzheimer's disease shares all of the same emotions and feelings as a person without cognitive impairment. The goal of* person-*centered care is to move the* person *from the feelings listed below in the left-hand column to the ones listed in the right-hand column. The shift may be only momentary, but* person-centered care *suggests that if we can link these moments together, then challenging behaviors will be reduced and the quality of life improved for the* person *with Alzheimer's disease.*

Loss	→	Fulfillment
Loneliness	→	Connectedness
Sadness	→	Cheerfulness
Confusion	→	Orientation
Worry/anxiety	→	Contentment
Frustration	→	Peacefulness
Fear	→	Security
Paranoia	→	Trust
Anger	→	Calm
Embarrassment	→	Confidence

Figure 4.1. The feelings associated with Alzheimer's disease and the goal of person-centered care.

stop the resident's behavior by letting him know that everyone was tucked in and had plenty of blankets. The staff also became more understanding when he fell asleep on the floor.

Feelings and Behaviors Can Be Changed by Meeting the Needs of the *Person*

Best Friends staff members can help move the *person,* even momentarily, from loss to fulfillment, loneliness to connectedness, sadness to cheerfulness, confusion to orientation, worry/anxiety to contentment, frustration to peacefulness, fear to security, paranoia to trust, anger to calm, and embarrassment to confidence (see Figure 4.1). Staff do this by helping the *person* feel connected, competent, useful, respected, appreciated, in control, successful, and loved (see Figure 4.2). This can be done in a very simple way, such as by asking an anxious resident or participant to help set up chairs for a group activity. When the task is finished, staff can offer praise and thanks for his or her work. This can help the *person* feel competent, useful, and appreciated.

To feel connected
To be respected
To be appreciated

To feel loved
To be known
To be understood

To experience belonging, community
To have a sense of still becoming
To share, to love, to give

To be compassionate, concerned, accepting
To be productive
To be helpful, useful, successful

To feel safe
To feel secure
To feel hopeful

Figure 4.2. The needs of persons *with Alzheimer disease.*

Beverly was admitted to The Fountainview Center. She was more cognitively intact and had more intact verbal skills than the other residents. She was able to tell staff that she was angry about her recent admission. "Before, I came and went as I pleased, and now there are lots of rules." Shirley Miller, director of nursing, noted, "I use her statement in my dementia class when I ask what fears learners have about growing older. The majority of staff answers the question with dependency as a major fear. Staff members have been able to look at their own fears in relationship to what a person with Alzheimer's disease experiences. They seem to understand that even giving limited choice can let a person stay in control for a while longer."

Staff members were able to learn directly from a resident about her needs and compare them with their own. She reminded staff members of the importance of helping every resident feel in control. When they allowed Beverly to make choices, they not only helped her maintain a sense of independence and dignity but they also prevented problems and outbursts before they occurred.

A participant at the adult day center Toca das Horttensias, Sao Paulo, Brazil, used to own a small shop. He was accustomed to constant contact with customers and still craved this social interaction. When he has moments of sadness or anxiousness, conversation and attention from staff can bring him back to a happy and relaxed mood. Lilian Alicke, president of the adult day center, noted, "We arrange for him to be near a woman who likes to sing, and they spend time singing together."

Persons need help to fulfill their needs; they usually cannot initiate ways to meet them. By matching up this (needy) shopkeeper with a gregarious participant, staff are meeting his needs and also freeing up a staff member to spend time with another participant.

Conclusion

After reading *The Best Friends Approach to Alzheimer's Care,* Joyce L. Feick, a student at Madonna University, used the elements of knack (see Chapter 1) to compose a poem about what it might be like to have the disease. It sums up what can happen when a staff member or caregiver learns to understand and empathize with the person with Alzheimer's disease:

If I Had Alzheimer's Disease

If I had Alzheimer's' disease I would forget things here and there and sometimes lose my way. I would feel confusion, frustration, and fear. I would want to be right. I would want this neurological, irreversible, progressive disease to stop and soon they'd find a way. Until that day, I would need you.

I would need you to be well informed, communicate skillfully to me, using your common sense, with finesse, maintaining your self-confidence, patience and flexibility, when setting realistic expectations with me.

With your caregiving integrity you would be nonjudgmental. You would plan ahead, knowing my full life story to know when to employ your empathy and optimism while valuing our moments together tied in humor.

I could count on you to stay focused while respecting my basic rights, while never forgetting to be spontaneous. But most of all, never neglecting to take care of yourself so we could walk through the rest of my life as Best Friends, knowing you have all the knack I will need.

This student went well beyond learning the coursework. She took the material into her head and heart to learn what good care is all about. She truly walked a mile in the shoes of the *person* with Alzheimer's disease.

The quality of care improves when staff members look at person-centered care from both sides. It is one thing to tell staff that *persons* with dementia want to be treated just as they would like to be treated; it is another thing to encourage staff to think about how they would like to be treated if they were the care recipient. Empathy allows the culture of care to change for the better. It helps staff make a better, more personal connection to the individuals they care for. It gives staff insight into what works and what does not. Empathy improves the level of job satisfaction by reminding staff of the importance of their work and the power that they have to reach and help an often-fragile *person* in need of warm hearts and helping hands.

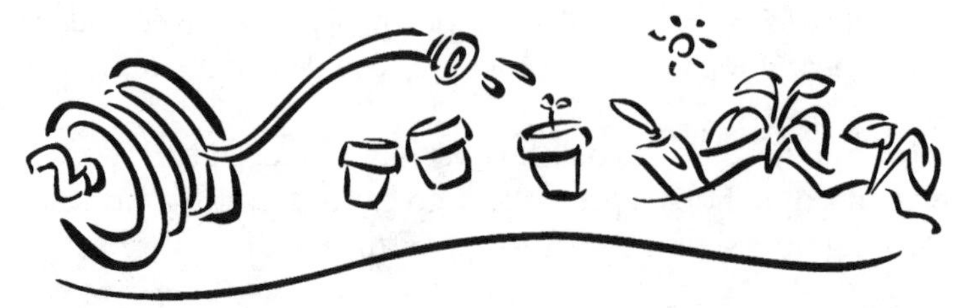

Training Tool Kit

Tool 4.0 / Warm-Up
Feeling Good

The purpose of this warm-up is to start your training with positive feelings and to make a point: that staff should understand how the residents or participants would benefit if staff could evoke the same positive feelings in them. This is what a Best Friends staff is always trying to do for the person with Alzheimer's disease.

Use this exercise as a way for staff to begin talking about themselves and their feelings. Tell staff that you are going to give them a few minutes to think about happy experiences or times in their lives. The list below should give you some ideas, or you can come up with your own:

Walking barefoot on a beach
Laughing with good friends
Being in a safe and warm living room during a winter storm
Winning a football betting pool
Celebrating your birthday and getting lots of nice presents

Invite the group to discuss how they felt during this exercise. You may need to provide cues (e.g., "How did it feel to win the football pool?").

Adapted from an exercise created by Cheryl T. Weidemeyer, program director, Christiana Care/Visiting Nurse Association, Evergreen Center I, Alzheimer's Day Treatment Program, Wilmington, Delaware.

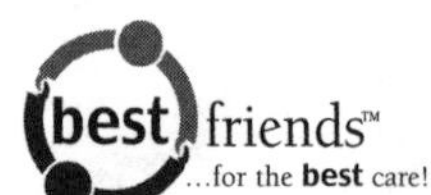

Tool 4.1 / Games for Learning
How Would You Feel If . . . ?

The purpose of this exercise is to get staff thinking about how persons *with Alzheimer's disease feel when they experience fearful or sad situations and to know that they can feel the same way.*

Use this list of questions to lead a discussion about difficult experiences and emotions. Take part in the discussion yourself so that everyone feels comfortable disclosing his or her feelings. Allow staff to share anecdotes or stories that are related to some of their statements; this will help staff members to get to know one another.

How would you feel if . . . ?

You just had your car keys in your hand and now you can't find them.

You found yourself home alone on your birthday.

Your spouse had just been fired from his or her job.

You were lost and, when you asked for directions, you found that they were too complicated to follow.

Your teenage son was 2 hours late coming home from a date.

Co-workers were whispering and kept looking at you.

You were about to park in a crowded parking lot and someone cut in front of you.

You heard a strange noise in the middle of the night.

You were at a family wedding and suddenly realized that you had on one black shoe and one brown one.

Discussion questions

Are these feelings justified or real?

Do you think *persons* with Alzheimer's disease ever have similar feelings? When and why?

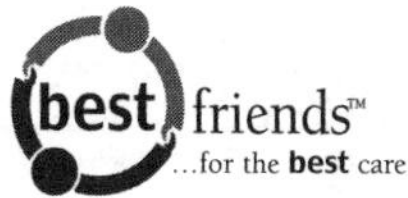

Tool 4.2 / Games for Learning
A Few of My Favorite Things

This simple and effective exercise can help staff begin to understand the losses felt by persons *with Alzheimer's disease.*

Hand out five index cards or pieces of paper to each staff member in the training group. Ask participants to write a favorite activity or an activity that gives meaning to their lives (e.g., taking a walk, going shopping, playing cards, visiting grandchildren, volunteering for church activities, driving) on each card.

Allow about 5 minutes and then ask each participant to pick up the first card, look at it, think about the pleasure that the activity gives them, and then throw it away as though they were giving up the activity altogether. Continue until all five cards are gone. Then lead a discussion about how it felt to give up these favorite activities.

Discussion questions

How did you feel when you threw away the things that you love?

Do you think *persons* with Alzheimer's disease ever have these feelings? When and why?

Variation from Debbie McConnell: The group leader randomly snatches the cards or pieces of paper from class members. This action reminds everyone that *persons* do not have a choice about what to give up and when.

Debbie McConnell is the director of education at the Alzheimer's Association, Santa Barbara, California.

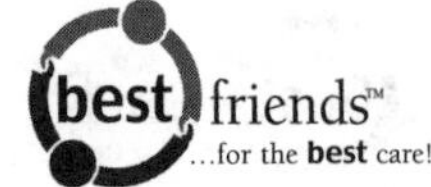

Tool 4.3 / Games for Learning
Walk a Mile in These Shoes

The purpose of this exercise is to develop empathy by practicing "walking a mile in the shoes" of persons with Alzheimer's disease.

Locate the largest pair of shoes possible; something oversized, colorful, eye-catching, or even goofy would be best. Ask for a volunteer from the staff to come to the front of the room and put on the shoes. Tell the group that the shoes have magical properties. When a staff member wears them, even for just a minute, he or she will become someone else.

Choose among the following names (or add your own names, perhaps a local celebrity) to make a point and have fun. Ask the staff member the following question:

How does it feel to know that you are now walking in the shoes of, in a sense becoming,

Michael Jordan
Sharon Stone
The President of the United States
Oprah Winfrey
An astronaut
Tiger Woods
Elton John
Tina Turner
Oscar de la Hoya
[name of a local celebrity]

How do you think the world perceives you as this individual? How do you want others to treat you?

Now ask the volunteer to imagine that he or she is walking in the shoes of, actually becoming, [name of a resident with dementia]. Ask the volunteer and the audience the following questions:

How does it feel to be [name of resident]?
How do you think the world sees you?
How do you want others to treat you?
What can make [name of resident] sad? Happy? Angry? Safe? Frustrated? Involved?

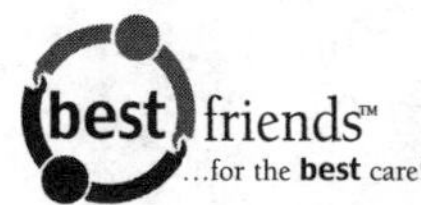

Tool 4.4 / Games for Learning
Making a Collage of Feelings

Debi Lahav explained, "These collages were made in supervision sessions at the day center. Students doing practicums at the center were asked to represent their impressions and images of the old people and themselves. All of the students spent 7 weeks at the center. What did they learn? How do they feel now? In this case, collage served as the perfect tool to reveal the students' underlying feelings. It was much better than a purely verbal supervision session."

1. The Puzzle of Life—The student saw herself as the hands holding the "pieces" of life that the members revealed. She viewed her job as helping them reveal more and more of themselves.

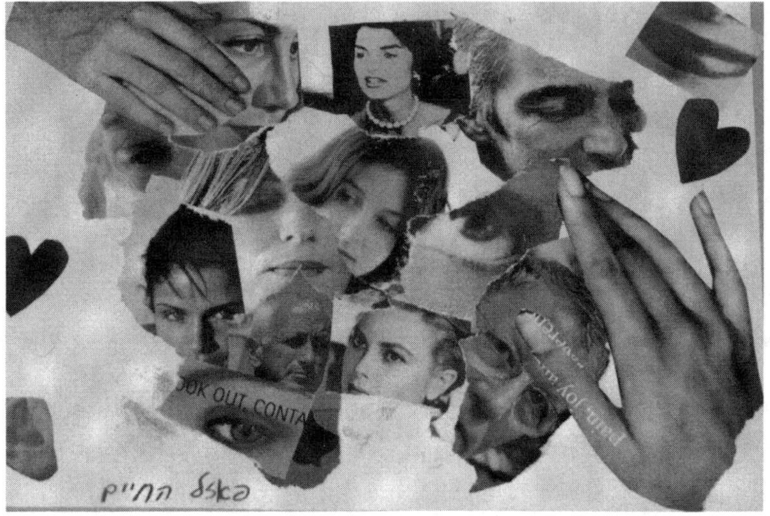

2. The First Week—After 1 week at the center, the student felt like the figure in the top left, with a veil partially covering her face. She saw caring hands, brain dysfunction, partial faces, communication, games, and more.

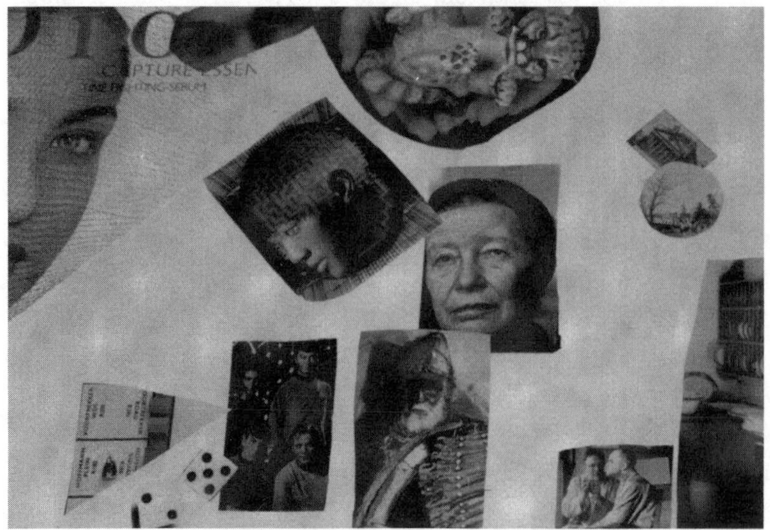

(continued)

3. The Last Week—The student felt as though she were walking in the desert, but there also were rainbows and feelings of accomplishment, like climbing a mountain. The man standing on the dark balcony is a symbol of the old people. The picture at the top right represents the chest of memories that the people have.

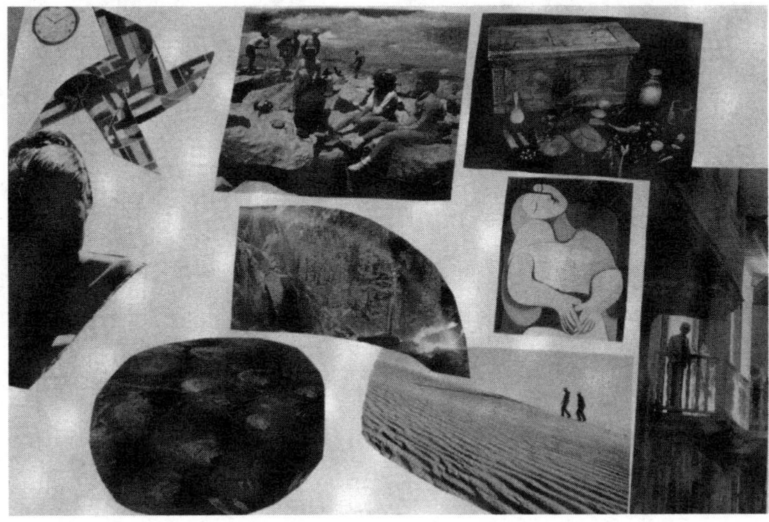

4. The Last Week—The footprint is like the difficulties and unpredictability in dementia. The student said that she often felt like a shepherd watching over her flock (helping the members go from activity to activity, to meals, to vans). Despite the difficulties, she discovered the possibilities of growth, as in the plant.

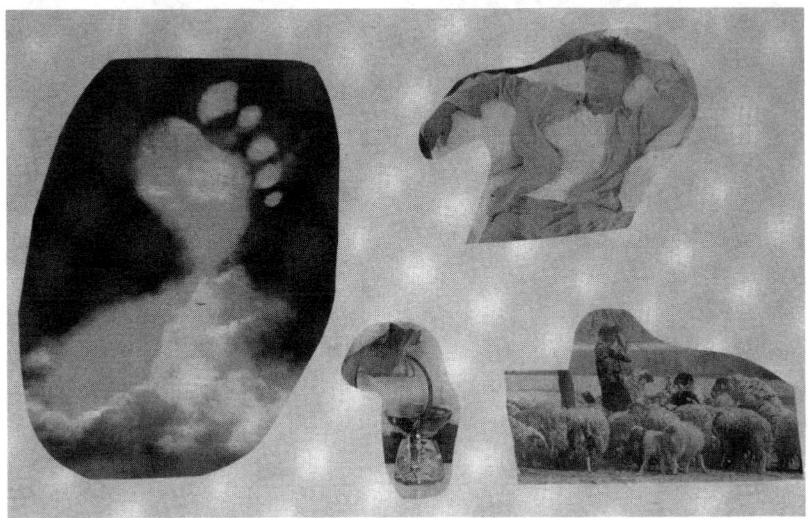

(continued)

5. Short Frames—The student saw herself in the middle, smiling a lot. Sometimes she took time out to sit and watch what was going on from the sidelines. The hands are the relationships, friendships, and the care that she gives and receives. Sometimes there are conflicts between members, as at the bottom. The blue and black clouds at left represent emotions and thoughts, which are sometimes optimistic and sometimes sad.

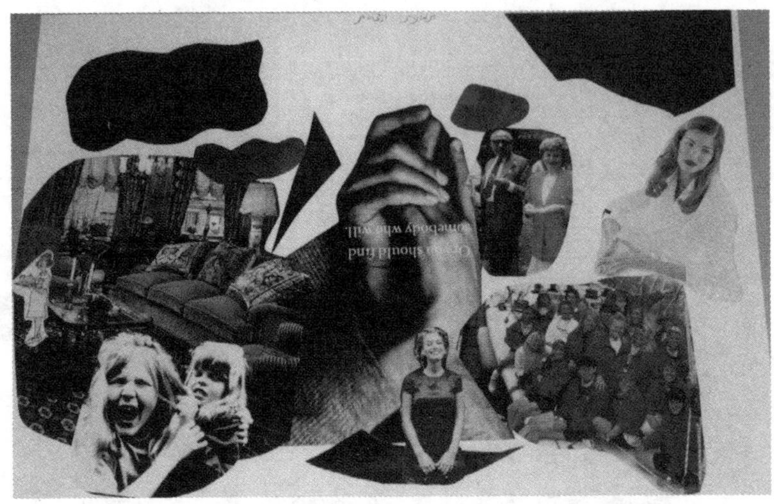

6. Behind the Lens—This student created a collage of how she learned about the life of the people at the center. She put together pieces of a puzzle starting at the upper left with childhood. Some of the people from the center were in the Holocaust in their early adulthood, which had a very strong effect on their lives. In old age, she realized, there can be happiness or loss.

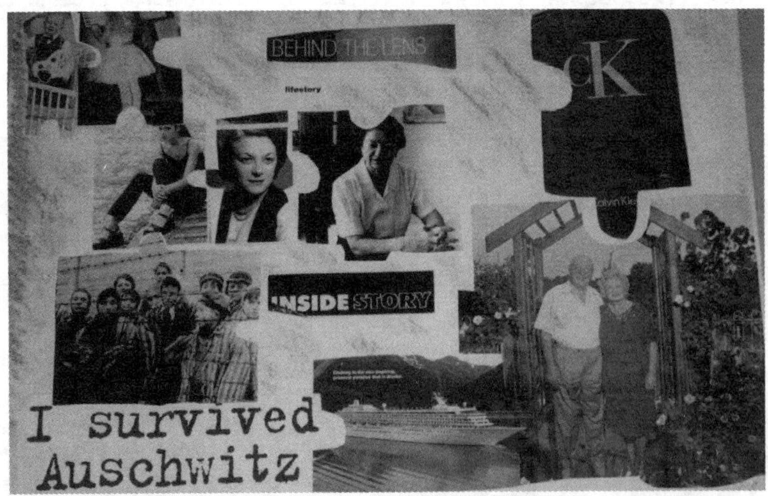

Courtesy of Debi Lahav, M. A., occupational and art therapist, Margolic Psychogeriatric Center, Tel Aviv Medical Center, Tel Aviv, Israel; reprinted by permission.

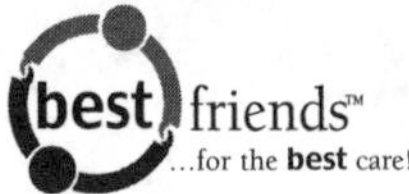

Tool 4.5 / Program Pointer

How Can We Be a Best Friend?

Distribute this handout to staff and ask them to complete the worksheet as completely as they can. Use it for a group discussion or for self-reflection. It also can be blown up and put onto a board or flipchart for staff to complete during the week following an in-service on this topic.

How can we be a Best Friend to the *person* when he or she exhibits any of the following distressing feelings? Fill in the blanks below.

Loss ____

____

Isolation and loneliness ____

____

Sadness ____

____

Confusion ____

____

Worry and anxiety ____

____

Frustration ____

____

Fear ____

____

Paranoia ____

____

Anger ____

____

Embarrassment ____

____

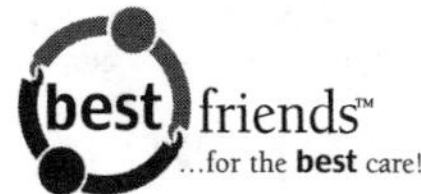

Tool 4.6 / Program Pointer
What I Perceive the Behavior to Be

The quotation at the bottom of this tool challenges us to look at the person's *behavior for clues and cues about how they are doing. Staff should always be on the lookout for warning signs of medical or behavioral problems. Prevention is always easier than treatment after the problem has occurred.*

Post this quotation on your Best Friends bulletin board (see an example in Tool 6.2) or use it in a newsletter. The title also can be used with the list of needs presented in Figure 4.2 to discuss how class members feel when their needs are or are not being met.

What I perceive the behavior to be . . . is just another expression of need.

—*Unknown*

Tool 4.7 / Program Pointer

The *Person* with Alzheimer's Disease as Teacher

The following are some suggestions on how to involve persons *with dementia in your training program. Although it must be done with forethought and sensitivity, there is often no better way to encourage staff empathy than to invite a* person *with early-stage dementia to speak at the training session. Many chapters of the Alzheimer's Association are working with diagnosed individuals for this very purpose and finding the results to be profound. It can provide insight and compassion to the audience. For the* person, *teaching others can provide self-esteem and feelings of accomplishment.*

Do

Discuss the session ahead of time with the *person* and his or her caregiver.
Let them know that you will be there to help or step in if needed.
Introduce the *person* properly, with warmth and dignity.
Have a friend or family member sit up front with the *person* for support.
Be flexible and patient.
Listen carefully.
Be very supportive if the *person* needs help.
Be aware that even if something goes wrong, it can be a learning opportunity.
Prepare a thank-you card for the group or class to sign.
Have a backup plan.
Use question-and-answer formats if you think that it would be helpful for the *person*.

Don't

Rush the *person*.
Stick to rigid deadlines.
Become anxious if the session doesn't go as planned.
Be overly solicitous or overly protective.
Keep the *person* engaged too long (stick to your agreed-on schedule).

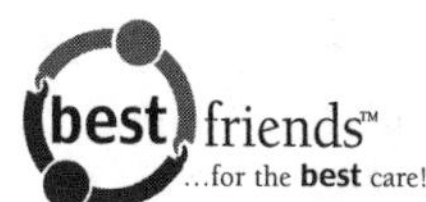

Tool 4.8 / Program Pointer
Hugs

This poem was created from answers given at the Helping Hand Day Center, Alzheimer's Association, Lexington/Bluegrass chapter, Lexington, Kentucky, to the question "what is a hug?" Create your own poem based on the answers of your program participants or residents. You can use this on a Best Friends bulletin board or newsletter. Read it at a staff in-service program to remind participants of how powerful hugs can be when given to the right person at the right time. Encourage staff to have fun role-playing or demonstrating types of hugs.

What Is a Hug?

A hug is warm and fuzzy and nice.
It is a friendly hello, an act of kindness and devotion.

A hug is reassuring and comforting, a kiss of life.

It is great, calorie-free, and costs nothing.

It is needed to survive.

You asked me when I like to hug?
Well, whenever I get a chance.

When you give me a hug, you get one back.
I like big, strong bear hugs that say,
"I love you."

I don't like crying hugs.

A hug is a way to greet a friend or a way to say,
"I love you."

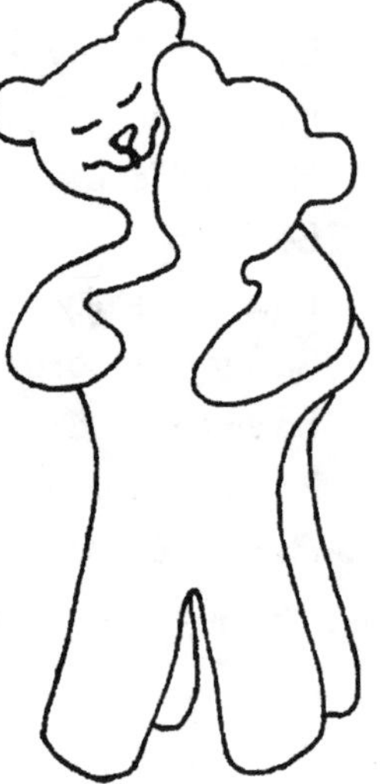

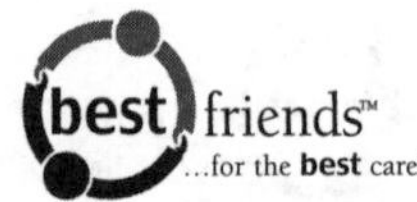

Tool 4.9
Turning No Knack into Knack

The purpose of this exercise is to show, with a dash of humor, the wrong way to do something. This is active learning that really sinks in, particularly when staff members themselves volunteer to take part in the role plays.

The following statements represent stereotypes or falsehoods about dementia. These examples of "no knack" can be used in a number of ways to explore staff attitudes and reinforce the lessons presented in this chapter. Draw the examples from a hat to discuss as a group or incorporate them in role plays. Invite staff to comment on the mistakes in the statements below. Then role-play or discuss the right way. The authors discuss the art of role plays in Tool 2.11. Use your creativity to have fun turning these examples of "no knack" into "knack."

Persons with Alzheimer's disease are always unhappy.

There is no way to figure out what a *person* is feeling.

Just keep a *person* warm, fed, and dry—that's about it. That's the best you can do.

If someone's personality changes for the better, then they don't have Alzheimer's. Mom seems much more happy-go-lucky now. This can't be Alzheimer's.

If he gets frustrated or anxious, just leave him alone. You can't change that in a *person* with Alzheimer's.

What's the use of giving him a hug when he'll just forget it anyway?

Gee, when I come to your day center, everyone seems so happy. Obviously they don't have Alzheimer's disease.

What a shame! There is nobody there anymore.

You can't embarrass her. She has Alzheimer's.

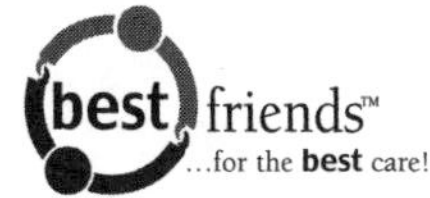

5

Assessment & Expectations

The administration of all long-term care programs requires paperwork, everything from financial responsibility forms to photo releases to important initial and ongoing health assessments and care plans. Paperwork and charting play an important role in any long-term care program, representing the outcome of a formal and, hopefully, carefully drawn assessment. When done with care and thought, these tasks give staff the information that they need to make decisions about admission, ongoing care, and, sometimes, discharge. It is a way of tracking the progress of the health and cognition of *persons* with Alzheimer's disease and a way of setting care goals and evaluating program success.

Paperwork also can be oppressive and endless. Even worse, it can keep effective program leaders locked in their offices when they could be out in the program, working with *persons,* helping staff, greeting families, participating in activities, giving feedback, solving problems, and even having some fun.

The goal of this chapter is to turn the "necessary evil" of paperwork into a "necessary good." This chapter also serves to suggest a Best Friends way of assessment, one that builds on existing or required forms to get a broader and more insightful picture of the *person* with dementia. A Best Friends assessment provides an ongoing picture of the *person's* underlying personality, beliefs, values, history, and traditions, not just his or her medical status. The following story reveals the cost of poor assessment in one fictional nursing facility.

Why Existing Assessments Often Fail

> Maryellen, the director of nursing, was busy reviewing records with staff. Thank goodness things were shaping up, she thought. The admission forms seemed to be complete in each chart, and care plan notes were being made on a regular basis. "I'm proud of these charts," Maryellen thought. "Things are going very well here at Happy View." As she took her morning walk down the corridors, her smile and mood began to change, however.

A staff member had called in sick, and this week's care management meeting had been canceled. "When did we have our last one?" Maryellen wondered to herself. "I think it's been 2, no, 3 weeks since we met."

Just then she saw one of the CNAs, Juan, sitting at a table doing an activity with a resident. "I'm so glad to see some one-to-one attention being given," Maryellen thought. Yet she couldn't help noticing that he was showing Mrs. Tate some pictures, and she was having trouble seeing them. "Didn't he think to find her glasses?" Maryellen wondered. She saw the glasses on the neighboring table and handed them to Juan. Another activity staff member was doing some gardening in the raised beds. "That's great," she thought, "but why isn't Louise letting the three residents get their hands into the soil? Didn't she remember that this group loves gardening?" She overheard the staff member say to them, "Great! Now that the weeding job is done, let's move on." Two of the women walked away from her at that point and wandered back into the facility. "I wish she would have read the care plan better," Maryellen thought. "If given the chance, I think they would have spent another half-hour outside gardening on this beautiful day."

As she walked inside, she saw a new volunteer sitting with a resident. She paused to listen in as the volunteer spoke, "So, John, tell me more about your daughter." John stared back blankly. Maryellen chimed in, "Oh, you must mean his son, Mike. John is so proud of him." The volunteer smiled and said, "Oh yes. How is that son of yours, Mike?" John laughed and said, "You are both so nice to me." Maryellen thought that this volunteer was doing a good job, but she wished that she had gotten the name and relationship straight. Hadn't she read John's biography sheet in the Psychosocial History Binder? Without Maryellen's cue, that conversation would have been over in a hurry. She thought some more about the experience of the last few minutes: "I have a lot of work to do!"

In general, long-term care programs succeed in creating a solid initial assessment and care plan. Maryellen probably documented the need that one resident had for glasses, the goal of involving residents directly in a gardening activity, and the fact that John loved to talk about his son. Unfortunately, there was no follow-through. Weekly care planning meetings were moved around, even canceled. Decisions were not communicated well to staff, changes in condition were not consistently noted, and, often, staff members were not reminded of the overall purpose of their jobs—to help residents or program participants achieve their maximum potential.

The fact that the staff at Happy View was not implementing Maryellen's hard work was not immediately obvious. On the surface, it appeared that the program was functioning well. Some one-to-one attention was being given, and residents were enjoying being outside. Yet, mistakes such as not putting on a resident's glasses or not letting residents take time to garden rob them of their dignity and keep them from experiencing successes. In this case, carefully executed care plans would have ensured that opportunities for quality were not lost. They would have turned a good program into a great one.

The Best Friends Assessment

The Best Friends assessment (Figure 5.1) is not intended to replace the tools being used to document medical and cognitive needs. Best Friends programs will use this document or create a similar one to add richness to the care planning process that will help staff set appropriate expectations of the *person*. What follows are key concepts that form the foundation of the Best Friends assessment.

Review Physical and Mental Health

Best Friends staff members know that the majority of *persons* with Alzheimer's disease are well into their 70s, 80s, and 90s. Many have age-related medical problems or chronic conditions, including arthritis, heart disease, and asthma. Making matters worse is that often *persons* with Alzheimer's disease have refused or been unwilling to continue going to doctors, dentists, and vision specialists. As a consequence, they may have a number of health problems that can be identified with a good assessment tool and dealt with in the care plan.

Mental health conditions must not be overlooked in the assessment. For example, depression often accompanies dementia and can be treated. A good assessment also looks at whether the *person* had or has other mental health disorders that can affect care.

All of this information helps staff members with knack avoid the common mistake of assuming that every problem presented by one of their residents or participants is dementia related. A *person* with Alzheimer's disease may be much more confused when he or she is dehydrated or sick with the flu. Best Friends staff members know that untreated medical conditions will make dementia much worse.

Review Cognitive Health

The Best Friends assessment also examines the *person's* cognitive health. It asks: What impact has dementia had on his or her ability to problem solve and initiate tasks? How diminished is his or her short- and long-term memory? What impact has dementia had to date on the *person's* speech, recognition of friends and families, and ability to follow directions? Dementia programs, in general, do a good job in this area of assessment. Program leaders should reinforce with staff that these cognitive losses, which are not always apparent to new staff and volunteers, are real. Not reinforcing this information can lead to many problems, including wandering, elopement from the program, and challenging behaviors.

Assess Who the *Person* Is

Best Friends staff members complete an assessment that looks at a *person's* qualities and personality. Someone with Alzheimer's disease will, for example, eventually have to retire from a career in teaching, but the qualities that made him or her a good teacher—generosity and caring—may be retained throughout the illness. Knowing this allows staff to evoke the *person's* social skills and graces and to determine when changes in personality should trigger alarms (e.g., the once-gregarious teacher becoming morose and agitated).

Best Friends Assessment

1. Check the boxes that apply to assess the *person's* cognitive ability.

	Poor	Fair	Good	Excellent
Memory	❑	❑	❑	❑
Judgment	❑	❑	❑	❑
Language	❑	❑	❑	❑
Initiative	❑	❑	❑	❑
Problem solving	❑	❑	❑	❑
Responsiveness to instructions/requests	❑	❑	❑	❑
Overall cognitive ability	❑	❑	❑	❑

2. Check the boxes that apply to assess the *person's* overall health.

	Poor	Fair	Good	Excellent
Vision	❑	❑	❑	❑
Hearing	❑	❑	❑	❑
Mobility	❑	❑	❑	❑
Overall health	❑	❑	❑	❑

3. Check the words that describe the *person's* personality before the illness and today.

Personality traits	**Before illness**	**Today**
Content	___	___
Extrovert	___	___
Fatalistic	___	___
Friendly	___	___
Happy	___	___
Introvert	___	___
Reserved	___	___
Serious	___	___
Suspicious	___	___
Timid	___	___

List which personality traits have changed. Can you name any triggers (e.g., people, places, time of day) or theories as to why the change occurred?

Change ______________________________ Reason ______________________________

____

Change ______________________________ Reason ______________________________

____

Change ______________________________ Reason ______________________________

____

(continued)

Figure 5.1. The best friends assessment. (From Bell, V., & Troxel, D. [1997]. The Best Friends approach to Alzheimer's care *[pp. 33–34]. Baltimore: Health Professions Press; reprinted by permission.)*

4. List the person's three most challenging behaviors.

____

Can you name any triggers (e.g., people, places, time of day) that cause these problems?

Problem ____________________ Trigger ____________________

____

Problem ____________________ Trigger ____________________

____

Problem ____________________ Trigger ____________________

____

5. List at least three things that the *person* seems to particularly enjoy or respond to:

____

____

6. List three qualities about the person that you would like others to know. (These qualities could include values, beliefs, traditions, or achievements.) How would the person have described himself or herself if asked to do so in just a few words?

____

____

____

What is the essence of this person? His or her core identity, his or her persona?

What is his/her self-worth and self-esteem based on?

What does this person value in his or her life and in relationships with others?

What is important to this individual? What are his or her passions?

What are the strengths, interests, abilities and preferences of this person?

What best describes how he or she would like to be known to others?

What is he or she known for among family and close friends?

What accomplishment is this person proudest of?

What roles and activities give comfort, meaning, pleasure, dignity and satisfaction and a sense of accomplishment in this person's daily life?

Figure 5.2. A new look at assessment. (Adapted from Seman, D., & Stansell, J. [1995]. Activity programming for persons with dementia: A sourcebook *[p. 12]. Chicago: Alzheimer's Disease & Related Disorders Association, Inc.)*

Dorothy Seman and Jane Stansell of the Alzheimer's Family Care Center in Chicago support this view and offer an insightful list of questions (Figure 5.2). This list can help any program develop a more effective, person-centered assessment form. The same material is laid out in an easy-to-use format in Tool 5.8. Seman, however, cautions against using this or any other list as the beginning or endpoint of assessment:

Many times the meaningful aspects of a person's *life story may not be conveyed to staff and others at the time of the initial assessment. Sometimes the* person *cannot recall these vital aspects of his or her own life because of dementia. The individual providing care may be too stressed out to be able to recount them or they may feel that the* person *is too far into dementia for these experiences to still have meaning. At other times, the current family contact may be unaware that certain rituals and traditions ever existed. With continued assessment, these meaningful aspects of a* person's *life may arise spontaneously, and thoughtful care will then make them a continuing part of the* person's *life.*

Thus, it is up to staff members to make an initial assessment and to continually add to the program's picture of the *person.*

Assess the Care Environment

Best Friends staff members understand that the environment can cause excess disability. There may be poor lighting, long hallways that lead to dead ends, poor acoustics, confusing wall treatments, or highly polished vinyl flooring that causes glare. All of these items can lead to discomfort and increased confusion, causing a *person* to function below his or her potential.

As part of her training program for staff members, Carly R. Hellen asks them to sit in a resident's room or program space for 15 minutes, taking note of the environment. They then share their findings and thoughts with the rest of the group.

This type of exercise allows staff members to judge whether the environment is helping them do their work or hindering it. How are the noise level, light, and overall comfort of the room? Would staff be comfortable spending time there?

Tool 5.6 contains a worksheet based on the principles of good dementia care design adapted from the work of Elizabeth C. Brawley, president of Design Concepts, Sausalito, California. Programs can use this tool to engage in an easy environmental assessment. It can be very helpful to know whether a program's environment is aiding in the delivery of good care or working against it.

Emphasize Remaining Strengths

Too often, charts and care plans emphasize negative aspects of *persons* with dementia. The pages are full of losses—what the *person* can no longer do. Clearly, charts and care plans contain important information, but they tend to emphasize losses as opposed to pointing out remaining strengths. Best Friends staff members emphasize the positive. Tool 5.1 shows strengths that all *persons* with dementia possess and strengths that can emerge with good care. When strengths are discovered, it helps everyone:

In the special care unit at The Olive Branch Senior Care Center in Tallulah, Louisiana, staff use the Best Friends philosophy to focus on residents' strengths. The administrator, Mary Jane Eiland, noted, "We decided not to take any losses for granted. The result was positive. For example, several residents who once were being fed are now feeding themselves. The quality of life of residents has improved greatly."

How can a meal be an opportunity for assessment? By sitting with a *person* during a meal, a staff member can assess the following areas:

Fine and gross motor muscle movements

Attention span

Problem solving

Sequencing

Perceptual abilities

Visual acuity

Socialization skills

—Carly R. Hellen, Director of Alzheimer's Care, The Wealshire, Lincolnshire, Illinois

It is important to spend time with staff to develop the art of looking for strengths.

—Karen Wyan, Assistant Administrator, Laurel Heights Home for the Elderly, London, Kentucky

This center's optimistic, can-do approach clearly is a success. Staff work hard to stay in a positive frame of mind, and the residents are the beneficiaries.

Do Not Overemphasize Stages

Best Friends staff members recognize that *stages* of illness have a place in clinical settings, but they should not be overemphasized in daily care. The authors began to rethink their views on stages of illness when a caregiver asked them, "When does the angry stage begin?" This reminded the authors of the danger of stages—in this case, a caregiver who is earnestly waiting for disaster to strike when it is possible that it never will.

The Best Friends staff does not dwell on stages of illness. Some people with Alzheimer's disease, for example, have a very difficult time behaviorally early in the disease, but they are easier to care for as time goes by. Others may start off with few behavioral challenges and eventually develop difficult problems such as sleeplessness or anxiety.

What is most valuable is for staff to evaluate each *person* as an individual, looking at his or her strengths and challenges. This approach avoids categorizing *persons*, discourages labeling, and challenges staff to take a fresh look at each *person's* care.

A resident was looking through various binders on my desk. I asked her, "Are you moving my books?" "No," she replied. "I'm reading." I stopped what I was doing and asked her to read a particular memo. She did so very elegantly and went on to talk about her days as a junior high school teacher of French and Spanish. This was a good lesson in not expecting too little from a resident!

—Mariegold Brown, L.P.N., The Fountainview Center for Alzheimer's Disease, Atlanta, Georgia

Leslie Congleton, program coordinator, Legacy Health Systems, Trinity Place Alzheimer's Day Respite Program, Portland, Oregon, uses the poem "My Favorite Sound" in staff training (see Figure 5.3). She reported, "It is full of images of all kinds of sounds. Its meaning and beauty is further enhanced by the fact that it was written by a group of 12 persons *with moderate to severe dementia. It is an example of the ability of a* person *with dementia to contribute and communicate their perception of things that have meaning for them."*

Looking for the positives, it was really uplifting.

—Kay Lloyd, Staff Educator, The Fountainview Center for Alzheimer's Disease in Atlanta, Georgia, about the Best Friends approach

Creative ability crosses the lines set by rigid staging. If Leslie had relied too heavily on stages, then she would have missed the opportunity for a creative and meaningful activity.

Individualize Care Plans

Best Friends staff members carefully individualize care plans. No two care plans should be alike. Each should tell a unique, compelling story. A care plan from Encore Senior Living Rediscovery™ Program is presented in Figure 5.4.

My Favorite Sound

My favorite sound

Is fifty dollars in change,

The sound of the waves,

The sound of Galli-Curci singing soprano,

The sound of my grandson's laugh,

Coyotes howling at the moon where the wind blows free,

People making noise at the table calling us to dinner.

I can't imagine the world without music.

Listen to everything!

The buzz of heat bugs in summertime,

The sound of something to eat,

Meat sizzling in a fry pan,

The soft flapping of wind in the birches,

The singing trees,

Crows and chickadees,

The trickle of water rushing over rocks.

Figure 5.3.

Note that it is detailed, concrete, and caring. It contains general information as well as an action plan. It covers personal care and activities. Above all, it is clearly individualized and does not use stock phrases or cookie-cutter approaches.

Assess Frequently as a Caregiving Team—*Persons* Vary from Day to Day

Best Friends staff members learn to recognize the daily ups and downs of *persons* with dementia. Experience teaches us that the losses of dementia do not take the form of a straight line downward. In fact, some *persons* seem to plateau for a period of time. They seem to have good days and bad, and good weeks and bad. Their moods and abilities often seem to vary

RESIDENT ACTION PLAN
She is a particularly sensitive individual with whom we want to build a trusting relationship. One way to build this trust is for all of us to be consistent in our approach. She gives definite clues when she doesn't like what you are doing. If she begins exhibiting some of these clues, leave and think of a different way to approach her. You may need to do this several times. When asking her to do something, try the following:

General Approach
•Be aware of your own level of patience. Realize this process could take a long time. If you are not able to give it the time and patience it needs, do it another time or ask someone else to do it.
•One person at a time is best. Have someone do it whom she trusts.
•Always be respectful as well as affectionate.
•Give her a warm greeting.
•Speak slowly with a smile, perhaps touching or holding her hand.
•Position yourself at eye level and give direct contact when looking at her.

Set the Tone
•Move slowly, speak slowly.
•Use a soothing tone of voice.
•Tell her what you are doing before you do it.
•Use gestures to demonstrate (e.g., when changing her sweater say, "We'll hang it up" and have the hanger in your hand; tug gently on her sweater to let her know what you're asking). Ask her, "Is this okay?" When changing her blouse, give her as much control as possible.

Help Her Relax
•Soak her feet.
•Try cream or massaging her legs and feet when changing her socks.
•Tap your foot when changing her shoes.
•Use lots of praise and touch to encourage her.

Create the Mood
•A.M.: Open her curtains and wake her gently, letting her know it's time to get up and that you'll be back in a few minutes to help her.
•P.M.: Walk her to her room and make sure that the lights are on in her room as you enter.

Handling Resistance
•If she begins using an angry or loud voice, stop. Reassure her (e.g., say, "I will not hurt you"). Use empathy: "It must be frustrating." Bow your head to communicate, "I'm sorry."
•If she continues to resist and becomes noticeably upset, leave and try again.

Closure
Be reassuring; don't just walk away when the process is complete but walk back with her to the living room, or say, "Good night, sleep well," and gently tuck the covers in and around her.

Figure 5.4. Sample individualized care plan developed by staff at Encore Senior Living Rediscovery™ Program, Portland, Oregon.

throughout the day. Long-term care programs should review care plans often, hopefully in the form of a team-approach weekly meeting. In small day center programs, it may be possible to talk about each *person*. In larger programs, these meetings ideally should occur with enough frequency so that over the course of several months, staff are taking an intensive look at each *person*. (See Tool 5.4 for a suggested format for weekly care planning meetings.)

The Fountainview Center's care plan team consists of the care plan coordinator, social worker, dietary manager, program director, and individual resident's family member. The group regularly asks all line staff for input in the development of care plans and their periodic reviews. "This has helped foster strong relationships between [sic] residents, families, and direct caregivers and made us all Best Friends with each other," according to Kay Lloyd, staff educator.

Staff members should learn the importance of what the authors call "checking the daily traffic" (see Tool 5.3). How is the *person* doing this week? Today? Are the planned activities appropriate and ones that might result in success? Has each *person* in the program been given a hug, a handshake, or a pat on the back during the day? During the last hour? Even when staff do simple things for residents, they still represent a very human connection being made. Checking the daily traffic also allows staff to observe or understand whether the *person* is doing well or is perhaps ill and requires attention.

Staff members at the Helping Hand Day Center program work hard to "stop, look, and listen" with each participant during each day. A participant who was almost always upbeat seemed unusually worried and anxious one day. Staff sensed this, made inquiries, and discovered that her husband had been hospitalized. Because of her dementia, she could not tell the staff what was wrong, but her behavior communicated the message.

When they discovered the problem with her husband, the staff at Helping Hand could give this participant extra attention and offer words of comfort and support.

Assess Combative Behavior Carefully

Best Friends staff members recognize that combative behavior is possible. Program leaders should encourage staff to not put themselves in harm's way and to remove themselves from sit-

The Four Roles of Assessment: Magician, Detective, Carpenter, Jester

The Magician sees problem behaviors as behavioral symptoms of unmet needs.

The Detective makes a "best guess" of underlying needs, their causes, and acceptable outcomes.

The Carpenter works to eliminate or reduce excess disability and to select appropriate approaches and interventions.

The Jester lightens the load with humor, freeing staff to think of more creative ideas and solutions.

—Joanne Rader, Associate Professor, School of Nursing, Oregon Health Sciences University (adapted from her 1995 book Individualized dementia care: Creative, compassionate approaches. *New York: Springer).*

uations that look threatening whenever possible. Giving the *person* time to calm down can sometimes do the trick. When combativeness does occur, however, staff should not overreact but instead look for triggers and potential solutions.

Combativeness stems from multiple, sometimes overlapping, causes. It can be caused by the impact of dementia on the *person;* lack of judgment, loss of memory, and other symptoms can contribute to frustration and anger. It also can be provoked by poorly trained or unempathethic staff; problems can happen, for example, when staff have no knowledge of the *person's* life story. The environment can cause undue stress; loud noise or poor lighting might frighten or even be physically painful to *persons* and convince them that they need to leave the premises. A poor activity program can cause boredom and restlessness, which can provoke a *person* to act out. Good assessment speaks to these potential problems and how they can be treated with a Best Friends approach. The assessment also can note when the judicious use of psychotropic medications proves helpful. (See Tool 5.9 for more tips on this subject.)

The adult day center at Sunshine Terrace in Logan, Utah, promotes a philosophy of healing and self-esteem through rediscovery of residual musical abilities. Music is the key that unlocks the door to once again finding joy in life.

—*Bonnie Baird Smith, Program Director*

Set Realistic Expectations

Best Friends staff members strike a balance between expecting too little and expecting too much of *persons* with dementia. When too little is expected of *persons,* staff members get what they expect. *Persons* should always be given a chance to finish a sentence, dress themselves, and help with cleaning up or gardening; if not, then staff may unknowingly rob them of their dignity and contribute to their decline. Alternately, if too much is expected of *persons,* then staff will fail. This can lead to staff frustration and declining morale. For *persons* with dementia, it can cause frustration, anger, and challenging behaviors.

A licensed practical nurse (LPN) on The Fountainview Center staff noted that one resident was nonverbal and wandered and initially appeared to be incapable of doing any activities of daily living (ADLs) on her own. After conducting a careful assessment, the LPN discovered that the resident still had fine motor skills, so she could be prompted to brush her teeth, feed herself, and help with her toileting and her grooming.

It is easy to overlook a strength that, once rediscovered and reinforced, supports dignity and makes a great difference to the daily life of the *person.*

Share Information with Families or Other Visitors

Best Friends staff members understand that although confidentiality must be considered, a program's goals should be shared with family members, visitors, and volunteers. This can be done through family conferences or even by modeling behavior when visitors are present. The importance of sharing information is that family members can be encouraged to work with the staff on common goals. For example, when staff members are trying to encourage a resident to walk or spend time outside, it can be harmful if family members say, "He can't do that anymore," or "Why bother pushing him?" The Bullet Card, introduced in Tool 7.4, is one method of sharing key goals.

Conclusion

A good assessment can prevent disaster. Consider the simple toothache: A *person* with dementia who is in unnoticed and untreated pain might begin to express anger, upset, and anxiety. He or she may not sleep well. He or she might strike out. These challenging behaviors could lead to the unnecessary use of psychotropic medications that might increase confusion. The *person* could fall into a downward spiral of being in pain → being overmedicated → becoming more gravely disabled. Careful assessment and ongoing care can prevent such a scenario from unfolding and instead keeps the *person* functioning at his or her best.

Carly R. Hellen of The Wealshire described well a staff with knack: "Good dementia care staff can sit down with a resident and over the course of a meal, or getting dressed, be able to get a holistic feel for the person's strengths and abilities." This is the Best Friends way at its finest.

Good ongoing assessment practices build staff confidence. When staff members grasp what a *person* is capable of—and not capable of—they can be more confident in everyday interactions and can learn ways of encouraging the *person* to achieve his or her best. It also can lead to many surprises (see Figure 5.5) about what the *person* may still be able to do, and, even more important, about who the *person* still is. And in looking for surprises in the *person,* staff will find surprises in themselves. Just like the *person* with dementia, the Best Friends staff sometimes can do more than they ever thought possible.

Music
Reminiscing
Creative art
Intergenerational experiences
Social graces
Mobility
Old skills
Old sayings and truisms
Eye–hand coordination
Rituals, sacred and secular

Figure 5.5. Surprises that may be found in the assessment process.

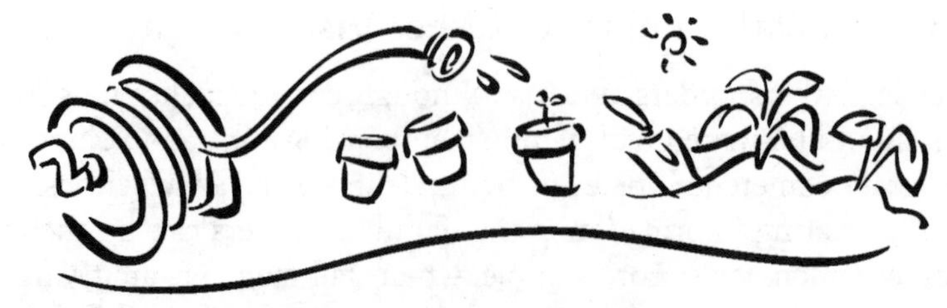

Training Tool Kit

Tool 5.0 / Warm-Up
What Do You See?

Have fun with this warm-up and note that Best Friends staff members look at their surroundings and try to see what is going on in the workplace.

Copy the survey in this exercise and hand it out to the class with pencils or pens. Take 10–15 minutes and ask everyone to walk around and try to complete as many of the questions as possible.

How many people in the room . . .

Have red hair?______Have smiled in the last 5 minutes?_____

Have brown hair?______Are wearing jewelry?_____

Have black hair?______Are wearing pants?_____

Have a ponytail?______Are wearing a skirt?_____

Have on earrings?______Are wearing glasses?_____

Have sneakers on?______Are wearing red clothing_____

Are more than 6 feet tall?______Are wearing a watch?_____

Are less than 5 feet tall?______Have frowned in the last 5 minutes?_____

Variation: Type up the questions, leaving room for staff members' names. Conduct the exercise like a scavenger hunt.

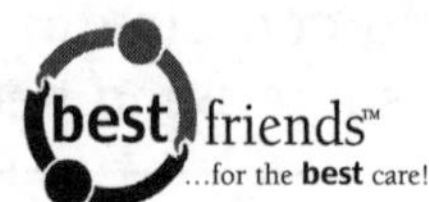

Tool 5.1 / Program Pointer
The Other Face of Alzheimer's Disease

Post on a bulletin board to share with staff and families.

Every individual with Alzheimer's disease is

A *person* with infinite value
A *person* with a name
A *person* with a spirit
A *person* with feelings
A *person* with will and personality
A *person* with a life story
A *person* who lives in the physical environment
A *person* who has the present moment

A careful assessment may reveal that the *person* with Alzheimer's disease may still be

A *person* who gives and receives love and affection
A *person* who can reminisce and respond to stories from others
A *person* who is compassionate and concerned
A *person* who enjoys verbal and nonverbal communication
A *person* who can be surprisingly flexible
A *person* who has a sense of humor
A *person* who is productive
A *person* with intact social graces
A *person* who maintains skills and talents
A *person* who responds to children and pets
A *person* who thrives on music and other creative arts
A *person* who is physically fit
A *person* who has excellent eye–hand coordination
A *person* who experiences all five senses
A *person* who responds to the experience of new information

From Bell, V., & Troxel, D. (1999). The other face of Alzheimer's disease. American Journal of Alzheimer's Disease, *14(1), 60–64; reprinted by permission.*

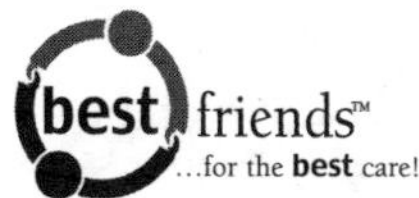

Tool 5.2 / Program Pointer

Encouraging Staff to Learn the Best Friends Assessment

This activity involves all staff in hands-on care planning, helping them build assessment skills. This exercise also can be repeated throughout the year to reinforce the importance of assessment, and even to update actual care plans.

Make copies of the Best Friends assessment form (pp. 90–91). Have staff break into small groups and use this form to assess a *person* of their choice. If the group discovers that they cannot answer a particular question, then ask them to talk about where they might go or how they might be able to find the information.

After 15–30 minutes, bring the groups back together and ask someone from each group to share the results of the work. As the staff member reviews the assessment, invite the entire class to comment and make additional suggestions. Also, remind staff of the importance of confidentiality.

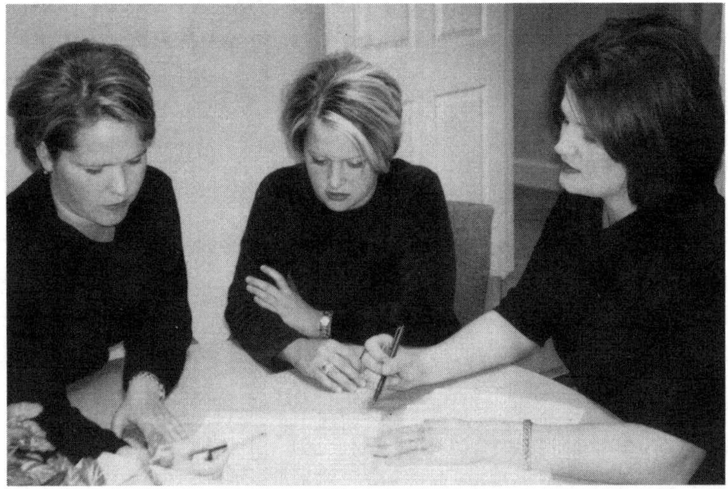

Staff members (from left) Tonya Tincher, Laurie Simpson, and Gwen Hutchinson of the Helping Hand Day Center, Lexington, Kentucky, review their Best Friends assessment forms.

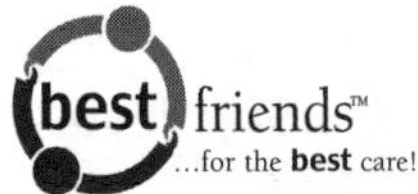

Tool 5.3 / Program Pointer
Check the Daily Traffic

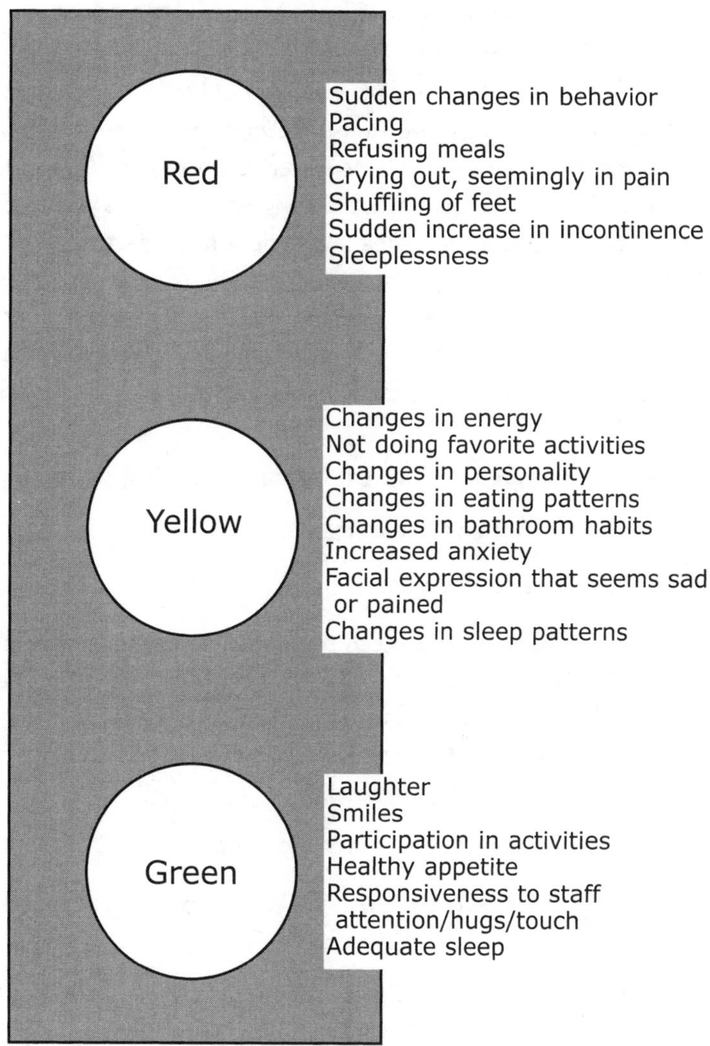

Use this handout to talk about the need to "stop, look, and listen" each day. A traffic light can be a good metaphor for this process, representing the concept that behaviors communicate messages. Red indicates behaviors that are of great concern and need immediate attention. Yellow indicates behaviors that need to be watched; they could be situational but may linger if a physical or environmental problem persists. Green represents behaviors that communicate "all is well."

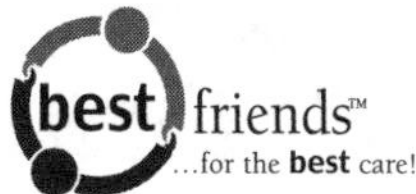

Tool 5.4 / Program Pointer
Suggested Staff Meeting Format

Every Best Friends program should hold a weekly staff meeting that includes key individuals who are responsible for a person's *care. A typical team in a larger facility might include staff members from nursing, nutrition, social services, activities, and CNAs.*

Weekly 1-hour meetings give staff a feeling of empowerment and connection with one another. It is vital that the hands-on CNAs be invited to participate. Often, they have the best idea of what works and what does not and what is going on in the lives of some persons. *Families also should be invited to participate when their loved one is to be discussed.*

If the long-term care program commits to weekly meetings, follow-through becomes important; every effort should be made to give this meeting the highest priority, perhaps even making it a mandatory meeting. There is never enough time to get everything done, but Best Friends programs do not fall into the trap of constantly moving, rescheduling, and canceling staff meetings.

Suggested Format and Topics: 1-Hour Meeting

5 minutes	Hellos and personal catch-up
10 minutes	Announcements
20 minutes	Review of selected *persons*. One staff member should take the lead and review the *person's* diagnosis and health status. The staff member should offer an opinion about how the *person* is doing in the program or residence and then ask for input and ideas. Specific problems or challenges that come up should be addressed.
10 minutes	Brief review of other residents
10 minutes	Brief review of past in-services or plans for future classes; use this as a time for reinforcement and reward.
5 minutes	End on a high note. Staff should give one another compliments about any special successes during the last week. Any special examples of knack in action also should be shared.

Adjourn

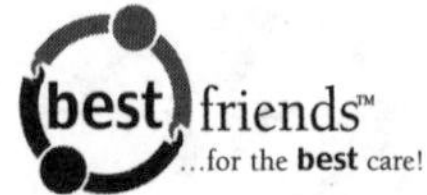

Tool 5.5 / Program Pointer

It's Important to Know . . .

Use this quote on your Best Friends bulletin board, in a newsletter, or in staff group discussion to point out that the person *is more important than the diagnosis.*

It's important to know what *person* the disease has, not what disease the *person* has.

–Sir William Osler, 1849–1919

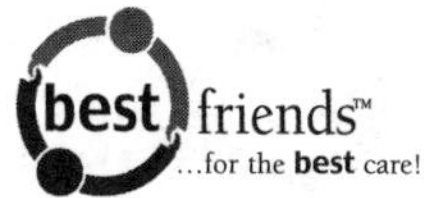

Tool 5.6 / Program Pointer
Environmental Checklist

Use this checklist to evaluate the design of your dementia care program and as a starting point when considering renovations.

Do:

- ❑ Locate programs on the ground level when possible.
- ❑ Provide bright light levels.
- ❑ Reduce glare, especially on the floor.
- ❑ Use contrasting colors for definition.
- ❑ Use large print for labels and signage.
- ❑ Create easy viewing in popular areas, such as art activity rooms.
- ❑ Create adequate, convenient storage space.
- ❑ Decorate with items that can be touched and investigated.
- ❑ Arrange and maintain furniture in one location.
- ❑ Use square tables with stable legs rather than pedestal-style tables (i.e., no folding tables).
- ❑ Provide safe, comfortable seating for residents.
- ❑ Use armchairs for dining and activity seating.
- ❑ Use rocking chairs that have a stable base.
- ❑ Provide easily accessible bathrooms.
- ❑ Use grab bars in place of towel bars.
- ❑ Provide a small working kitchen, including microwave and refrigerator.
- ❑ Provide safe, secure, and easily accessible outdoor environments.
- ❑ Create visually accessible outside areas for easy staff viewing.
- ❑ Create destination areas in the outdoor environment.
- ❑ Provide an area that is protected from weather in the outdoor environment.
- ❑ Provide chairs and benches with comfortable cushions and back/arm supports.
- ❑ Use handrails on outdoor walking paths.

Don't:

- ❑ Locate the entrance where program participants can congregate and easily slip out.
- ❑ Create walkways that have no destination.
- ❑ Use abstract artwork.
- ❑ Call attention to the doors.
- ❑ Allow a corridor to end at an exit door, unless it opens onto secure outdoor space.
- ❑ Use multiple types of floor covering to break up floor areas.

Courtesy of Elizabeth C. Brawley, president, Design Concepts Unlimited, Sausalito, California.

Tool 5.7 / Games for Learning

The Assessment Game

The purpose of this exercise is to help staff gain hands-on practice in talking about and putting together the pieces of an assessment (see also Tool 3.8).

Prior to the training session, cut art foam board into puzzle pieces and glue Velcro on each piece. On a sheet of paper write the phrases from the possibilities listed below. Cut out each phrase and stick one on each puzzle piece. Divide the class into groups and give each group one or more pieces. Ask them to discuss the content of the piece or pieces and how each relates to assessment. At the end of the discussion, ask for a volunteer to come to the front of the class and put the piece back into the puzzle. (You can create a master outline of the puzzle to lay on the tabletop for guidance.)

Review overall health.
Everyone has remaining strengths.
Who is the *person,* and what can he or she still do?
Set realistic expectations.
Individualize care plans.
All staff contribute to the assessment.
Assess the care environment.
Don't rely too much on stages.

Emphasize that . . .

We make assessments all the time.
All staff members can participate in assessment
Staff who are with the *person* the most often probably have the best ideas for the assessment.
The more complete the assessment, the more ideas that staff can use for high-quality care.

Courtesy of Susan D. Berry, Alzheimer's disease consultant and trainer, Warsaw, Indiana.

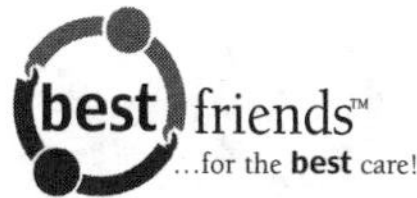

Tool 5.8 / Program Pointer
The Real Me

Complete the following set of questions regarding a participant or resident. Afterward, discuss as a group.

What is the essence of this *person* (i.e., his or her core identity, persona)? ____________

____

What is his or her self-worth/self-esteem based on? ____________

____

What does this *person* value in his or her life and in relationships with others? ____________

____

What is important to this *person*? What are his or her passions? ____________

____

What are the strengths, interests, abilities and preferences of this *person*? ____________

____

What best describes how he or she would like to be known to others? ____________

____

What is he or she known for among family and close friends? ____________

____

What accomplishment is this *person* proudest of (e.g., good cook)? ____________

____

What roles and activities bring comfort, meaning, pleasure, dignity, and satisfaction and a sense of accomplishment to this *person's* daily life? ____________

____

From Seman, D., & Stansell, J. (1995). Activity programming for persons with dementia: A sourcebook *(p. 12). Chicago: Alzheimer's Disease & Related Disorders Association, Inc.; reprinted by permission.*

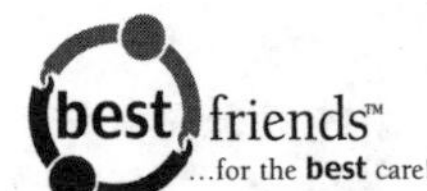

Tool 5.9 / Program Pointer
Handling Combativeness

Use this handout for discussion.

If the *person* is prone to combativeness, do:

Look for triggers (e.g., needs to go to the bathroom, is in pain, does not like being rushed).

Chart time of day and incidents to look for patterns.

Keep the *person* physically active with light exercise.

Spend time outdoors.

Look for favorite activities, rituals, and traditions and incorporate them in the intervention plan.

Use positive verbal as well as body language.

Ask staff whether any particular members are particularly successful with the *person.*

Discuss the *person* more frequently at care planning/staff meetings.

Evaluate the frequency of personal care tasks: Are they absolutely necessary? How often should they be carried out?

Don't:

Immediately label the *person* as combative—look for solutions.

Overmedicate.

Force the *person* to perform a personal care activity or other action against his or her will; don't try to reason with him or her or argue about it.

Overreact.

If the *person* is combative:

Ask the *person* what is wrong so that you can gather information as to the reason for the behavior; sometimes the *person* can tell you.

Ask him or her to stop and gauge the *person's* response; it can improve matters.

Encourage staff and volunteers to stay out of harm's way.

Give the *person* space and as much control of his or her situation as possible.

Use psychotropic medications judiciously.

Engage in honest communication about the behavior with family members.

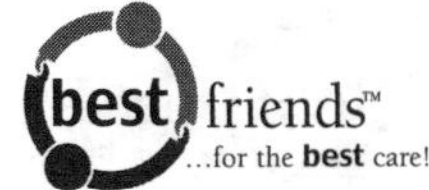

Tool 5.10

Turning No Knack into Knack

The purpose of this exercise is to show, with a dash of humor, the wrong way to do something. This is active learning that really sinks in, particularly when staff members themselves volunteer to take part in the role plays.

The following statements represent stereotypes or falsehoods about dementia. These examples of "no knack" can be used in a number of ways to explore staff attitudes and reinforce the lessons presented in this chapter. Draw them from a hat to discuss as a group or put them into role plays. Invite staff to comment on the mistakes. Then role-play or discuss the right way. The authors discuss the art of role plays in Tool 2.11. Use your creativity to have fun turning these examples of "no knack" into "knack."

All you need in an assessment is the medical information.

The *person* would do better if he or she just tried harder.

A *person* should not have any stimulation at all—it's just too stressful.

Trying to keep up with glasses and hearing aids is just too hard. Why bother when the *person* has Alzheimer's?

You tell me the behavior and I'll tell you what stage the person is in.

The less that the family and staff talk about the diagnosis, the better.

When will Mother hit the angry stage?

Even when they ask, I don't let residents help clean up or sweep the floor. They're not very good at it.

She told me she was born in Oklahoma, but I knew differently. I explained it to her so that she'll get it right next time.

I'm sure that they all like gospel music. That's why I play it every day.

She grew up in Japan, but I doubt that she remembers anything now about her heritage or background. We can just treat her like everybody else.

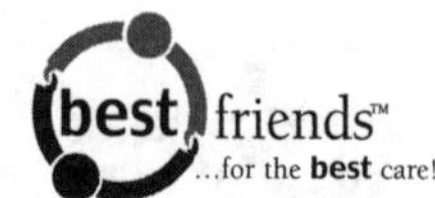

6

Friendship

What *persons* with Alzheimer's disease need most of all is a good friend, a Best Friend. This philosophy is not based simply on altruism. Evoking elements of friendship in Alzheimer's care brings out the social graces of *persons* with dementia. It creates a more joyful caregiving atmosphere or milieu that gives them increased feelings of comfort, happiness, and security. The result is fewer challenging behaviors and an optimum quality of life for the *person*. That makes a staff member's job easier and more rewarding.

At one in-service taught by the authors, a number of staff members raised their hands to ask about specific problem areas (e.g., wandering, striking out, activities not working). With each question, the authors replied, "What do you think? How could you be a Best Friend to that resident? What would a Best Friend do in that situation?"

At first, this strategy was met with resistance. Staff members wanted "the answers." We repeated the question, "What would a Best Friend do in that situation?" The staff began talking and brainstorming some excellent ideas:

Maybe I could stop and think why he's doing this.

I could come back and try again later. I have bad days sometimes, too.

A friend would be more patient.

I could listen more carefully.

I think I pressured her to move too fast. That's why she got angry.

I'd also be bored just sitting there. I'd want to leave, too.

Almost all of the staff members present participated in the discussion, despite their varying educational backgrounds, job categories, social and economic circumstances, cultural and ethnic backgrounds, and language skills. Friendship was something that everyone could understand. They were not called on to remember the neurobiology of dementia. The exercise asked them to imagine being a friend. Their answers, we thought, were really quite expert.

The Serenity Nursing Home, a residential home in Johannesburg, South Africa, embraced the Best Friends model in an innovative way. Everyone on the staff chose at least one resident to be his or her own Best Friend. They were expected to spend at least 1 hour each week with this resident.

Staff members began to form relationships with their Best Friends. They did their regular jobs well, but they kept a special eye out for their resident; some even visited their Best Friends after hours. Staff members made the effort to learn more about the backgrounds of their Best Friend, and they swapped stories. Lessons were learned; if care improved when staff members learned one life story, then it would certainly improve if they learned more life stories. If care became easier because of the special attention that they were giving their Best Friend, then would a similar effort pay dividends with other residents?

Serenity's administrator, Michael Livni, allowed the lowest-paid, most inexperienced workers to choose first from among the residents—a housekeeper could choose first and, in theory, could choose the most sparkling, fun, interesting resident. As the highest-ranking employee, Michael Livni got the person *whom no one else had chosen. This approach accomplished two things: 1) It allowed the lowest-level workers to be exposed to residents who might enrich those staff members' lives, and 2) because the administrator did his part in spending time with perhaps the most challenging resident, he was demonstrating the importance of giving every resident the best care.*

Every road is rough to me that has no friend to cheer it.

—*Elizabeth Shane*

Being a friend is what geriatric nursing is all about.

—*Kelli Martin, geriatric nurse, West Park Long Term Care Center, Cody, Wyoming*

I praise the way Best Friends approaches the staff and encourages them to become friends with the residents. So often I see staff treat residents as objects and not people.

—*Rachel L. Everett, student, Madonna University, Livonia, Michigan*

Tell them to look after my Best Friend.

—*Senior night sister, Serenity Nursing Home, Johannesburg, South Africa, from her hospital bed after being severely injured in a car accident some 400 miles away from the facility*

Livni said that the Best Friends model changed the culture of care at Serenity Nursing Home. Staff morale and retention have improved, and workers tell their friends and family members that Serenity is a good place to work and live.

The authors have formulated a number of key concepts of Best Friendship, which follow.

Friends Know Each Other's History and Personality

Best Friends staff members know their residents or participants as well as they know their personal friends. They can tell you key facts about a *person's* life, something about their family, and something about their personality. They know about the *person's* achievements, jobs, and values.

At Omahanui Private Hospital in New Plymouth, New Zealand, a change in location of the nurses' station and work assignments helped staff and residents get to know one another better:

The nurses' station was moved into a corner of the lounge area so that nursing staff members were able to mingle with patients at all times. Each nurse/caregiver was given a small group of four to five patients to care for, so that the same nurse works with the same group of people from the time of admission until their deaths. When that nurse has a day off, she is relieved by the same nurse each week, thus reducing the number of nursing staff involved with each patient and allowing a relationship of trust and friendship to develop among the resident, his or her nurse, and family members.

When staff and residents get to know one another, dementia care is easier. In the Omahanui case, patients' agitation and challenging behaviors were reduced. Staff also took greater pride in how their patients were doing. It worked well to regularly match staff to the same *person*. Another example follows:

At Karrington Cottages, a Sunrise Assisted Living Community in Rochester, Minnesota, five to seven residents live in an apartment and share a kitchen, living room, and dining room. Care managers share all of the housekeeping duties and help with personal care as needed. The care managers and residents get to know one another in a special way as they live, work, and play together. "An environment of friendship is obvious," noted Linda O'Connor, the executive director.

Many dementia care programs have embraced the concept of universal workers, perhaps because it mirrors home and family situations and encourages residents and staff to get to know one another well.

Friends Do Things Together

Best Friends staff members engage in activities with *persons* in their care. The activities include everything from structured group activities to one-to-one activities that might take only a few seconds (e.g., see Tool 9.5). As in most friendships, activities do not have to be planned or formalized. For example, no one calls a friend and says, "Let's program a movie Saturday night."

A resident at Laurel Heights Home for the Elderly does not stay on one subject, but she does respond to the words "Best Friends" and a hug and praise for being a good mother, homemaker, and church worker. She explained to staff member Dorothy Bailey, "I love having a friend. We can do lots of things together. Yes, I need a friend with me a lot. We can walk. We can go to church."

I could not pick just one Best Friend; I chose two. I look forward to visiting with them each day. I feel like we are really getting to know each other in a way we never thought about. I look forward to it as much as they do.
—*Carol Gregory, Business Office, Laurel Heights Home for the Elderly, London, Kentucky*

With our dearest friends, we don't have to explain why we are afraid of thunderstorms, they just know we are.
—*Herman Melville*

What Is Being a Best Friend to the Person with Dementia?

To know as much as you can about the person.

Do things for him or her, and do things together.

Work on the relationship and look after the person.

This may build up their self-esteem and yours.

Become his or her advocate.

Perhaps both of you will have fun.
—*Michael Livni, Administrator, Serenity Nursing Home, Johannesburg, South Africa*

Just a simple touch or moment of attention from a passing staff member enriches this resident's day.

Best Friends programs encourage staff to bring their own hobbies, interests, and enthusiasms to their work. Doing so can be particularly beneficial when a staff member discovers common interests or a shared background with a resident (e.g., both growing up in Wyoming, a shared love of horses).

Dana E. Newquist, the administrator of Alzheimer's Four Seasons, owns a 1940s–era Seagraves fire engine. He enjoys bringing the colorful truck to the facility for the residents to enjoy and occasionally ride in. Newquist admits that he enjoys the activity as much as or more than the residents, responding to the fun and nostalgia of the old fire engine. He even drives it in the local Fourth of July parade each year, often with residents enjoying the ride as passengers.

Friends are experts in caring. This is what friendship is all about.

—Gayle Pennington, Program Director, Riverside Adult Day Program, Wilmington, Delaware

A staff member and a resident have become very good friends at The Fountains. They seem to understand each other's personality and moods. Although the resident is unable to call the staff member by name, she looks for her and often slips her arm around her waist and gives her a big smile. They compliment each other: "You look pretty today." "You look pretty, too!" There is a friendship, a bond, a relationship that is close, playful and loving.

—Diane Will, National Community Life Director, The Fountains Continuum of Care, Inc., Tucson, Arizona

We are all travelers in the wilderness of this world. And the best that we can find in our travels is an honest friend.

—Robert Louis Stevenson

Friends keep us going through rough times.

—Anonymous

Friends Communicate

Best Friends staff members value communication with *persons* for whom they care, using both verbal and nonverbal communication. They learn to speak and listen skillfully. Most important, staff members need to encourage *persons* with dementia to communicate when they can; even when language is impaired, *persons* often have a strong desire to communicate, to connect with another person.

Laura Stewart, an employee in the billing department at Laurel Heights Home for the Elderly, is a Best Friend to a resident. She told the authors, "My day is not complete unless my Best Friend and I visit. I just cannot go by her door without going in and seeing how she is doing, and if she has slept well or needs something. Being her friend is my favorite part of the day."

Why not give all staff, even those not directly involved in resident care, an opportunity to benefit from a Best Friends program?

A staff member from Serenity Nursing Home sent home only one postcard from a recent trip overseas—to her Best Friend.

The gesture of the card probably meant the world to the resident. Communication can occur even a long way from home.

Friends Build Self-Esteem

Best Friends staff members know that dementia can shatter self-esteem. A skilled staff member gives compliments often and offers encouragement. Even the simple act of asking an opinion, such as, "Do you like my outfit today? Does my blouse match my skirt?" can evoke a positive feeling. The resident senses that you value his or her opinion.

A resident at Toca das Horttensias lived in Spain during his youth. Knowing that he was proud of his background, staff would play Spanish folk music and prepare a traditional Spanish meal when he seemed sad. These efforts would lift his spirits, and he would tell stories of his happy childhood in Spain.

The smell of the Spanish food and the melodies of the Spanish music evoked joyful memories in the resident.

Friends Laugh Together Often

Best Friends staff members understand that life has its comic moments. A good-natured staff member is not afraid to laugh when funny situations occur or when someone tells a joke, pun, or amusing story. Clearly, it would be wrong to laugh *at* the *person*, but it is okay to laugh *with* him or her.

Staff at Evergreen Center I share the view that "maintaining an enthusiastic, friendly, and humorous tone provides all of us with many great moments. Our day involves a lot of fun, 'color,' and laughter together. Laughter is our recreation," said Cheryl T. Weidemeyer, program director.

Laughter really is the best medicine.

Friends Are Equals

Best Friends staff members act with authority, but they never talk down to a *person*. Mariegold Brown, a LPN at The Fountainview Center, told the authors that she and a resident both liked to read:

The resident reads to me from magazines and always gives me her comments at the end of each reading, which are very comical at times. We also talk on different subjects, and I'm always delighted with the resident's wit and smarts. . . . She also helps me with my spelling.

Brown had a friendly give-and-take relationship with the resident. By asking the resident for help with her spelling, the staff member is creating an environment of equality that will enhance the *person's* self-esteem.

Friends Work at the Relationship

Best Friends staff members are not overly sensitive. They do not wear their emotions on their sleeves. Any friendship takes work, and staff are not afraid to gently tease and encourage activity and involvement.

For 4 years, a participant in the Helping Hand Day Center had been a very outgoing and jolly person, loving dancing, working puzzles, and making bracelets from assorted beads. She gradually lost her verbal and fine motor skills and has grown frustrated, even angry, at these losses. Staff and volunteers have learned to be flexible to adapt to her changing condition and to understand when her frustration is directed toward them.

The Best Friends staff keep this *person* engaged and a part of the adult day center. It is difficult for the staff to witness her losses, but, as she declines, the staff's love and care increase.

Friends Show Love and Affection

Best Friends staff members offer love and affection often. They are masters of the handshake and the hug. Their faces wear more smiles than frowns. For less-effusive staff members, some kind words such as, "Mrs. Johnson, you are a good friend," or, "I really enjoy spending some time with you. We're friends, aren't we?" can evoke a similar response.

In Brazil, the culture encourages and supports the frequent exchanges of hugs and kisses among friends:

Nancy was born in southern Brazil, where there is a diverse community of people of Portuguese, Polish, German, Spanish, and Italian descent. She enjoyed a close relationship with her family and friends, in which hugs and kisses were given frequently. At the Toca das Horttensias, staff dealt with her aggressive spells or bouts of confusion with these same hugs and kisses.

These acts of love and affection helped Nancy feel safe and secure again.

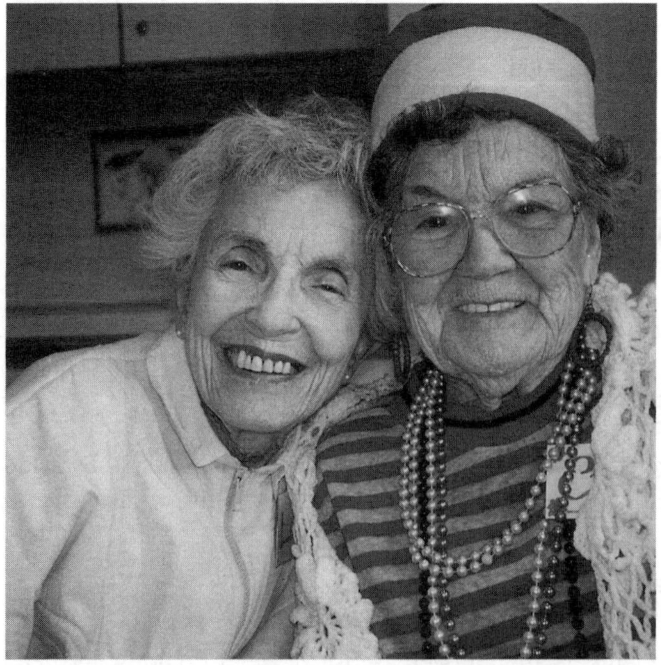

Volunteer Lorraine Lollis (left) and her Best Friend, Eva Powell, share many smiles and hugs throughout the days that they are together at Helping Hand Day Center.

Friends Can Overcome Social Barriers

In adult day centers and long-term care communities, *persons* often form friendships with one another. Staff in many programs have told the authors of the formation of unlikely friendships: For example, a former bank teller now jokes and holds hands with a former bank president.

The members of the early-stage Alzheimer's support group in Santa Barbara, California, come from all walks of life. The group is cosponsored by the local Alzheimer's Association and the Friendship Adult Day Care Center. Initially, most of the support group members did not use day center services, but, as the group continued, many became candidates for the Friendship Center. Three members of the support group finally agreed to attend if they could go together on the same days. Notably, they help one another, do things together, and enjoy one another's company.

This interesting example demonstrates that an early-stage support group has the potential to encourage sustained friendships among its members and that a group like this can provide an important transition to day center care.

The West Park Long Term Care Center has found that the Best Friends model is not just staff and resident relationships. Many residents help and become friends with other residents with dementia.

Persons often form friendships with one another, sometimes even helping one another throughout the day.

Conclusion

A volunteer in the Helping Hand Day Center reflected on the death of a participant in the program to whom she had been a Best Friend. Jane Owen had spent one morning a week with this participant for more than 4 years. "I knew her better than most of my other friends

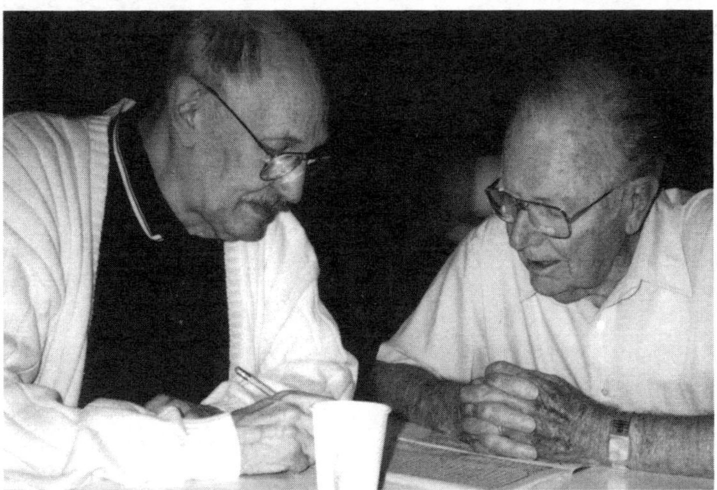

George Smith (left) and Charles Tate are Best Friends at the Helping Hand Day Center, Lexington, Kentucky.

and family. I had a sense of her moods and personality as she did mine. We had spent that much time together. She was as much a Best Friend to me as I was to her."

Another volunteer from Helping Hand Day Center inspired the authors with his wise thoughts about friendship. When T.J. Todd reflected about being a Best Friend to a participant, he said that they had developed a warm and special relationship. When she died, T.J. said, "I miss her very much. We were friends ... the best of friends."

Both Jane and T.J. said that they felt immeasurably enriched by their time at the Helping Hand Day Center. Both believed that they gained as much as they gave. The authors also were struck by a story from Deanna R. Pham, the director of social services at The Fountainview Center for Alzheimer's Disease:

Deanna always believed that she did a good job relating to the 120 dementia care residents at the center. Even though it was a challenging task, she tried to know the needs of each person *in the facility. When the director of staff education introduced the Best Friends model, however, Deanna realized that many quiet residents or those who stay in their rooms did not get as much attention as the outgoing, active residents. She realized that they were waiting for staff to "make the first move" and decided that, in addition to her daily interactions, she would pick one resident each week to single out. She would initiate activities with these residents; take strolls in the courtyard; and talk about the past, their dreams, and even their regrets. "Each week, I feel I have one more 'friend' in the building and one less 'resident.' "*

Robert Louis Stevenson wrote, "A friend is a gift you give yourself." A Best Friends program builds a caring community that enriches all who are involved. Deanna realized that the weight of her responsibilities would make it challenging for her to be a Best Friend to everyone during the course of a typical work week. Yet her creative and life-affirming solution is one that will have great impact. Changing the culture of a long-term care program happens in small steps. Imagine that every staff member at a large facility took the same initiative as Deanna and singled out a new resident each week. A wave of change would occur, from an institution to a home, from a place to work to a community, and from a group of strangers to a group of friends.

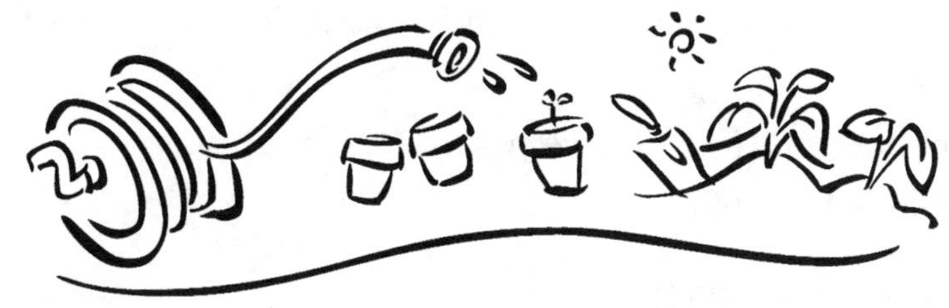

Training Tool Kit

Tool 6.0 / Warm-Up
Your Best Friends in Life

This exercise gets staff thinking about the link between friendship and the work that they are doing. It has proven quite popular in various workshops around the United States.

Use a flipchart or board to record the group's answers. Ask the class to take a minute or two, close their eyes, and think about a close personal friend. Tell them that you will be asking them to say aloud the friend's first name. You will also ask them to name a quality about that friend or something else that makes it a friendship (e.g., John—he's a listener, Mary—she sticks by me through good and bad, Margarita—we laugh and go shopping together).

As the names are read and qualities assigned, write them down on the chart or board, putting the first name on the left-hand side and his or her qualities on the right-hand side; for example:

John	Listener
Mary	Loyal
Margarita	Laughing/shopping/doing things

Try to get everyone to participate. Review the list of qualities. Compliment group members on their great friends.

Ask the participants whether these qualities would also be good ones for staff. Ask whether they think that the *person* would respond better to us if we created this same relationship (e.g., humor, trust, support, listener, patient) with them.

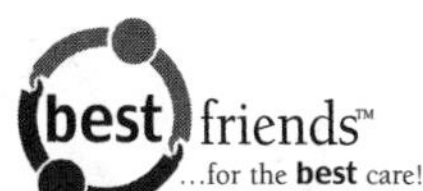

Tool 6.1 / Program Pointer
Elements of Friendship

Use this list in teaching staff, or use parts of it to include regularly on the Best Friends bulletin board or in the newsletter.

Friends Know Each Other's History and Personality

In Alzheimer's care, a Best Friend—

Becomes the *person's* memory
Is sensitive to the *person's* traditions
Learns the *person's* personality, moods, and problem-solving style

Friends Do Things Together

In Alzheimer's care, a Best Friend—

Involves the *person* in daily activities and chores
Initiates activities
Ties activities into the *person's* past skills and interests
Encourages the *person* to enjoy the simpler things in life
Remembers to celebrate special occasions

Friends Communicate

In Alzheimer's care, a Best Friend—

Listens carefully
Speaks skillfully
Asks questions skillfully
Speaks using body language
Gently encourages participation in conversation

Friends Build Self-Esteem

In Alzheimer's care, a Best Friend—

Gives compliments often
Carefully asks for advice or opinions
Always offers encouragement
Offers congratulations

(continued)

Friends Laugh Often

In Alzheimer's care, a Best Friend—

Tells jokes and funny stories
Takes advantage of spontaneous fun
Uses self-deprecating humor often
Enjoys the humor of the other person

Friends Are Equals

In Alzheimer's care, a Best Friend—

Does not talk down to the *person*; he or she shows respect
Always works to save the dignity of the *person*, to "save face"
Does not assume a supervisory role
Recognizes that learning is a two-way street

Friends Work at the Relationship

In Alzheimer's care, a Best Friend—

Is not overly sensitive
Does more than 50% of the work
Builds a trusting relationship
Is creative

Friends Show Love and Affection

In Alzheimer's care, a Best Friend—

Initiates affection and shows it often
Employs physical touch, including handholding and hugs

Friends Can Overcome Social Barriers

In Alzheimer's care, a Best Friend—

Looks for surprises
Understands that we sometimes have many things in common
Recognizes that old attitudes and prejudices sometimes diminish or disappear
Enjoys unlikely friendships

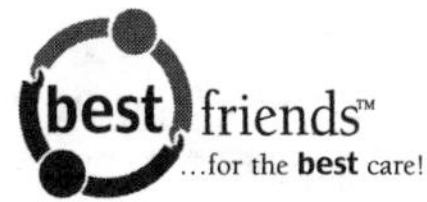

Tool 6.2 / Program Pointer
Best Friends as Volunteers

The Helping Hand Adult Day Center program of the Lexington/Bluegrass Alzheimer's Association (Kentucky) has been praised for its innovative use of volunteers. Volunteers include students and octogenarians. Many have worked weekly in the program for more than 10 years. The program attributes its success to its Best Friends philosophy. Most of the volunteers are assigned to be regular, weekly Best Friends with the same participant. This allows them to develop a long-lasting relationship with their Best Friend, which adds meaning and satisfaction to the volunteer service.

The program offers the following tips for success in your volunteer program:

- Take time to assess your need. Have you made a commitment to use volunteers in your program? Is someone available to coordinate the program and provide supervision?
- Consider some of these volunteer assignments: Be a Best Friend to one participant for several hours each week, play the piano, plan or lead programs, lead an exercise, be a mentor to a student, or enjoy an art project.
- Write job descriptions (one page or less) for each volunteer position.
- Recruit a group of volunteers to start a class together and build camaraderie.
- Schedule a thorough orientation and training program. Continue monthly in-services, scheduling time for socializing. Encourage volunteers to attend area educational programs and conferences.
- Encourage volunteers to get to know well their Best Friend's life story and use it often.
- Schedule volunteers to work with the same *person* or *persons* each week (try to schedule more than one *person* because his or her attendance may vary, depending on physical or mental condition). This makes the volunteer experience meaningful; keep in mind that many programs fail because volunteers are willing to help but are not challenged or given meaningful assignments.
- Evaluate the program often by asking the volunteers to provide feedback regularly.
- Establish a volunteer newsletter, even if it is very simple. Use it for program news and to highlight the backgrounds and achievements of your volunteers.
- Thank volunteers often. Be specific. For example, "You said just the right thing to your Best Friend when he was singing along with the soloist!"

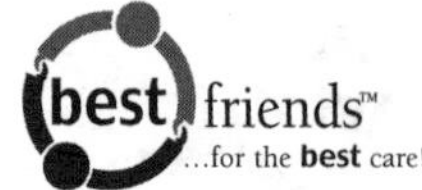

Tool 6.3 / Program Pointer

Suggestions for Creating a Best Friends Bulletin Board

Many Best Friends programs create a weekly or monthly bulletin board, apart from the activity calendar. The authors encourage this because it reminds all staff and volunteers about the goals of the program, describes successes, and can be enjoyed by all who are part of the community or program. (The bulletin board in the photograph is the Best Friends bulletin board from the Helping Hand Day Center in Lexington, Kentucky.)

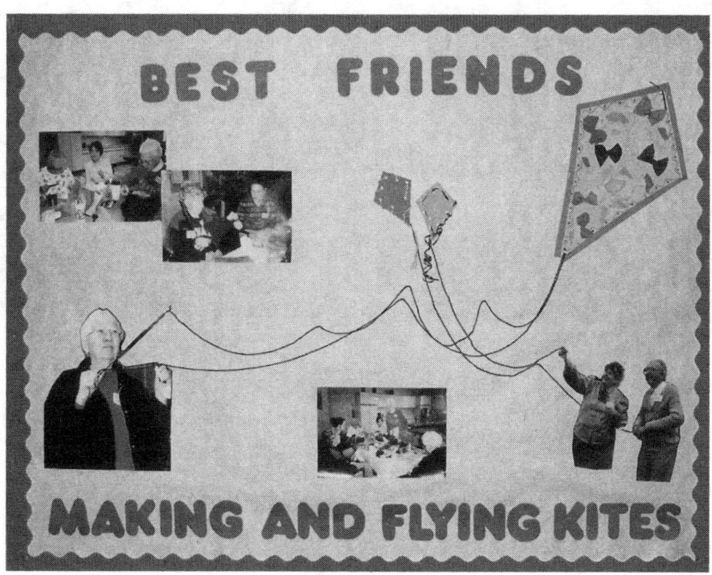

A Best Friends bulletin board gives equal importance to staff, volunteers, and residents/day center participants and builds the sense of community.

Items that you can include in your Best Friends bulletin board:

Pictures of residents, staff, and volunteers
Sayings about friendship
Creative art, including drawings, collages, and poetry
Weekly/monthly birthdays (again, don't forget staff and volunteers!)
"Did You Know?": trivia or facts about residents, staff, and volunteers (e.g., current events, including new grandchildren or great grandchildren, weddings, new family pets; past successes, awards, old skills, jobs, and other talents)
Highlights of Best Friends activities (e.g., pictures or descriptions of Best Friends' taking walks, enjoying an ice cream cone, sitting in the sun, making favors for a children's hospital, visiting another resident, playing cards, just enjoying each other's company)

(continued)

Variation: Lynn Ritter, Professional Education Coordinator of the Dementia Specific Training Institute, Northwest Ohio Chapter of the Alzheimer's Association, developed a display describing the elements of friendship in the Best Friends model. This is used for staff training and to reinforce the lessons learned when teaching the Best Friends model (see below).

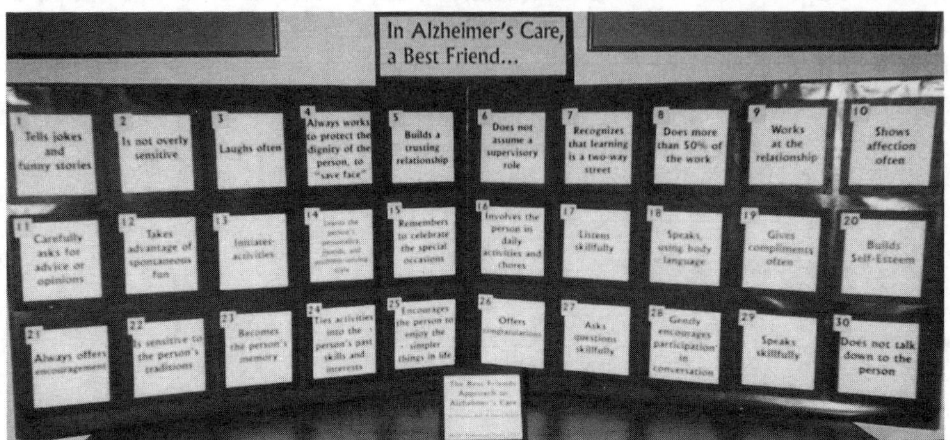

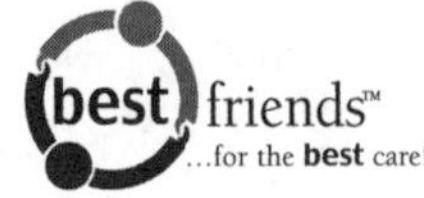

Tool 6.4 / Games for Learning
Friendship Is Multicultural

Adapt this game as a quiz or trivia contest, or ask staff to translate the word friendship *into as many languages as they can. For example:*

Friend	English
Amigo/Amiga	Spanish
Ami/Amie	French
Fruend	German
Amico/Amica	Italian
Tomodachi	Japanese
Khauer	Hebrew
Prieten/Prietena	Romanian
Amicus/Amica	Latin
Kamarad	Czech

Add some of your own:

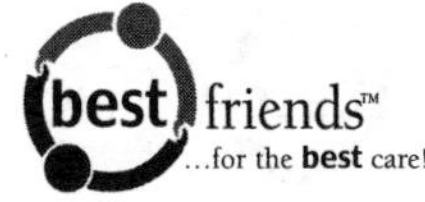

Tool 6.5 / Program Pointer
Quotations on Friendship

Let families and staff know that you are collecting sayings about friendship. One fun source is greeting cards—many are devoted to friendship.

The only way to have a friend is to be one.
—Ralph Waldo Emerson

It's a good thing to be rich, and a good thing to be strong, but it is a better thing to be beloved of many friends.
—Euripides

Two persons cannot long be friends if they cannot forgive each other's little failings.
—Jean de la Bruyere

Your friend is the man who knows all about you and still likes you.
—Elbert Hubbard

Under the magnetism of friendship, the modest man becomes bold; the shy confident; the lazy active; and the impetuous prudent and peaceful.
—William Makepeace Thackeray

Friendship that flows from the heart cannot be frozen by adversity, as the water that flows from the spirit cannot congeal in winter.
—James Fenimore Cooper

A friend is a person with whom I may be sincere. Before him, I may think aloud.
—Ralph Waldo Emerson

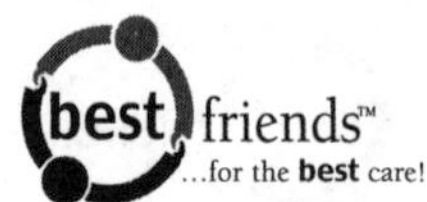

Tool 6.6 / Games for Learning
Being a Best Friend

What does it mean to be a Best Friend to a person *who is a resident in a community or a participant in a day center? This exercise will help staff draw their own conclusions.*

Divide the class into small groups, and ask each group to choose a resident or participant and think about the following questions:

- What can the two of you do together that you both enjoy? [walk, hold hands, people-watch, talk about sports or fishing, feed the birds]
- Do you have anything in common in your life stories? [born in same month, like cats, enjoy being outdoors, like chocolate]
- What makes the *person* smile? [a joke or pun, your smile, a compliment, cookies]
- Do you ever reminisce together? [talk about weddings, flying a plane, old cars, military service]
- Have you found any skills in the *person* that were a surprise to you? [knitting, spinning a top, cooking, painting, playing piano]. Have you shared any of your skills with him or her?
- What kind of displays of affection does the *person* enjoy? [hugs, back rubs, handshakes]
- Does the *person* ever show affection to you? If so, how?
- Can you share personal thoughts and feelings with one another? [successes, feelings, problems that need a solution]
- Do you ever talk about personal values to each other—what is most important in life to both of you? [friends, family, careers]

Variation: Ask each staff member to think of a particular resident and answer the questions for that resident. Discuss the process and results as a group.

Variation: Ask the class to do this exercise with a *person* whom they really enjoy being with. Then do the exercise with a challenging resident or participant.

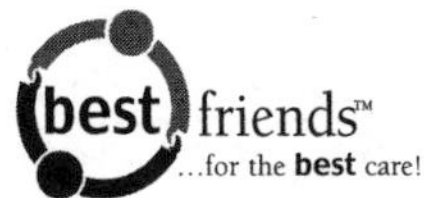

Tool 6.7 / Program Pointer
Best Friends Reminders

Use this summary sheet of Best Friends' ideals in staff training or orientation. It also can be the basis of an in-service training session.

Approach your residents as you would your Best Friend, demonstrating that they are respected and valued.

Take advantage of the principles of friendship to help you gain new ideas for handling day-to-day care in a more natural and positive way. Your residents will respond to the positive feelings that they receive from you.

Try to prevent a difficult or a challenging behavior rather than to deal with it when it happens.

Start each shift by forming a new relationship with your Best Friend based on getting the most out of your time together.

Encourage your co-workers to replace the stress and strain of caregiving with satisfaction by using the Best Friends approach to care.

Make it your team goal that each resident will receive three hugs per shift.

Courtesy of The Fountainview Center for Alzheimer's Disease, Atlanta, Georgia.

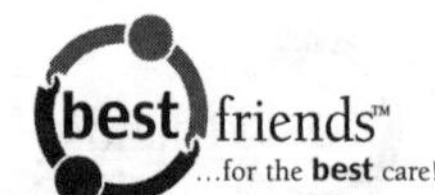

Tool 6.8 / Games for Learning
Friendship Quiz

Use this quiz for staff training.

Choose from this list of elements of friendship the one that you think best matches the description and write it in the space provided. (Some are used more than once.)

Elements of Friendship

Friends know each other's history and personality.
Friends do things together.
Friends communicate.
Friends build self-esteem.
Friends laugh often.
Friends are equals.
Friends work at the relationship.

1. Does more than 50% of the work ______________________________
2. Involves *persons* in daily activities and chores ______________________________
3. Gives compliments often ______________________________
4. Becomes the *person's* memory ______________________________
5. Has spontaneous fun with the *person* ______________________________
6. Gently encourages the *person* to participate in conversation ______________________________
7. Does not talk down to the *person* ______________________________
8. Works to preserve and protect the dignity of the *person* ______________________________
9. Speaks slowly to the *person* using simple terms and listens skillfully ______________________________
10. Builds a trusting relationship and shows affection often ______________________________

Courtesy of The Fountainview Center for Alzheimer's Disease, Atlanta; based on materials from Bell, V., & Troxel, D. (1997). The best friends approach to Alzheimer's care. *Baltimore: Health Professions Press.*

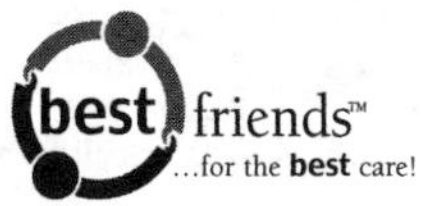

Tool 6.9 / Program Pointer
Friendship Week

One week every month is Friendship Week at Laurel Heights Home for the Elderly. Below is a sample from a January 1998 newsletter distributed by the staff. Staff collected quotes from various sources, including family members who are always on the lookout for new material. Create a Friendship Week of your own in your Best Friends program.

Between Best Friends

Some people are so special that, once they enter your life, it becomes richer and fuller and more wonderful than you ever thought it could be.

January 12 Friendships aren't perfect, and yet they are precious. For me, not expecting perfection all in one place was a great release.

January 13 We have something very precious. I am reminded of that whenever I am away from you, busy doing something; you drift into my mind, making me smile.—Gary LaFollette

January 14 The friend given to you by circumstances over which you have no control is God's own Gift.—F. Robertson.

January 15 A friend is one to whom one may pour out all the contents of one's heart, chaff and grain together, knowing that gentle hands will take and sift it, keep what is worth keeping, and with a breath of kindness blow the rest away.—George Eliot

January 16 Friends are an important part of sharing the burden and worry of each day. Too often the "I-can-handle-it-myself" society we live in seems to promote loneliness rather than friendship.—Sheri Curry

January 17 I breathed a song into the air; it fell to earth, I know not where … and the song from beginning to end, I found again in the heart of a friend.

January 18 I thank my God upon every remembrance of you.—Philippians 1:3.

January 19 Snowflakes are one of nature's most fragile things, but look what they can do when they stick together.—Vesta M. Kelly

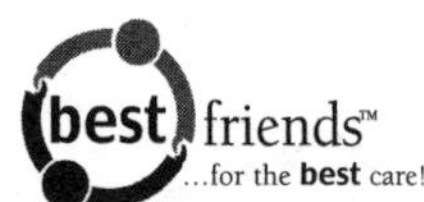

Tool 6.10 / Program Pointer
What Is a Friend?

Use this alphabetical list for your Best Friends bulletin board, for your newsletter, or in staff training.

A Friend . . .

Accepts and loves you as you are
Believes in you
Calls you just to say "hi"
Doesn't give up on you
Envisions the beauty of you
Forgives your mistakes
Gives unconditionally
Helps nurture you
Inspires you and is inspired by you
Jokes with you
Keeps you close at heart
Loves to hear you laugh
Makes a difference in your life
Never judges
Offers support
Picks you up
Quiets your fears
Raises your spirits
Says nice things about you
Touches your heart
Understands you
Values you and really listens to you
Walks beside you
X-plains feelings honestly and kindly
Yearns to participate in your well-being, and
Zaps you with rays of appreciation

Revised by Jim Dickman from an anonymous source. Contributed by Julie Johnson and Marcia Nielsen, Oregon Trails chapter of the Alzheimer's Association, Portland, Oregon.

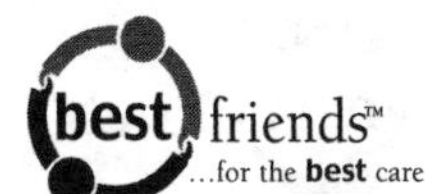

Tool 6.11

Turning No Knack into Knack

The purpose of this exercise is to show, with a dash of humor, the wrong way to do something. This is active learning that really sinks in, particularly when staff members themselves volunteer to take part in the role plays.

The following statements represent stereotypes or falsehoods about dementia. These examples of "no knack" can be used in a number of ways to explore staff attitudes and reinforce the lessons presented in this chapter. Draw them from a hat to discuss as a group or put them into role plays. Invite staff to comment on the mistakes. Then role-play or discuss the right way. The authors discuss the art of role plays in Tool 2.11. Use your creativity to have fun turning these examples of "no knack" into "knack."

I want the residents to know that I'm a staff member here at all times. That way they'll know I'm in charge.

There is no one here who can say a complete sentence. It's impossible to be a friend with someone if you can't talk.

I don't think she likes me, so I'm not going to put myself out for her any more.

I'd love to be friends with this resident, but I think the facility would frown on it.

It feels phony to give compliments unless I really mean them, so why bother?

I don't have time to laugh and make jokes when there is such a long list of things to be done.

I don't think it's professional to give hugs or hold hands.

It's only worth it to me to be a friend to the residents who are fun and easy to be with.

I've tried to be a friend to Mrs. Weber but it didn't work, so why try again?

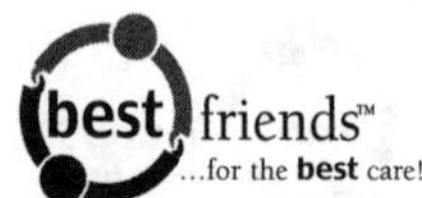

7

The Life Story

Friends know a lot about one another. They typically know one another's personality, family history, values and traditions, job(s), hobbies and interests, political views, and spiritual beliefs—their life story. This knowledge and shared history allow friends to feel comfortable together, improve communication, and create a fairly deep level of intimacy. This is what friendship is all about.

An Alzheimer's disease care staff with knack know the life stories of the *persons* for whom they care as well as they know their own friends. But not all programs have knack; not all programs are special. In fact, when we visit a so-called special care unit or program, we employ a simple test to determine whether it really is "special." We ask staff to tell us something about the residents. When staff can paint a rich portrait, there is reason to believe that it is a good program. Conversely, when staff seem to know very little about the residents, it is unlikely that high-quality dementia care is being delivered, as in the following example.

> The Stretched-Too-Thin Day Center had a fun afternoon planned. The activity director, Michael, had read that most older people liked to dance and had found some big band cassette tapes at a garage sale over the weekend. "I know this will be a great new activity. I hope it will fill those troubling late afternoons at least a few times a week," he commented to the program administrator.
>
> After lunch and a short break, Michael and the other staff members put the chairs into a circle and announced the dance. The activity seemed to get off to a great start, with several staff members dancing with participants; some participants even danced with each other. Then Michael noticed that Louise was still sitting in her chair. He approached her, smiled, and took her hands, saying, "Come on Louise, let's join the group. Dance with me!" Louise frowned. She was not able to say much, but Michael was sure he could get her in the mood to dance. "Come on, I'm sure you are a wonderful dancer."
>
> As he gently pulled, she pushed. A volunteer chimed in, "Louise, you don't want Michael to think you don't like him." Michael tried again. Louise stood up, and Michael felt successful. He looked forward to telling the administrator that there had been 100% participation in the activity. In the midst of his self-

Life stories can help the caregiver become a strong anchor for the person in the sometimes stormy seas of seeking recognition of self.

—Diane Will, National Community Life Director, The Fountains Continuum of Care, Inc., Tuscon, Arizona

To know that one uses five sugars in his oatmeal can be the key to having a peaceful breakfast or any breakfast at all. To know the name of a spouse or a pet can change a moment of overwhelming panic into a much calmer mood or even lead to a time of reminiscing.

—Karen Wyan, Assistant Administrator, Laurel Heights Home for the Elderly, London, Kentucky

During our training, we celebrate the life stories of each resident. What an opportunity we have to help people succeed by remembering their achievements, reminiscing about days gone by, to laugh, to love, and to lighten the load of their disease. Together we discovered that residents, although unique in experiences and personality, were not unlike ourselves. Their lives, too, have been filled with joys and sorrows, plans for the future, accomplishments, and heartaches. We talked about specific residents' histories—Meg, the world traveler; Jack, the hard worker who loved the outdoors; Rachel, the caregiver

congratulatory dialogue, Louise took her hand out of Michael's, made a fist, and punched Michael right in the jaw. Pandemonium ensued. As one activities staff member took Louise to another room, Michael admitted that he was more embarrassed than hurt. Unfortunately, the administrator rushed in, yelling, "Call the family! Tell them that our program cannot handle combative people! She's out of here!"

As this terrible scene unfolded, Louise's sister arrived at the facility. Staff told her what had happened. Flushed and upset, her sister said, "Don't you know? Louise and I were raised in a religion that thinks dancing is a sin!"

When the Best Friends staff get to know participants or residents well, caregiving becomes much easier, activities are more fulfilling, communication is enhanced, and problems are prevented before they occur. If the staff at the Stretched-Too-Thin Day Center had developed a comprehensive, written life story on Louise and taken steps to ensure that staff and volunteers had learned it, then the upsetting incident never would have happened. Of course, a staff member with knack probably could have avoided the incident altogether by watching Louise's body language and taking her expressed feelings seriously.

At the center, the administrator's first response was to label Louise as combative. It should have been to "stop, look, and listen" and think about what caused such a response. Further research might have revealed her past and allowed the administrator to understand that Louise's response was understandable, even justifiable. Louise could no longer verbalize her beliefs, but deep down she knew that dancing was wrong. She got her point across.

Program leaders are encouraged to review their existing social history forms: How complete are they? Were they completed in a timely fashion compared with the date of admission? Are they accessible to staff? Are staff referring to them? The life story can add immeasurably to the social history form, but it must be comprehensive to capture information like that revealed in the story of Louise. It is also important that the information go beyond biographical facts to get an idea of the *person's* attitudes, beliefs, values, and traditions (see Tool 7.9). For example, several questions that can be asked during an initial assessment include: What were her attitudes toward money? Was he a part of a faith

Childhood	**Adolescence**
Birthdate and birthplace	High school name
Parents and grandparents	Favorite classes
Brothers and sisters	Friends and interests
Early education	Hobbies and sports
Pets	First job
Young adulthood	**Middle age**
College and work	Grandchildren
Marriage(s)/relationship(s)	Hobbies
Family	Work/family role
Clubs and/or community involvement	Clubs and organizations
First home	Community involvement
Military service	
Older adulthood	**Other major ingredients**
Life achievements and accomplishments	Ethnicity
Hobbies	Religious background
Travel	Awards
Family	Special skills

Figure 7.1. Elements of the life story. (Adapted from Bell, V., & Troxel, D. [1997]. The Best Friends approach to Alzheimer's care *[p. 68]. Baltimore: Health Professions Press.)*

community? Where did she like to spend New Year's Eve? Does he have other traditions that are meaningful?

The *person's* written life story gives staff unlimited tools for providing high-quality care. Diane Will, national community life director of The Fountains, said, "It is important to know the life story so you can give back pieces of memory. When you help *persons* remember, you give them their life." Elements of the life story are featured in Figure 7.1 to guide the creation of life stories at your facility or program.

The following are key concepts that can help any program more effectively collect and use life stories to provide high-quality dementia care.

Every Program Should Obtain a *Person's* Life Story Before Admission

Best Friends staff members understand that programs need as much information about the *person's* life story as they do

for her own ill family members—roles so engrained within them and still very much a part of who they are today.

—Briana Melom, Director of Education and Family Services, Alzheimer's Disease Center, Mayo Clinic, Rochester, Minnesota

I am fortunate to have shared many special moments with "friends" who have Alzheimer's disease in my work. Every person is unique and teaches me to value the moments we have in life and the times we have together.

—Carole A. Bromgard, Manager, Brighton Gardens Community special care unit, Lakewood, Colorado

The life story is very useful and expands the "customary routine" of the MDS (Minimum Data Sheet). It gives staff vital information to use on a daily basis to assist *persons* with dementia to remain connected with as much of their memory as possible.

—Karen Wyan, Assistant Administrator, Laurel Heights Home for the Elderly, London, Kentucky

Because of a note on a bullet card, a LPN learned that she shared Hungarian heritage with a resident. The two sing folk songs together, entertaining themselves and other residents.

—Kari Staron, Social Services Director, Hennis Care Center of Bolivar, Bolivar, Ohio

Olivia Fischer's love for animals was deeply engrained within her. She'd had an affinity for strays, taking them in as pets when she could and even putting out boiled chicken for the neglected cats that would collect at her door for meals.

When I first met her, she was living in a small, rural senior housing facility. Because her home was no longer able to meet her needs, I was coordinating her admission to the assisted living facility where I worked. As I approached her to conduct the pre-admission assessment, Olivia was waking from a dream. She had been riding horses, she told me, and had fallen off just before I awakened her.

"Oh my, what a dream!" she exclaimed as she came out of her sleepy haze. Her face and hands held the lines of a woman who had worked hard, but her smile came easily and her laugh bubbled up from within her as she told me about the horses.

When she was nearing the end of her life, Olivia became the first resident in a new hospice home, which was nestled in the woods on the edge of Rochester. Staff soon began noticing a small stray cat hanging around the back door. Hospice workers began putting dishes of food outside for the

about his or her medical condition. Both are essential to delivering high-quality care. A dietary plan could not be made for a new resident without knowing whether she has diabetes. A *person* could not be admitted without knowing his medication needs. Similarly, the staff of a Best Friends program understand that without obtaining a complete life story, staff will have few tools to help the *person* feel safe and secure and to manage behavior challenges.

The Helping Hand Day Center will not enroll someone until the life story is completed. Program manager Gwen Hutchinson said, "Before we had this policy, we were always chasing after families for the information. Now we meet with them or interview them on the phone to write the life story together, before the person is enrolled." This policy gives the program vital information, but, equally important, it also demonstrates to the family that staff have a desire to get to know their loved one well.

The Life Story Should Be Accessible to Staff and Volunteers

Best Friends staff members work hard to ensure that important life story information does not gather dust in the chart. Program leaders should be aggressive and innovative in developing strategies to get the staff and volunteers to learn participants' life stories.

Staff at Wellington Parc of Owensboro take a detailed life history prior to and on residents' admission to the facility. Portions of new residents' life histories are placed on a form called an admission alert. Before admission, the alert is reviewed by staff. The completed life history is placed in the resident's medical record, but not before a copy is made for the life history book, a three-ring binder containing the residents' life stories. "Hopefully the transfer from home to facility is smoother when the staff already know pieces of the life story," explained Holly Cecil, the facility's administrator.

The Wellington Parc program keeps its life history book in a staff break room, which is not open to the public. Limited access respects confidentiality, allows staff to review the stories at their leisure, and makes the book available for quick reference.

In her dementia training work, Dee Carlson encourages programs to use "bullet cards," which contain a short summary on each resident that is readily available to all staff members (see Tool 7.4). Bullet cards are another way that life stories can get off the charts and into the hands of staff who need them. Facts about *persons* are highlighted by bullets and can work wonders for students and volunteers or new staff who may not have had a chance to read and review the longer life stories.

Every Dementia Care Program Should Have on File a Written Life Story on Each Staff Member or Volunteer

Best Friends staff members enjoy sharing some aspects of themselves with their residents, including family or cultural traditions, special recipes, hobbies, funny stories, family pictures, and more. A good program encourages sharing by asking staff about themselves and then sharing this voluntary information with the community.

The self-esteem of staff members can be enhanced by pointing out their accomplishments and letting each staff member have his or her "moment in the sun." As discussed in Chapter 9, staff can lead an activity or activities during the year. Perhaps the head cook is also a painter or the gardener collects World War II memorabilia. Maybe the administrator loves dancing the tango and the bookkeeper plays drums. These interests bring excitement and variety to a residential community or day center.

At Hotel Pawnee, part of the Urban Group, each staff member prepares a memory book of his or her life. Unexpected friendships form across department lines as staff learn and enjoy one another's stories. People who live in a community form bonds. This is happening at Hotel Pawnee and in other programs that encourage staff to get to know one another as people, not just as employees.

Use the Life Story to Greet the *Person* and Improve Recognition

Best Friends staff members greet the *person* with knowledge of his or her life story. When a staff member says, "Hello, Marjorie. How is your son Peter?" an immediate connection is established. It suggests to the resident, "this staff member must know me."

little cat, but were cautious about doing anything more. It was Olivia's life story, her lifelong love for animals, that finally convinced the staff to bring the cat indoors to become the house pet. During the last days of Olivia's life, the cat slept on her bed. For a woman who, in her 90s, still dreamed of horses, it seemed a fitting completion to her compassionate life. To this date, the cat is living in the hospice. Her name is Olivia.

—Briana Melom, Director of Education and Family Services, Alzheimer's Disease Center, Mayo Clinic, Rochester, Minnesota

A male resident at Wellington Parc of Owensboro had been responsible for signing the payroll at his former place of employment. On weekends, he seemed to be looking for something to do. Because he had been in management, he wanted to sit behind the nurse's station. The nurse allowed him to do so and gave him a pen and pencil. The resident asked for figures as though he were writing a check. This continued until he remembered that he was not making a copy for company records. Staff secured carbon paper for him to make the required copies.

The Alzheimer's Four Seasons is a small residential home where residents and staff get to know one another well. Dana E. Newquist, the owner/administrator, always uses information from the person's *family life or past in his daily greetings. For example: "Hello, Mr. Wartella. When are you going to show me that golf swing you are famous for?"*

A small touch like this goes a long way in dementia care.

Use the Life Story to Introduce and Reintroduce Residents to Individuals Around Them

Best Friends staff members frequently use the technique of "introductions." By introducing residents to one another (often, repeatedly) using facts from *persons'* life stories, a social atmosphere is created that is comforting to all present. Introductions also gently cue *persons* about where they are and who is around them. Finally, it is an opportunity for staff to remind *persons* of some special accomplishment or a pleasant memory from their past. An example might be, "Mike, do you know Larry? Larry was Little League Coach of the Year." This immediately establishes a connection between residents and builds self-esteem by pointing out a past accomplishment.

The Helping Hand Day Center staff introduces persons *who share a table over lunch. "Theodore, this is John. Look—here are two truck drivers sitting side by side! I want you both to meet Henrietta, the best nurse in Lexington."*

Introductions help turn a meal into a more meaningful activity. The participants feel that they are at a social occasion or party instead of a routine meal. Something special is happening and it is appreciated by all. (See Tool 8.8 for more on making the most of mealtimes.)

When a *person's* life is celebrated by naming accomplishments, it helps staff members recognize that a full life was lived before the onset of dementia. It can be all too easy to focus on the *person's* current state of disability. When staff learn that a frail, somewhat uncommunicative resident was a former skiing champion or chaired the annual community church bazaar, it can help them remember the importance of care with dignity.

Use the Life Story to Reminisce About the *Person's* Life

Best Friends staff members mine life stories for material to use to reminisce with *persons*. Clearly, when one can talk about experiences from a resident's life (e.g., "your parents really survived the sinking of the *Titanic*?"), many doors are opened for sharing that can be enjoyed by the resident and staff alike. When little information is available, one can still reminisce. For example, simply knowing that a *person* grew up in Sweden can invite conversation about Swedish food, the weather, skiing to school as children, reindeer, and other topics. Figure 7.2 shows a volunteer and a resident reminiscing over the older man's life story book at Laurel Heights Home for the Elderly.

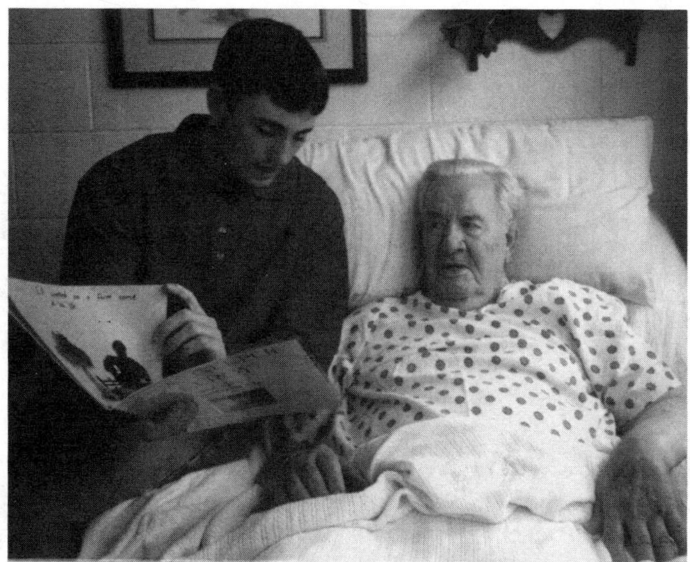

Figure 7.2. Dustin House, a volunteer, and resident E.A. Gilpin reminisce over the older man's life story book, which Dustin made for him as a student project, at Laurel Heights Home for the Elderly.

Scrapbooks or memory boxes made especially for each resident can help remind staff of the *person's* life story and stimulate reminiscence. Dee Rucker created a life story book of Hazel Kennamer to stimulate reminiscence. Dee was a student in the occupational therapy program at Eastern Kentucky University and Hazel's Best Friend (see Figure 7.3). This life story book is particularly effective because it features photographs and uses simple language.

There are many ways to cue people to reminisce, as in the following example:

Hannah Herward, administrator of Eden Pines, Lynchburg, Virginia, created a "life experience" quilt in which each square represents the symbolic life story of a resident. Individuals were interviewed and a beautiful quilt created (see Figure 7.4) that serves as a legacy for future generations. "I often talked about all the things these hands have done to help jog memories—like woodworking, sewing, and praying. This helped each person decide what his or her quilt square would show."

This project was not only an innovative and interesting way to evoke residents' life stories but it will also become part of the region's living history.

Use the Life Story to Provide One-to-One Comforting Care

Best Friends staff members are present for *persons* when they are sad, anxious, or just having a bad day. A life story can provide tools for working with a *person* during these times, deciphering a problem, or offering some appropriate distraction.

Carole A. Bromgard, manager of Brighton Gardens Community special care unit, Lakewood, Colorado, wrote, "When one new resident became anxious, we started to look at a photo album and talk

Hazel's Story

by Dee Ann Rucker

Hazel is the oldest of five Turner children [*ask her about responsibility of first-born*]. She was born on November 29, 1911 in Evarts, Kentucky. Evarts is a small coal-mining town, in Harlan County, at the foothills of the Appalachian Mountains in southeastern Kentucky. Harlan County was, for many years, known as "Bloody Harlan" because of the many feuds involving the unions of the coal mines.

Hazel lived in Evarts with her **mother**, Desdemona ("Dezzie") [*ask about nicknames*], her **father**, James Howard (J.H.), and her four younger siblings. The Turner family attended the Congregational Church [*strong ties to this church; enjoys hymns*].

J.H. was a merchant in Evarts and did many kind things for his customers, mostly coal miners, when he could. Hazel's paternal grandfather came from the other side of the Appalachian Mountains in Virginia to settle in Kentucky just one generation before. Hazel has two younger brothers and two younger sisters. After Hazel came **Eugene**, then **Berenice**, Orin, and **Frances**.

Hazel recalled that she and Eugene always fought about who should be the boss [*identifies personality traits—strong-willed, leader*]. Hazel thought she should be the boss because she was the oldest, and Eugene thought he should be the boss because he was the oldest boy. They loved to play tricks on one another and to get Berenice, Orin, and Frances to choose sides. One time, the children were playing a game where one was blind-folded and led around the yard. This particular time Hazel led Eugene right straight through a pile of fresh cow manure (a "cow pie" it was then called). [*Enjoys telling stories from childhood.*]

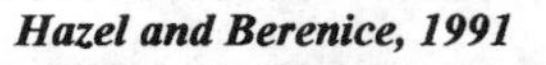
Hazel and Berenice, 1991

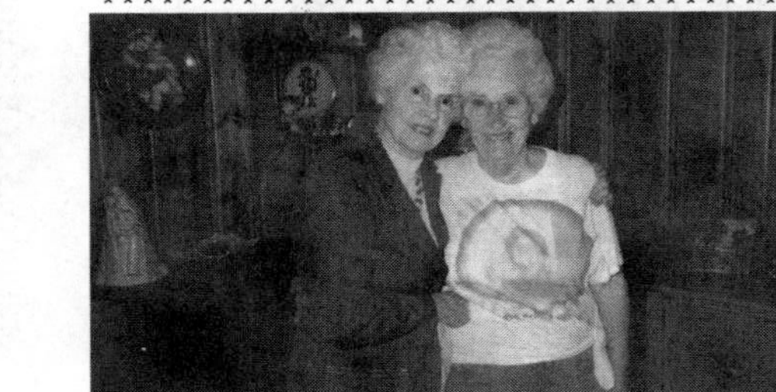

A

Figure 7.3. A) Selected pages from Hazel Kennamer's memory book and life story. B) Photographs and memories from Hazel's life, compiled by Mynga Futrell, Hazel's daughter. (Courtesy of Mynga Futrell.)

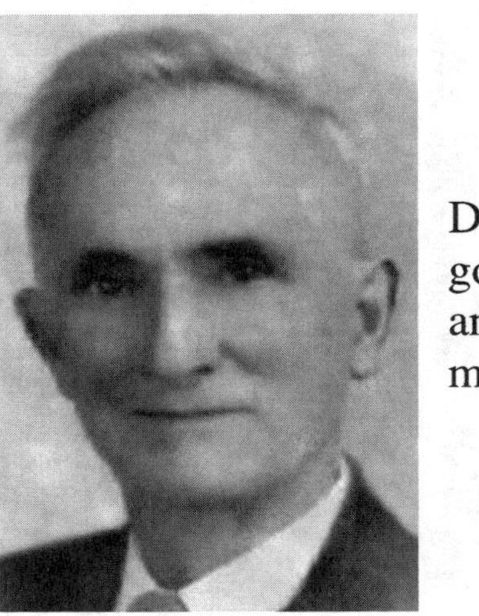

This is my beautiful mother.

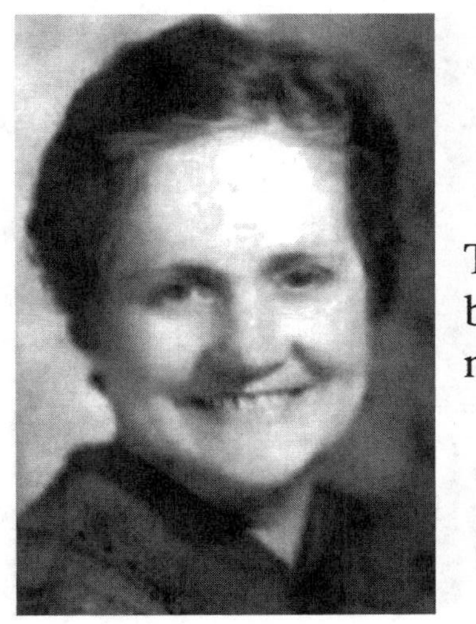

Dad—a good-hearted and honest man.

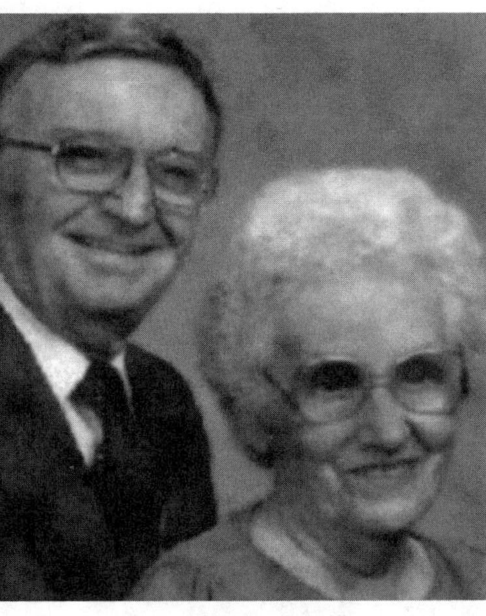

Niece and I are very close. Billy was like a brother.

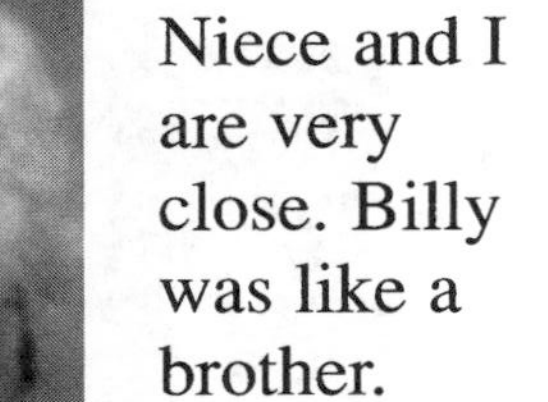

Aunt Fannie loved having us children to visit.

Figure 7.3B

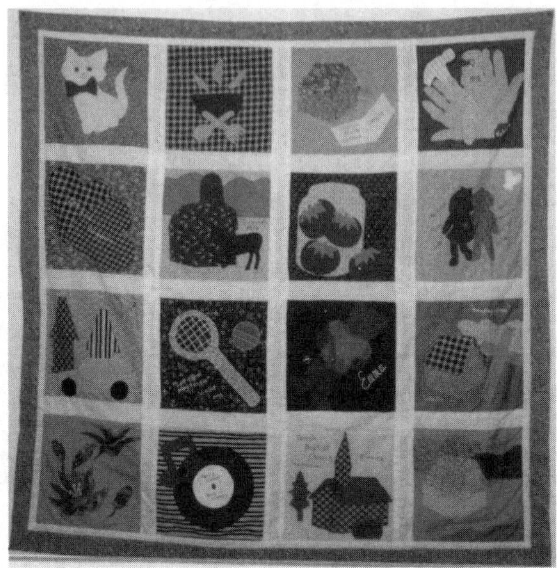

A

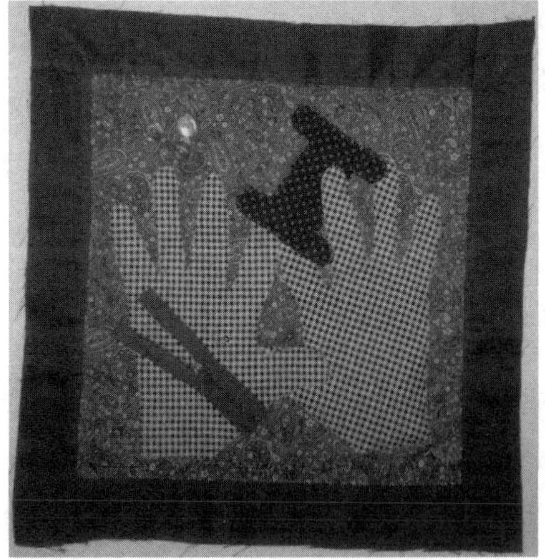

B

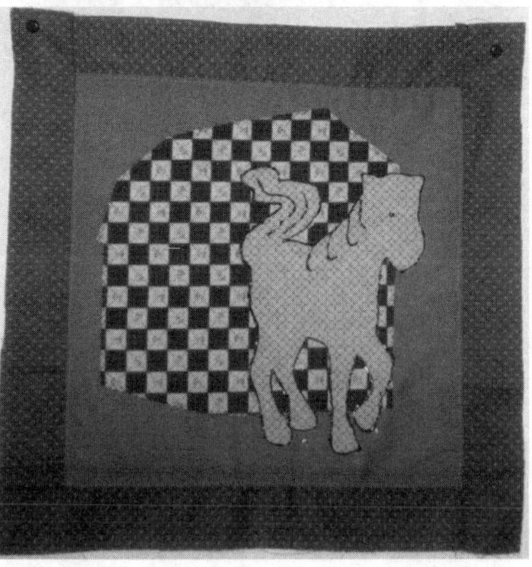

Figure 7.4. Eden Pines' life experience quilt and selected squares. (Photographs courtesy of Hannah Herward, Eden Pines, Lynchburg, Virginia.) A) This square was made by an 82-year-old African American woman who spent most of her life taking care of others. She sewed most of her clothing and those of her relatives. She fondly remembers sewing a red dress for her sister; the zipper had to be sewn in perfectly: "I took that zipper out so many times, I didn't think the seam would hold up." It was important for her sewing to be the best that she could do. B) This quilt square was completed by Norris Covington, an 84-year-old man who spent most of his life on his farm in Appomattox, Virginia. He grew tobacco and corn and raised five children. Mr. Covington remembers his horse, Stonewall Jackson. He would ride Stonewall for 1 hour every day, no matter what the weather was like. "I loved that horse. He was my best friend. He loved the woods, he did!" Norris loves to talk about his adventures as a cook on a tugboat in the Gulf of Mexico and about the beauty of Mexico's land and people.

about her wonderful history—her husband, the railroad, and all their fun trips. Soon the panic faded. Looking at her pictures with her, as a friend, always seemed to calm her."

Carole used reminiscence to evoke feelings of happier times. Consider how difficult the task of cheering the resident would be if the staff member knew little about her personal history and background. This staff member could indeed make matters worse.

Knowledge of the life story can take away much of the fear and anxiety that some staff and volunteers feel over spending time one-to-one with the *person.* When staff and volunteers have some knowledge of the *person's* past, as well as likes and dislikes, it makes spending time with him or her much easier.

Use the Life Story to Improve Communication Through Clues and Cues

Best Friends staff members use their knowledge of the *person's* life story to fill in the gaps when communication flags. A day center participant waiting for his or her ride home might say, "I'm waiting for, for that person, for my . . . ." A Best Friends staff member will be able to fill in the blank by mentioning the relative by name or providing other information that may help the participant finish his or her thought. *Persons* always should be given a chance to finish the sentence; a helpful clue or cue can make that possible.

One project resulted in a tool that all staff could use to provide clues and cues regularly:

The South Laurel High School Family Life Skills Class in London, Kentucky, adopted a local residential community and created life story booklets, describing important life events with pictures and artwork, for each of the 60 residents in the Laurel Heights Home for the Elderly. The residents' responses were emotional and joyous. They shared the booklets with staff, family, and friends. Resident Milton Kidd exclaimed in the Knack for Best Friends newsletter (see Tool 2.5), "Look at my life story that the student wrote for me. I've got to show it to my Best Friend. She will be interested in all these facts about me."

This creative project not only improved communication among staff and residents but it also brought communitywide attention to the facility and to the school. Chapter 8 discusses this and other techniques for improved communication.

Use the Life Story to Improve Activities

When Best Friends staff members know a *person's* hobbies or interests (e.g., stamp collecting, horses, quilting, journalism, woodcarving), they can introduce these activities into group and one-to-one programming. In some cases, a staff member with similar interests might make a special connection with a resident. This can allow for some individualized activities, a highly desirable commodity in dementia care. In other cases, the resident may still be able to "show and tell." For example, a resident who was a master weaver might take pride in showing the group her work.

One resident at Encore Senior Living Rediscovery™ Program who was a retired teacher seemed restless and anxious. Her life story provided clues to working on design activities that center around a school setting, including curriculum planning books and children's books. This allowed her to use her nervous energy in a productive way. "Her disruptive behavior has now been eliminated thanks to an understanding of her life story," noted Delores M. Moyer, senior vice president.

Use of this resident's life story empowered her to feel that she has a role or job to do at her new home—to continue her work as a teacher.

Use the Life Story to Point Out Accomplishments

Best Friends staff members honor residents and participants by remembering their successes. When appropriately cued, *persons* often remember awards and special honors. Staff should make certain that the life story lists them. Everything from early childhood awards to lifetime achievements or other sources of pride (e.g., raising four successful children, community volunteer work, even just hard work all of his or her life) should be included.

A participant in the day center at Wellington Parc of Owensboro worked as a groomer at Churchill Downs Racetrack, home of the Kentucky Derby. He loved being reminded about his time at the famed track. As a tribute to him, the staff planned a special party with a Kentucky Derby theme, complete with derby hats and nonalcoholic mint juleps.

It is important to respect each individual's life story to promote his or her self-esteem and find meaningful moments for the *person.*

Use the Life Story to Prevent Challenging Behaviors

Best Friends staff members cleverly use the life story to prevent challenging behaviors. For example, reading life stories often unearths subjects or situations to avoid. They can reveal that a *person* was bitten by a dog early in life and therefore becomes agitated around animals.

A life story also can reveal tips for diffusing anxious moments. A *person* who loves animals can be comforted by a dog when he or she is feeling sad. In the following case, a life story revealed an unusual waking and sleeping schedule:

A nurse at The Fountainview Center discovered that one of her residents had always awakened at 3:30 A.M. to be on time to a 5:30 A.M. job. When this early riser continued her long-time pattern, it was at first upsetting to the staff. After learning about this through the life story, however, staff were more accepting and stopped the frustrating battle to change her sleep pattern.

The best dementia care communities are able to work with individuals' habits and idiosyncrasies. If a *person* always slept until noon, then hopefully the program can figure out a way to let him or her sleep in and get the family to support this decision as well.

Knowing a life story well can ensure that the language used to provide a distraction or positive message is as grounded in the truth as possible. One resident at The Fountains asked where her husband was, and a new staff member guessed, "He's out fishing." The resident knew that her husband was not fishing; he was, in fact, afraid of the water and had never fished in his life. This seemingly in-

nocuous answer backfired and caused the resident anxiety and stress. If the staff member had known the resident's life story, then she might have been able to offer a more appropriate answer, such as, "He's at the college preparing his lecture."

There can be danger in not knowing a resident's life story. A stock phrase such as "gone fishing" might evoke a very negative response.

Use the Life Story to Incorporate Past Daily Rituals

Best Friends staff members encourage the continuation of rituals that were practiced by the *person* before his or her illness. By their very nature, rituals provide individuals with structure, order, and comfort. A *person* who always took a daily walk may be comforted by continuing this ritual in his or her new home or day center. *Persons* also can be comforted by religious traditions, as in the following story provided by Dorothy Seman:

Josephine, a Catholic woman, had advanced dementia. She had a very short attention span. She often sat with her eyes closed and made vocal sounds that were difficult to understand. While Josephine made these sounds, she moved her hands in a repetitive circular motion. Staff were puzzled, until someone ventured, "If I didn't know better, I'd say she was praying the Rosary." The next time Josephine made the hand movements, a staff member placed a rosary in her hands. Josephine began fingering the beads. With tears in her eyes, she beamed at the staff member and put the crucifix to her lips to kiss it. Josephine's daughter later confirmed her mother's devotion to her faith, but she thought her mother's condition too advanced to maintain her traditions. In fact, reconnecting her with this tradition seemed to give her comfort.

Daily rituals—sacred or secular—are important. For some individuals, morning coffee or afternoon tea is essential.

Use the Life Story to Broaden the Caregiving Network with Volunteers

Best Friends staff members know that comprehensive life stories can be a gold mine of potential volunteers. Using the life story, a list can be made of potential organizations or volunteers who can provide help to a dementia program. For example, the local fire department can be asked to bring their mascot Dalmatian to visit a retired firefighter, a church organist can be asked to play for a church member and others who no longer attend services, or a local Elks Club chapter can be asked to raise funds for the program in honor of a past member.

A participant in the Helping Hand Day Center had been active in a women's community chorus. When this fact was revealed in her life story, staff contacted the chorus and were able to recruit volunteers to spend time with her at the center.

The life story can be the starting point of a successful drive to recruit more volunteers to a dementia care program.

Conclusion

William M. Small, Jr., president and owner of The Fountainview Center, wrote the authors a compelling letter about how the Best Friends model changed his facility's perception of the life story:

Under our old model of care, a dementia resident's life story was briefly covered by our social worker during the initial care plan and then filed away in the chart. Thinking back, many times someone bringing in a resident's obituary column from the newspaper prompted the next discussion on his or her life story. Many times this discussion would involve the staff that had directly cared for the resident, pointing out all the interesting things that they never knew about the resident. These discussions would reveal a personal dimension to the resident that our staff had never been privileged to see.

This vignette dramatically contrasts with how we view our residents today and how we relate to them. We use the Best Friends approach to each resident's life story and find it useful in conveying the difference in our philosophy of care from others. It also reminds us that we want to get to know our residents, our best friends, while they are with us, not through reading newspaper clippings after they are gone.

COLLINS, Charles
95, a Montecito resident for 30 years, passed away on June 26, 1999 at Saint Francis Medical Center from complications of pneumonia.
He was a happy, kind, and gentle man whose dimpled smile lit up every room and life he entered.
Charley was born on January 7, 1904, as he loved to recount, "in a half-dugout near Manitou in the Oklahoma territory before it became a state". He was the fifth son of Mark and Elizabeth Collins.
His father had homesteaded a quarter section of land on which he raised cotton. Charley liked his life on the farm and often joked about welcoming rainy days on which he didn't have to hoe cotton.
He wanted to go to agricultural school and become a farmer. But his mother begged him to attend business school, after which he moved to Oklahoma City at 16 and became a bookkeeper for Antoine Clausen, a pioneer Oklahoma City developer. Charley worked diligently by day but filled his nights with song and dance through performing with a small band where he played the saxophone and learned to tap-dance. His early amateur efforts finally became his profession. He studied to lose his accent and perfected his dancing.
He eventually worked his way to New York where he played The Palace, the ultimate goal of every vaudevillian. He shared billing with the young Bob Hope. He later won the juvenile lead in "Ripples," a Broadway show starring Fred Stone. It was there he met Fred's actress daughter, Dorothy.
Charley spent a couple of years performing in London where he and Dorothy were married in 1932. They worked both separately and together through the years. They starred in a revival of the "The Red Mill", which had a very long run on Broadway in the late 40's. Charley's career included the lead in a 1936 musical comedy film, "Dancing Pirate," in which he showed off his dancing skills. His last professional appearance was on television in the 80's as a guest star in a segment of "The Master Series."
Charley and his wife worked in musicals, comedies and reviews until the mid 1960's. They retired to Santa Barbara, CA, in 1969, where Dorothy died in 1974.
Charley, a new and enthusiastic resident of Santa Barbara, learned from the late Walker Thompkins that the irregularities of Santa Barbara's streets were attributed to an early surveyor's errors. He composed the following rhyme, entitled

"Haley's Jig:"

Carrillo, Cabrillo,
Castillo, and Haley
Conferred at Ortega
and Soledad daily.
Santa Barbara surveying
held much of their thought
And Haley sold a deal that
the other three bought.

They told him
to take his good chain
and his compass
And lay out the streets
to avoid any rumpus,
But Haley just wanted
to go for the ride
And his short chain
was lengthened with
stretchy rawhide.

When the sun was real hot
on the rawhide
t 'would beat
And the next block was
short by a number of feet
But early at morn,
with dew on the rock
The rawhide would stretch
and lengthen the block.

So if streets
don't quite jibe
Then haul in your jib
And tack when you should
Or you'll fracture a rib!

Charley was an avid and vocal political participant and a member of the Channel City Club. He had a long exchange of letters with Ronald Reagan, a former colleague in the Screen Actor's Guild.
He often said that he had had a long and wonderful life.
For the past 26 years, he has happily resided with his beloved and devoted Catherine Good Garvin, who survives him. From his large group of siblings, only one sister, Elma of Charley wanted no formal services to be held, but friends who wish may remember him with a contribution to the Friendship Center, 89 Eucalyptus Lane, where he spent many pleasant hours.
Arrangements by Welch-Ryce-Haider Funeral Chapels.

Figure 7.5. Obituary of Charles Collins, a participant in the Friendship Adult Day Care Center, Santa Barbara, California. Staff knew him well, and even showed his old films. Does your program capture this depth of information, or would you discover these things only after your resident or participant had died? (Article courtesy of Catherine Good Garvin.)

The last statement is one that resonates with many program leaders in long-term care. Facilities that embrace the Best Friends model and a revitalized life story will find that obituaries are a way to celebrate the *person's* life, not to meet him or her for the first time.

Figure 7.5 contains one such obituary, that of Charley Collins, well known in the Santa Barbara community and a participant at Friendship Adult Day Care Center. The authors offer this obituary as a tribute to Charley and as a demonstration of the rich details that are included. Friendship Adult Day Care Center was not surprised by the details of his colorful life. The authors believe that any dementia program that embraces the life story to its fullest will have the same experience.

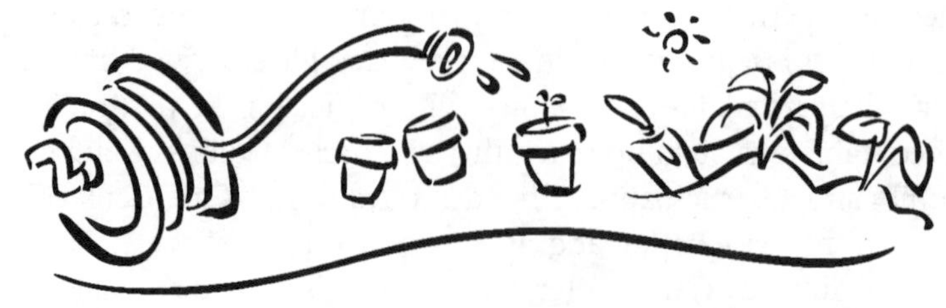

Training Tool Kit

Tool 7.0 / Warm-Up
Getting to Know One Another

This fun exercise helps staff learn more about one another's life story (and subsequently, residents or participants) and helps build relationships in the community.

Pass around index cards to each staff member in the room, and ask them to answer one or more of the following questions. (Use these as suggestions or create your own, as appropriate. For example, in some urban communities many staff members may not own a car or drive.)

Tell the audience that you will be reading from the cards, and everyone must guess who the story is about. Therefore, they should not write down things that they do not want to share with the group.

Collect the cards, and encourage staff members not to show their cards to a neighbor. Choose one or more cards at random and begin reading some facts. Ask the group to guess whom the facts are about. For each "winner," award a prize of a small item such as candy.

Questions for Cards

If you could have dinner with anyone famous, dead or alive, who would it be?
What kind of car do you drive? What kind of car do you wish that you could drive?
Do you like cats or dogs, or neither?
What is your favorite music or singer/group?
Who would you most like to be stuck in an elevator or stranded on a desert island with?
What is your favorite food?
If you could go anywhere on a vacation, where would you like to go?

Variation: Ask staff to create a bullet card or other quick and easy technique about themselves. Have them do it for their own reference or perhaps to share with another staff member in the room.

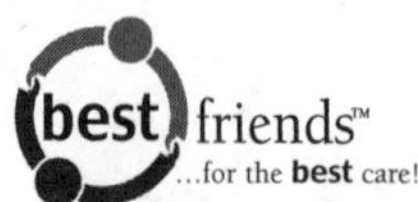

Tool 7.1 / Games for Learning
Your Best Friend in Life

This is a fun game that helps class members think about the life story. It is similar to Tool 6.0, but this tool asks for biographical information instead of personal qualities. Use a flipchart or board to record the group's answers.

Ask the class to close their eyes, take a minute or two, and think about a close friend or best friend. Tell them you will ask them to say aloud the friend's first name and that you will ask them to name two or three facts about that person (e.g., his or her place of birth, hobbies, religion, interests, job).

As the names and facts are read, write them down on the board, putting the first name on the left-hand side and facts on the right. An example of this is:

Sergio	carpenter, trumpet player, soccer player
Rosa	shopper, quilter, born in Walla Walla, three sons
Daryl	Southern Baptist, traveler, antique collector

Try to get everyone to participate. Review the list of facts. Note that we know a lot about our friends.

We should strive to know as much about the life stories of *persons* in our care as we do about our friends. Discuss how care improves when you know the residents or participants well.

Variation: Pass out index cards and invite the group to write three things about themselves that they would like to share. Ask participants to pass the cards to you when they are finished writing. Read the information on the cards or conduct a guessing game about the items on the cards. Discuss how fun it can be to learn more about one another.

Tool 7.2 / Program Pointer
Encouraging Staff to Learn the Life Story

Several programs have devised ways to encourage staff to learn the life stories of program residents or participants:

Life story presented to the staff by the *person* or family the first week of admission.
—Laurel Heights Home for the Elderly

Life story available in staff lounge for staff to review at leisure.
—Wellington Parc of Owensboro

Create a life story book for each *person.* Examples include "This is Your Life" book *(Omahanui Private Hospital),* "Life Story Booklet" *(Laurel Heights Home for the Elderly),* "Life Storybook" *(Porterville Senior Day Care).*

Present a "This is Your Life" tribute to *persons* on special occasions, such as birthdays.
—Helping Hand Day Center

A staff member takes one life story per week and presents a 10-minute summary at a staff meeting.
—Laurel Heights Home for the Elderly

Introduce *persons* using one bit of information from the life story whenever a group activity convenes.
—Helping Hand Day Center

Share some articles from a *person's* life story to be included in the topic for the day, such as a WAC or Wave uniform belonging to a participant, when uniforms of all kinds is the topic.
—Helping Hand Day Center

A life experience quilt project; squares depict the lives of residents.
—Eden Pines

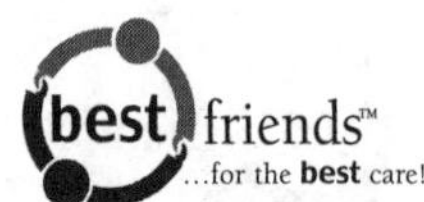

Tool 7.3 / Program Pointer
Ways to Use the Life Story

The life story can be woven into your program every day. Here are some suggestions:

Greeting the *person* and improving recognition

Introducing the *person* to others

Reminiscing

Providing one-to-one comforting care

Improving communication through clues and cues

Designing appropriate activities

Pointing out accomplishments

Helping to prevent challenging behaviors

Incorporating long-held daily rituals

Broadening the caregiving network and resources

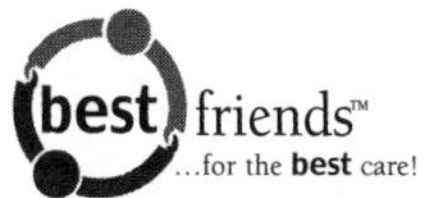

Tool 7.4 / Program Pointer
Bullet Cards

Bullet cards on each resident should be created following placement and updated regularly. Bullet cards can be index cards or sheets of paper that are filled out by the staff member who is responsible for each resident and document 10–15 unique things (e.g., likes, dislikes, preferences, values, habits, interesting tidbits) about him or her. It also is a good idea to include on the card the resident's picture to personalize it. The following bullet card is presented as an example:

Resident's name: John R.

Primary care provider: Amy Smith

Admission date: 11/2/99

- Prefers to be called J.R.
- Likes his coffee before he gets dressed; little cream, one sugar
- Had a son who died in an auto accident—a source of great sadness
- Loves to hear jokes and can tell a few
- Was the principal of a large elementary school; loves to discuss teaching
- Tends to pace when upset or angry
- Will do anything for a Snickers bar!
- Enjoys baseball games
- Daughter Lisa likes to hear about her dad's day and get pictures of him doing activities
- Hates lima beans, okra, and spinach
- History of right leg pain; treated well with aspirin. Doctor says John should take a daily walk.
- Is very private while bathing; keep a towel around him

Developed by Dee Carlson, president, ACCET, Inc., Lexington, Kentucky.

(continued)

Bullet cards should be kept in a place that is accessible to all staff. Each month, a supervisor should check to see that current information is maintained on the cards.

Variation from Dee Carlson: Ask each staff member to make a card for him- or herself and share it with the rest of the group. Consider this activity for staff training; it is a good team-building exercise.

Variation from Helping Hand Day Center: Prepare cue cards for new staff or volunteers to use in a one-to-one session. Cards should contain at least six things that a *person* enjoys throughout the day. Make the cards available for the asking or put on one side of the card the *person's* preferred name and tack it on a bulletin board in the office.

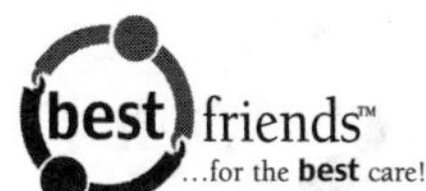

Tool 7.5 / Program Pointer
Life Story Quick and Easy

Here are nine more ways to get the life story into daily use in your program:

Prepare a life story poster on each person with important facts on the back for quick ideas for things to do or tips for individualized conversation.

—Porterville Senior Day Care

Take pictures of each *person* for a picture gallery and label each picture with the *person's* preferred name.

Feature a "resident of the week" or "resident of the month" in the newsletter or on the bulletin board.

Create trivia questions based on information in the life stories and use them in group settings for guessing "Who am I?"

—The Fountainview Center

Look for things that residents or participants have in common, such as being born on the same day, and use the information in newsletters or make a guessing game to see who has the answer first.

Encourage staff to adopt a Best Friend.

—Helping Hand Day Center, Laurel Heights Home for the Elderly, and Serenity Nursing Home

Prepare a brief script about the articles in the memory box or the reminiscence basket to help facilitate conversation when visiting with the *person.*

Prepare a life story card with a familiar picture and a brief descriptive paragraph for the *person* to read or for someone to read to the *person.*

—Cindy Lynch, dementia care consultant and researcher, New Concord, Kentucky

Feature a life story on the monthly activity calendar.

—Hotel Pawnee, The Urban Group

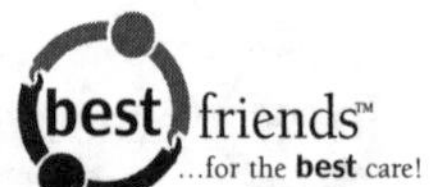

Tool 7.6 / Games for Learning
Creating a Real Life Story

The most effective learning comes from using actual case studies or conducting hands-on learning in a long-term care program.

Affix a sheet of butcher paper to a wall. Ask class members to name as many facts about one resident or participant as they can. See how many you can name (25? 50? 100?). Provide cues such as *family, spirituality, pets, favorite activities, colors, hobbies,* and *jobs.* Write the facts on the butcher paper.

Repeat the exercise several times with different residents or participants.

Variation from Kay Lloyd—Who Am I?: This is a fun game in which the group leader can prepare lists of some unusual facts about specific residents or participants (e.g., Who studied art in Paris? Who helped make the largest pizza ever made? Whose favorite color is purple?). These can then be read to the group, who must guess which person it is.

This game reminds staff that surprises can always be found and of the rich lives of many *persons* in their care.

Variation: Brainstorm how staff members can find out more about the *person* (e.g., where to find information in the charts, how to ask families for more information, how to get information from the *person*).

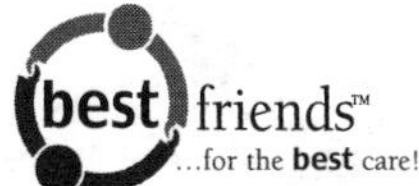

Tool 7.7 / Program Pointer

Involving Families in the Life Story Process

Families almost always appreciate a Best Friends program's interest in writing a thorough life story, but because they are often overwhelmed by caregiving, getting the needed information can be challenging. Here are some ideas for gathering initial and ongoing life story information.

✓ Make a telephone appointment before the *person* is admitted and interview a family member about his or her loved one. You will get more information in an interview process. Many families are too busy or overwhelmed to fill out forms themselves.

Variation: Assign this task to a line staff member, volunteer, capable resident, or other family member.

✓ Remember that some families may not know much about the relative or friend in question. Do your best and take on the challenge of expanding the amount of information given to you.

✓ Write a letter to family members asking them to consider making a photo album or scrapbook of their family member for the staff. (*Note:* Many families will not have the time to complete this task, but some will. At least you will have more information on some of the residents.)

✓ Ask the families to bring five photographs depicting memorable scenes from the *person's* life or family. When they come in, paste the photos on an 8 inch × 11 inch card and immediately write captions with the help of the family member. Visitors or staff can use these photographs to start conversations or reminisce.

✓ Ask the family to bring in several articles that reflect important times in the *person's* life (e.g., uniforms, books, travel souvenirs). Use them in activities or to share with staff.

✓ Schedule a family member or members to speak at the facility; even school-age children can do this, and staff respond to intergenerational efforts.

✓ Start a monthly scrapbook club for family members and interested residents and participants.

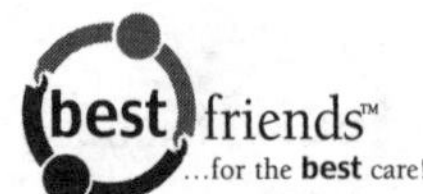

Tool 7.8 / Program Pointer

Knack for Best Friends Newsletter

Create your own newsletter similar to this example from Laurel Heights Home for the Elderly.

Since we learned that one of our residents used to insist that her kids and husband clean up as soon as they came in from working on their farm, we know that it is important to her to be neat and clean. She is much calmer and happier when we act on this and talk with her about it.

—Buffy Nichols, LPN

We love to have pictures of their family, home place, church, etc., to look at with our residents.

—Jennifer Callansa, CNA

I love to laugh and sing and be happy with my residents. It helps to get them dressed.

—Candy Smith, CNA

When I see a resident looking sad and I say, "I'm sorry you're feeling blue today, I feel that way now and then, too," I can see a response almost immediately.

—Carol Miller, social worker

The other day an Alzheimer's resident was wandering and pacing big time. We would take turns holding hands, singing "Jesus Loves Me" (a favorite song of hers), and even dancing with her. It seemed to calm her down some, but it took all of us taking turns for quite a while to get her relaxed enough to rest.

—Tracy Brown, CNA

When we find one of our Alzheimer's *persons* crying, it usually helps to take a few minutes to talk with her about her daughter and that she is at work, and that her daughter washes her clothes, and comes for breakfast. It only makes her cry more to tell her not to cry.

—Wilma McDowell, CNA

Knack can be ...

Knowing a resident's life story. Those little things that make a bath something to look forward to.

Letting our face and smile show how glad we are to see him or her. Joy all over our faces is a great hello to a friend.

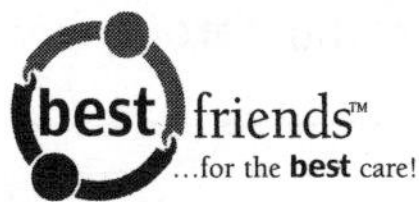

Tool 7.9 / Program Pointer
Recipe for a Life Story

Copy or adapt this life story form for use in your program.

Alzheimer's Care at Aspen Ridge: Recipe for a Life Story

Name ______________________ Birthdate __________
Birthplace ______________________________
Nickname/Terms of endearment ______________________
Marital status __________ Spouse's/partner's name __________
No. of children ___ No. of grandchildren ___ No. of great-grandchildren ___

Name of children	Age	Spouse	Children's names	Age
1) ________	___	________	________	___
2) ________	___	________	________	___
3) ________	___	________	________	___
4) ________	___	________	________	___

CHILDHOOD

Mother's name __________ Birthplace ________ Occupation ________
Father's name __________ Birthplace ________ Occupation ________
Brothers/sisters ______________________________
Pets ______________ Early education ______________
School days, memories, favorite or humorous events ______________
____
Honors/awards/proud moments ______________________
____

ADOLESCENCE

Name of high school ______________ Favorite subject __________
Name of best friend ______________________________
Hobbies/sports/interests ______________________________
First job ______________ Favorite clothing ______________
High school memories/favorite or humorous event(s) __________
____
Honors/awards/proud moments ______________________
____

YOUNG ADULTHOOD

Name of college ______________________________
Clubs/community involvement ______________________
Marriage(s)/partner(s) ______________ Wedding anniversary __________
First date w/spouse/partner ______________________
Wedding-day memories ______________________________
____
____
First home ______________ Military service __________
Work years' memories/favorite or humorous event(s) __________
____

(continued)

Tool 7.9 / *(continued)*

Special memories about children ______
Honors/awards/proud moments ______

______

MIDDLE AGE
Hobbies ______
Clubs/organizations ______
Community involvement ______
Honors/awards/proud moments ______

______

Special memories about grandchildren, favorite or humorous event(s)

______

______

______

OLDER ADULTHOOD
Life achievements and accomplishments ______

______

Hobbies ______
Travel ______
Special memories about family/favorite or humorous event(s) ______

______

OTHER MAJOR INGREDIENTS
Ethnicity ______ Religious/spiritual background ______
Awards ______
Special skills ______
Favorite movie actors/actresses ______
Favorite music style ______
Favorite sports personality ______
Favorite color(s) ______
Favorite book(s) ______

______

Other favorites ______

______

______

Traumas/tragedies to be aware of ______

______

How does the *person* like to spend New Year's Eve? ______

______

If stuck on a desert island, what 3 things would he or she bring (assume food, water, shelter are already provided) ______
Would his or her desk (or kitchen shelves) be neat or messy? ______
Is the *person* an optimist or a pessimist? ______
What was his or her attitude toward money? ______
Finally, I would like you to know the following about this *person*:

______

______

Tool 7.10
Turning No Knack into Knack

The purpose of this exercise is to show, with a dash of humor, the wrong way to do something. This is active learning that really sinks in, particularly when staff members themselves volunteer to take part in the role plays.

The following statements represent stereotypes or falsehoods about dementia. These examples of "no knack" can be used in a number of ways to explore staff attitudes and reinforce the lessons presented in this chapter. Draw them from a hat to discuss as a group or put them into role plays. Invite staff to comment on the mistakes. Then role-play or discuss the right way. The authors discuss the art of role plays in Tool 2.11. Use your creativity to have fun turning these examples of "no knack" into "knack."

She doesn't know who she is, so why bother with the life story?

I don't like to talk about myself at work since I don't think anyone would be interested.

I just greet everyone the same way: "Hi, sweetie." It works just fine, and it is easier that way.

Why can't they talk about today's events? I get so tired of hearing about things that happened so long ago.

I think it is better to do the same activity with everyone. They like to be in a group, and I don't think they really need that much one-to-one attention.

I know he used to be an auto mechanic, but he wouldn't be interested in cars now.

I know that she lost two of her brothers years ago in a boating accident, but she wouldn't remember that anymore. I think it will be okay to take her on the boat trip.

If she doesn't get the names of her children right, be sure to correct her. It's important that she remember their names.

I wonder why she gets so aggravated with me when I set her straight. I'm only trying to help her.

Her granddaughter said that she was not born in Oklahoma, so be sure to correct her when she talks about being born there.

Everybody loves dogs, so bring in your two pit bulls!

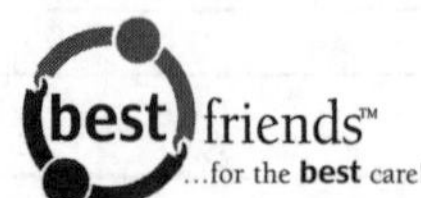

8

Communication

Communication brings us together. It is part of a healthy and full life to have friends and family to whom we can talk and who will listen to us. Friends may spend hours every week (or day) on the telephone. They may exchange written notes, letters, and e-mails. They may talk over coffee at a cafe. They may look across a crowded room and exchange gestures and facial expressions that are as easily understood as words.

Because it attacks a *person's* ability to communicate, Alzheimer's disease threatens this important link between the *person* and his or her caregivers. As the disease progresses, *persons* experience increasing difficulty understanding written and spoken words and directions. They also struggle to communicate their wishes and needs (see Chapter 3 for more on language and Alzheimer's disease). Yet, throughout this process, most *persons* retain the desire to communicate. Best Friends staff respect this desire and strive to keep the *person* connected to life. This chapter shares ideas and methods for making this possible.

The following vignette illustrates what can happen when staff are not well trained in effective communication techniques:

> "The Echo Heights Residence for the Confused seemed aptly named this Thursday," thought Anna, an activity assistant at the 30-bed nursing facility. "Why is everything so hard lately?" she thought, frustrated. She looked at her watch and realized that it was time for the group activity. She called out to Pam, "Let's get them together in the lounge for bingo and other games."
>
> Gradually, about 15 people assembled in a small, darkened room (several of the light bulbs were burned out in the old ceiling fixtures). Pam said hello to the group but commented, "I hope you won't mind me too much today. I'm in a bad mood. I had a huge fight with my boyfriend last night. All he wants to do is watch TV."
>
> "That's terrible, Pam, but let's try to have some fun today," Anna replied, trying to change the subject. Just then, the wandering alarm began to chirp; two of the CNAs went to investigate, leaving Anna by herself. As the alarm droned on, one resident complained, "Why doesn't someone answer that phone?" Others frowned, and one new resident, Mrs. Perlstein, began rubbing her forehead.

Anna realized that she had forgotten to get the bingo cards off the shelf in the hallway. She looked at one of the residents and asked, "Mr. Spencer, would you go get the bingo cards—you know, the ones in the hallway, next to the big plant on the fourth shelf from the bottom?" Mr. Spencer smiled and got up and walked in that direction.

Dr. Rose stood up. He seemed somewhat agitated. "Who are these people?" he demanded. Trying to maintain calm, Anna said, "Don't get up, Dr. Rose. Just sit down. I know you will want to stay here."

Mrs. Perlstein began to speak, but it came out as a string of words that were not connected together. Anna looked puzzled. "I'm sorry, honey. I can't understand what you're saying. What are you saying? Can you tell me what you want? What do you need?" Mrs. Perlstein suddenly burst into tears. Several other residents looked alarmed, and, while one comforted Mrs. Perlstein, another began to cry.

"I'm sorry, honey." Anna said, realizing her mistake. "Let me get you some coffee." Just then, Mr. Spencer returned to the group with a potted plant instead of the bingo cards. "Here it is!" he announced proudly. With that, Anna began to cry, too.

Although the example above is extreme, colleagues in long-term care tell us that all of these elements happen far too often in dementia programs. Most staff members are caring people. Unfortunately, poor training, particularly in the vital area of communication, contributes to a dementia program's spinning quickly out of control.

In the example above, many parts of the whole worked against good communication. The environment was working against the staff (poor lighting and lots of distracting noise). Staff failed to set an upbeat tone (did not smile; brought personal problems into the discussion). Staff failed to greet the residents in a friendly fashion (call them by name, smile, give a compliment) or to make introductions (explain why they were together, introduce themselves and each other using elements of the life story). They also did not demonstrate a desire to communicate with residents (repeatedly telling Mrs. Perlstein that they could not understand her, not noting her body language; giving Mr. Spencer overly complex directions). Finally, staff did not demonstrate respect for the residents (calling the new resident "honey" and issuing orders in the way in which they dealt with Dr. Rose).

With all of these negative aspects working against them, staff were not likely to have created a successful group activity. Never was any attempt made to point to the purpose of the gathering or to encourage participation. The residents internalized the sour and chaotic mood.

What could have saved the Echo Heights Residence for the Confused? Let's review the key concepts concerning the Best Friends approach to communication.

Check the Environment

Best Friends staff members recognize that the surrounding environment can facilitate communication or make it nearly impossible. Even the best efforts to communicate can be thwarted when there is ambient noise or other distractions. With poor lighting, the *person* may not be able to see a staff member's face, hindering understanding. When the space is cluttered, conflicting stimuli can confuse or distract the *person*.

Heritage Court at The Samarkand Retirement Community completely remodeled its facility to evoke feelings of home and to move away from the typical environment of a skilled nursing facility. Staff discovered that the changes in the environment—improved lighting, cheerful colors, new furnishings, open spaces, and a discovery garden—had a dramatic, positive impact on residents' functioning. Communication seemed greatly improved and activities more successful. The program director, Val Maxey, observed, "There now seem to be more spontaneous interactions between residents and staff. It seems more like a family home, with lots of give and take."

Heritage Court's administrator, Steven Anderson, said that the goal of Heritage Court is not to be homelike but to be a home. He commented, "The environment is more than bricks and mortar; it's people, too." (See Tool 5.6 for an environmental checklist.)

Remember the Basics of Good Communication

Best Friends staff members apply the principles of good communication to every encounter with a *person.* Communication is enhanced by good eye contact (although not in every culture; in some cultures, eye contact can be considered inappropriate, rude, or worse); specific, descriptive language; good volume and tone; and use of appropriate gestures.

Christian Health Center was the home of Rebecca Riley (read more about her in the Dedication at the front of this book), who was diagnosed with Alzheimer's disease in 1984 and featured prominently in The Best Friends Approach to Alzheimer's Care. *Before Rebecca's death, staff were aware of the importance of continuing to communicate with her. They approached her using eye contact and a big smile and called her by name. She always responded with a smile. Often, a staff member would rub her hand, give her a hug, and massage her shoulders. Because Rebecca had been a nurse, they talked to her about nursing. When she could no longer respond verbally, her eyes still lit up when staff connected with her.*

Eye contact, touch, and using the *person's* life story for conversation add up to a staff with knack. Of note is the staff's desire to continue communication even late into the illness.

Use the *Person's* Preferred Name

Best Friends staff members always start from a place of respect, using more formal salutations (e.g., Dr. Simpson, Mrs. Weaver). They also recognize that *persons* sometimes recognize a different name. A *person's* first name, for example, often is better recognized late into the illness because it has been with him or her since birth.

Mary Katherine, a participant in the Helping Hand Day Center, suddenly started asking everyone to call her "Kitty." Even her family had forgotten that this was an early childhood nickname. Staff followed her wishes, and she always brightened when she heard her nickname. Perhaps hearing it evoked an earlier, happier time for her.

Some programs prohibit the use of first names. We believe that rigid rules do not complement good-quality dementia care. If the *person* wants to be called by his or her first name, then program leaders should allow it.

Make a Good First Impression

Best Friends staff members understand that first impressions are everything in Alzheimer's care. Because the *person* may not remember the name of a specific staff member, his or her role, or even that they have already met, it is important for staff to get into the habit of identifying themselves. They should also approach the *person* from the front, smile, even offer a friendly handshake. A cheerful disposition and a friendly greeting go a long way.

A male resident at Wellington Parc of Owensboro receives assistance from staff in every aspect of care. The activity director decided that the resident might enjoy a foot massage. As she rubbed his feet, he spoke. He had not been able to verbalize an understandable word for a long time. It was a wonderful moment for the staff member to know that she was able to relate to him on some level. When she left the room, she immediately called the resident's wife.

A CNA at West Park Long Term Care Center works to create a good first impression when she wakes a resident in the morning. She is careful not to shine the light in her eyes. She calls her by name in a soft voice, gives her a gentle back rub, and offers a cup of juice or coffee.

A smile and a sensitive "good morning" get both CNA and resident off to a good start.

Keep Language Simple

Best Friends staff members realize that seemingly simple, everyday conversations can be full of complex, even conflicting, words and directions. This can be overwhelming for *persons* with dementia, who need to be communicated with in simple and direct language and instructions.

Quite often I just cradle her face with my hands, and she knows I care about her.

—Lisa Snyder, Director of Special Care, West Park Long Term Care Center, Cody, Wyoming

A resident at West Park Long Term Care Center was brushing his teeth, and a staff member told him to shave with his electric razor when finished. A few minutes later, he was observed wandering from his room with blue gel toothpaste spread over his face like shaving cream.

The human face is a picture show of expressions. We can often communicate more with our eyes than with words.

—Anonymous

The staff member realized her mistake immediately; she had given too many instructions at once. Fortunately, she remedied the situation with a hot washcloth and some gentle reassurances.

When using repetition, staff can take steps to help the listener understand better. Add some descriptive detail each time. An example might be, "Give me your purse, that brown purse, that nice brown leather purse on the chair."

Ask Questions Using Discretion

Best Friends staff members realize that *persons* with Alzheimer's disease face very real memory losses. When asked a question that they do not know the answer to, *persons* may experience feelings of anxiety, sadness, frustration, and anger. Even worse, they know that they should know. When questions are asked, they should be broad enough not to require specific facts and details. A staff member also can provide appropriate cues and clues. When a question cannot be answered, a staff member with knack will not leave the person hanging. (See Tool 8.9 for more on "do's and don'ts.")

Employ Good Timing

Best Friends staff members have a good sense of timing. Sometimes a *person* simply will not cooperate with a request. Rather than try to pressure the *person* to do something that he or she simply does not want to do, a staff member with knack learns to listen to the *person's* refusal and respect it. If the task or request is really important and in the *person's* best interests, then the staff member can use finesse to encourage him or her to comply. Sometimes just bringing up the matter later works well.

Cindy Stancil, director of operations, Liberty Commons Assisted Living, Wilmington, North Carolina, employs good timing in her work: "For some residents, I know never to ask them to do anything before their first cup of coffee in the morning."

Be Conscious of Nonverbal Communication

Best Friends staff members recognize that as language and words fail the *person,* he or she looks to them for nonverbal clues and cues. The *person* gets messages from a staff member's tone and volume of voice, posture, and hand gestures. When he or she sees a smile and positive body language from staff, the *person* many times will respond in kind. Conversely, when staff seem disinterested, tense, or troubled, their mood can affect all aspects of care. Best Friends staff members learn to leave their problems at the door and project a positive message and tone whenever they are with a *person.*

A sink was installed at the nurses' station, and the ladies often "prepare" vegetables for the evening meal. Suppertime is spent around the table or in front of the fire and is a sociable time, with hot, frothy chocolate; coffee or tea; and cookies and conversation.

—Patricia Wesley, Omahanui Private Hospital, New Plymouth, New Zealand

We try to encourage warm welcomes at The Fountainview Center. A CNA entered one military veteran's room with a salute, saying, "Reporting for duty, sir, at your service." As this resident is a highly decorated military man, this greeting made his day.

—Anne M. Helmly, Director of Community Relations, The Fountainview Center for Alzheimer's Disease, Atlanta, Georgia

Do Not Argue With or Confront the *Person*

Best Friends staff members understand that it is virtually impossible to win an argument with a *person* with Alzheimer's disease. The *person* often remains convinced of a particular fact or point of view. Trying to dissuade him or her of it would be akin to trying to convince an administrator that he or she really is a resident. Arguing only leads to frustration and failure. Also, confrontation can cause the *person* to become defensive and angry.

Remember to listen to the music, not the words.

—Meredith Gresham, writer and consultant, Avon, Connecticut

Staff at Villa Alamar are trained not to argue with persons. *If a resident says the grass is blue, then staff do not disagree. They will add, "What a pretty color!"*

Having the ability to let go of the "right" answer allows staff to develop the knack.

The director's office at Karrington Cottages Assisted Living, in Rochester, Minnesota, is on a corner wall, and each time one of the residents rounds the corner, he stops in and tells the director that he has just come into town and has just stopped by to say, "Hello." The director always responds by saying, "Have a nice day!"

Remember that Behaviors Communicate a Message

Best Friends staff know that early in the disease, the *person* can communicate feelings and problems in words; later, his or her behavior articulates what words cannot. Yelling or striking out can signify that the *person* is in pain. Wandering can be triggered by boredom. Tears can suggest loneliness. Laughter or humming may mean that the *person* is happy.

We transformed our very institutional-looking bathroom into a marine sensory room, where aromatherapy baths are routinely enjoyed by many of our Best Friends.

—Barbara Susan Dicker, Facilitator, Action Learning (Dementia) Team, Carinya Village Nursing Home, Perth, Western Australia

Staff members at the Sunshine Terrace Adult Day Center in Logan, Utah, were concerned that their afternoon participants who stayed on after most of the participants had already left for the day were becoming anxious and worried. The older adults looked out the window and door constantly, fearing that they had been forgotten and would be left behind.

The Center's staff paid attention to the restless behavior and solved the problem by holding a special music session at the end of the day. Singing and the tapping of feet replaced worry about being forgotten.

Cindy Lynch, a dementia care consultant and researcher, used her problem-solving abilities to understand better her grandmother's behaviors and to look for solutions:

Grandmother sat hunched over in her wheelchair, unable to read or talk about her favorite topics. She flailed and muttered, communicating her agitation. I believed that something written simply and clearly about her favorite things might encourage her to speak and read again. Carolyn Read, a friend and reading specialist, prepared a beautiful set of 9 inch × 12 inch reading cards with a colorful picture of one of Grandmother's favorite topics on each card. A descriptive large-print paragraph is written on each one. The first time Grandmother read aloud from the cards was a wonderful experience for both of us. Grandmother succeeded in an activity that had been lost to her. Instead of her becoming agitated, I got to see her look into my eyes and smile for the first time in months.

Not giving up means making efforts like this granddaughter did.

Treat the *Person* as an Adult

Best Friends staff members never talk down to the *person* or treat him or her as a child. Baby talk never should be used. The authors also discourage the use of the "royal We." Saying, "Let's take our medicine now," or "Let's take off our pants," is demeaning to the *person* and can lead to some unintended results and confusion; the *person* might be expecting the staff member to do all of these things with him or her.

When a new volunteer at the ADCare Adult Day Service Center asked a participant to read aloud to the group, the participant found the request absurd and refused to do it. A staff member stepped in and said, "I left my glasses at home, and I'm interested in today's paper, but I can't read it. Would you read it to me?" The participant immediately helped out.

A task that at first seemed purposeless became meaningful when put in a more adult context. The participant believed that she was helping the staff member, not having to perform for a group.

Use the Life Story Often

Best Friends staff members use the *person's* life story in almost every aspect of communication. Staff use it to greet the *person,* to engage in conversations giving clues and cues, to

The sense of touch creates bonds not seen before between the staff and residents.

—*Dana E. Newquist, Director, The Alzheimer's Four Seasons in Santa Barbara, California, about introducing massage therapy in the residential home; massage gives the staff another means of communication and reduces agitation in* persons.

I think the most difficult thing about caring for the *person* with Alzheimer's disease is communicating with them. After reading your book, I found myself reading the expressions on my residents' faces and applying that to what they were trying to say. It was easier than I thought.

—*Rachel Everett, student, Madonna University, Livonia, Michigan*

The desire to be understood, not just heard, is universal and the people we count on to understand us are our friends.

—*Herman Melville*

give compliments, to reminisce, to provide appropriate distractions, to introduce the *person* to others, and to note what subjects to avoid.

One resident of Heritage Court at The Samarkand Retirement Community is prone to anxiety attacks. When staff notice her becoming anxious, they talk with her about a pet mouse that she had when she was a little girl. This memory always brings a smile to her face, and she launches into a description of the mouse that lived in the woodpile on her back porch.

This use of the life story brings this resident back to happier days. It rarely fails to take her out of her anxious mood.

The Helping Hand Day Center staff and volunteers are always impressed and amazed to learn that one participant at the center was one of the few women pilots in World War II. She beams when reminded about this rare achievement and loves being teased about how such a petite individual could have flown such a big plane. Because of this and other honors, she is listed in a book as one of the Outstanding Kentucky Women of the 20th Century.

Using past successes and present accomplishments often facilitates communication and enhances participants' self-esteem (see Tool 8.3).

Maintain Caregiving Integrity

Best Friends staff members act in the best interests of the *persons* in their care. The same principle holds true in communication, in which staff should not pretend to understand the *person* if they do not. They may use finesse to make an affirming statement such as, "I really enjoy being with you." If a *person* seems to be making a strong statement about something, a staff member can reply with integrity, "You always have such good ideas."

Dee Carlson has noted that the technique of distraction is widely used and often is successful (e.g., "Let's have an ice cream cone," "Join me for a walk"). She reminds staff to proceed with caution in some cases. For example, if a teenager were still out hours past curfew and her father said to her anxious mother, "Don't worry! Let's have an ice cream cone," it would be inappropriate and could provoke anger. The anxious mother might have believed that her husband was not respecting her concerns or, worse, did not care.

The same principle holds true in dementia care; distractions or diversions need to be appropriate to the situation and executed with finesse. Ice cream cones or other distractions can sometimes save the day, but on their own they may not calm the *person* who is upset about memories of a mother's death or afraid of being abandoned. Staff always should pay attention to the *person's* concerns and respond when possible; distractions should be used appropriately and as a next step.

Respond to the *Person's* Emotional Needs

Best Friends staff members provide an empathetic shoulder to lean on. Work with early-stage Alzheimer's support groups has taught the field much about the emotional needs of *persons* with dementia; *persons* have a need to share their feelings. The simple words, "It's been hard for you, hasn't it?" or, "Tell me more about that," are life affirming.

When a resident who spoke only Greek came to The Fountainview Center, staff learned to communicate with her on an emotional level. They experienced and shared her frustration, grief, and delight. They became more in tune with her because they had to rely on something other than the spoken word. Deanna R. Pham, the social services director, observed that staff related to her in the same way that they relate to many residents who cannot communicate verbally, "through the understanding that comes only with friendship."

It took a resident who could not speak English to show that caregivers often are overreliant on words. The situation forced staff to get more in touch with the emotional life of the resident. These lessons helped them communicate better with all of their residents.

Screen Out Troubling Messages or News

Best Friends staff members know that a little worry can grow into a big one for *persons* with dementia. When possible, screen out sad, violent, ominous, or controversial messages. This is not always possible with communitywide tragedies (e.g., major fire, tornado) or in cases of personal loss (e.g., the death of a friend or loved one). When losses do occur, staff should make sure that the *person* feels safe, is offered reassurance, and is given an opportunity to share his or her feelings.

As part of the Helping Hand training program, volunteers and staff practice sharing upbeat, positive stories and news. They read the newspaper with the participants, looking for stories and ads with a positive message that can lead to pleasant conversation. Looking at supermarket ads, staff can say, "Can you believe that you can buy strawberries right here in Lexington, Kentucky, when there is snow on the ground?" or ask, "Do you like strawberry shortcake?"

Persons cannot always be protected from bad news, but when we have the opportunity to screen out bad news, it is usually a good decision. With *persons* already being vulnerable to worries, we should try to accentuate the positive.

Speak Using Positive Language

Best Friends staff members know to speak to *persons* in positive language. An example is, "Let's go this way," instead of, "Don't go that way." The technique of having staff "walk a mile in the *person's* shoes" can be effective. Most staff members will admit that they do not like to be told "no." Neither do *persons* with dementia.

Cheri Taylor, the executive director of Porterville Senior Day Care, enthusiastically greeted an arriving participant by name. When the person *said she wanted to leave, Taylor assured her in a kidding tone that everyone would miss her if she left. "Miss me? You don't even know me!" the woman replied. Taylor said, brightly, "Everyone in Porterville knows you. You've lived here for a long time. I love you. I don't want you to leave." The participant's mood suddenly changed. She paused for a moment and said, "Leave? I'm not leaving."*

The use of positive language in adult day centers often makes the difference between having participants stay in their cars or come into the center.

Employ Humor

Best Friends staff members make artful use of humor. Sharing a joke or pun evokes laughter, and laughter is communication at its finest. We all tend to laugh when someone tells a joke. Even if we do not understand the punch line, just hearing someone tell a joke can be funny in itself.

Staff at the Care Club day center use a joke book to lighten up on life. "All of the staff and volunteers are encouraged to bring funny stories to tell to the group. We usually can bring a smile to even the sourest face."

Humor seems to transcend dementia, and *persons* pick up the good mood and happy spirit from those around them. Laughter really is the best medicine.

Turn "No" into "Yes"

Best Friends staff members honor a *person's* right to say "no." But if it involves the best interest of the *person,* then staff should avoid giving him or her a chance to refuse. For example, when giving medication, it would be a mistake to ask whether he or she wants the pill now. A staff member aiming for a "yes" might say with finesse, "Here's your favorite juice and the pill the doctor ordered. Bottoms up!"

When *persons* with dementia are given a chance to say "no," they most often do. This happens for the simple reason that the decline in cognitive skills in dementia makes it harder to absorb information and make decisions. *Persons* do not fully understand what it is you are asking them. When in doubt, a safer choice for all of us is to say "no." Here is an example of changing "no" to "yes" from Villa Alamar:

A Sophie Tucker look- and soundalike, Izzy did not come to Villa Alamar with a vibrant attitude. Although she had sung for years in a famous choral group, she said "no" to all of the invitations to join the music activity. The staff made frequent room visits, gave her lots of hugs, and talked about the fun everyone was having singing and dancing. It took time, but eventually she left her room, cast her walker aside, and danced the shimmy, laughing and enjoying herself immensely.

Turning "no" into "yes" through gentle, friendly, and persistent one-to-one attention can pay big dividends. Just keep in mind that residents' rights must always be respected.

Do Most of the Work

Best Friends staff members are not afraid to do most of the work in conversation. It is up to staff to initiate verbal and nonverbal communication. Asking a simple question of a resident or participant who has been silent for a period of time or walking up to someone and offering an arm or shoulder for him or her to hold onto are types of appropriate communication.

Best Friends staff do this throughout each day. A good training program stresses that staff do not want *persons* ever to feel or be ignored.

A staff member at Heritage Court at The Samarkand noted that one woman often sat by herself in the hallway. When approached by staff and others, she always expressed contentment and said that she did not need anything at all. Staff decided to be more proactive and began to pull up a chair beside her to ask her opinion about some topic or, in one case, to ask her to help pick out a teddy bear to give to a child. Even though she had poor vision, she could feel the stuffed bears and picked the softest one as the gift. Staff also learned more about her fascinating life overseas. Even just a few minutes of communication at a time enriched her life and gave the staff a sense of satisfaction.

It takes work to initiate conversations, but the payoff can be great. Most *persons* have a desire to communicate. It is up to us never to give up and to find the key that opens the door.

CONCLUSION

Best Friends staff members always ask, "How can I be a friend to the *person* in my care?" One way is to practice effective and genuine communication. Words and language often fail us, yet nonverbal communication can bridge the gap. When staff project a sense of warmth and welcome, it can make *persons* feel more secure and happy.

Staff also should be encouraged to remember the benefits of improved communication. Not only will staff experience less frustration but they also will be able to complete their jobs sooner and easier. The often-challenging job of bathing, for example, can go better when staff use elements of the life story and provide careful instructions along with dashes of humor.

There is another benefit to training staff in how to communicate with *persons* with dementia. It also helps them communicate better with other staff members. This enhancement can pay dividends in the areas of team building, staff morale, and the accomplishment of goals. It can help staff resolve conflicts and learn assertiveness. It also can help bring together staff from diverse cultures.

Staff with knack learn that communication brings us together across time and generations. *Persons* with dementia retain many long-term memories. The authors have learned much from them about history and culture. We have learned herbal recipes from a woman who was born in a covered wagon. We have "seen" Lindbergh land in Paris. We have "traveled" in dozens of countries. We have learned about discrimination in the rural South of the 1950s. Communication connects us to one another.

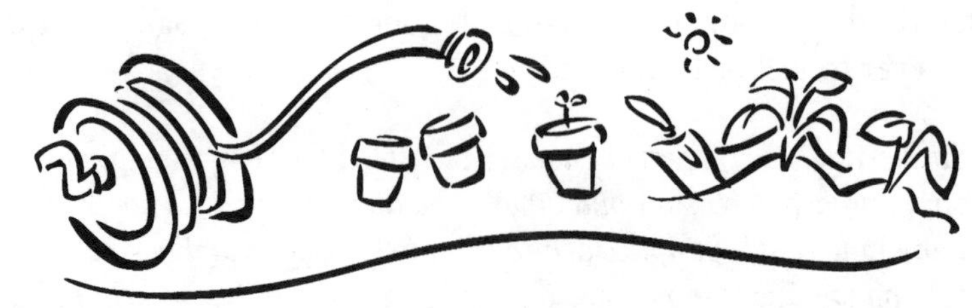

Training Tool Kit

Tool 8.0 / Warm-Up
Communicating Without Words

Use this warm-up to make the point that you can communicate successfully, even without words, especially when language skills diminish in persons with Alzheimer's disease. Gestures and facial expressions can be magical. Creativity also counts!

Ask the group to stand and line up by month and date of birth (e.g., January 1–December 31), but not by years. Participants must do this without speaking at all. Any form of communication (e.g., hand gestures, written notes, driver's licenses) that they can think of besides using words is acceptable.

Depending on the size of the group, give participants 5–15 minutes to line up. Then, starting from the front of the line, ask everyone to state verbally the month and date of his or her birth. Move participants around as needed to obtain an accurate result.

At the end, ask the group members to take their seats. Discuss how it felt to communicate without words.

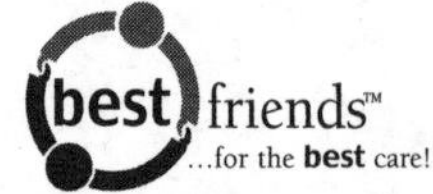

Tool 8.1 / Games for Learning

Role Plays

Role plays are one of the best techniques for teaching communication because they help staff members truly understand what works and what does not. The following role play has been scripted for you. Use the examples in Tool 8.10 to write more.

Topic: Using the Life Story in Communicating a Message

Scene: Jake, a participant in an adult day center, is sitting at a table that needs to be moved for an evening event. He is immovable and uncooperative. What can staff do to move Jake?

The Wrong Way

STAFF MEMBER: I need to move this table.
JAKE: Go along. I'm staying here.
STAFF MEMBER: (*somewhat disgruntled*) C'mon, let's go. I'm in a hurry.
JAKE: I'm staying here!
STAFF MEMBER: They're waiting on us to move (*takes Jake's arm and pulls*). We have to take these tables down to make room for the next activity. Can't you understand that we need to move? Let's go!
JAKE: (*getting agitated*) Let them get going!

Discuss with the group what is wrong with this example (Jake's being rushed, physically pushed; overexplaining; no introduction).

The Right Way

STAFF MEMBER: (*making eye contact and smiling*) Hi, Jake! How is that great golf game of yours going?
JAKE: Oh yes, golf. I like it.
STAFF MEMBER: (*leaning close as if sharing a special secret*) I wanted to let you know the meeting is about to begin next door.
JAKE: Meeting? Yes, the meeting.
STAFF MEMBER: I have reserved a special seat for you up front, just like you always ask for.
JAKE: Oh, that! Yep, can't beat that!
STAFF MEMBER: (*extends an arm*) Let me show you to your seat. I know you don't like being late!

Discuss with the group what is right with this example (introduction, use of life story, positive body language such as extending an arm, short simple sentences, repetition, optimistic and respectful attitude).

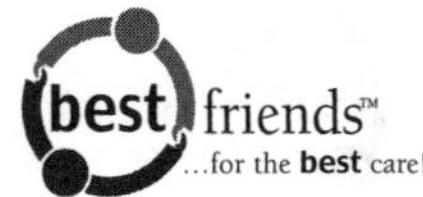

Tool 8.2 / Games for Learning
The Greeting Game

Here is one program's effective example of training using role plays.

Two caregivers [staff members] walk toward each other. Each caregiver takes a turn using different body and verbal language. (Scenarios can spring from what caregivers have seen, done, or experienced, so that the role play comes from real-life situations.) One has a slight scowl, walks fast, seems preoccupied, does not speak, or says a perfunctory hello (or whatever examples are given). The other caregiver is the resident.

After the participants pass each other, they discuss how each of them is feeling—sad, not welcome, upset, ignored, more lonely, and so forth. Then they practice welcoming smiles, open arms, handshakes, eye contact, a touch on the shoulder. This is followed by a moment of activity-based care such as, "Lucy, I love that pink blouse you put on today," or, "Margaret, you always wear such unusual jewelry. Would you tell me about this bracelet?" or, "Fred, are you ready to finish painting that birdhouse today?"

The group discusses the feelings—happy, welcomed, safe, included—that caregivers felt by using this technique. The "homework" assignment from this exercise is to try three positive greetings the next day and report the results at the next training session. Past reports have demonstrated positive results, including smiles, big hugs, and kisses from the residents and a window opened to engage *persons* in conversation and activity-based care.

One caregiver learned that a particular resident did not like to be hugged and needed a firm handshake. The caregiver believed that the lesson helped her to become more of an equal friend to the resident because they had communicated and she had become sensitive to the resident's moods and needs. The resident, who had avoided any contact with her, was now able to look the caregiver in the eye as they vigorously shook hands. She believed that they had begun to form a friendship.

Courtesy of Diane Will, national community life director, The Fountains Continuum of Care, Inc., Tucson, Arizona.

Tool 8.3 / Games for Learning
A Little Fact Goes a Long Way

The entire class will see, through role play, how conversation becomes easier and more rewarding when we know even a few facts about the person *with dementia. The group leader role-plays a* person *with dementia who is communicating with an audience member.*

You (the group leader) should write facts about yourself on 5–10 index cards—one fact per card. For example, you might write:

Born on a farm	Enjoy making quilts
Have twin brother and sister	Love country-western music and opera
Won a spelling bee	Father was a coal miner
Love cats	First one in family to go to college

Stand in front of the group and ask a class member who does not know you to come to the front of the class. Ask the group member to engage you in conversation. In almost every case, the conversation flounders because the class member does not know the life story of the *person* and finds it difficult to choose subjects to talk about. (You should role-play refusal to participate in the conversation and gradually appear increasingly confused or agitated.)

After a few minutes of difficulty, hand the class member a descriptive index card. Do this one card at a time. Hopefully he or she will use the information on each card to enhance the conversation. (You should now respond to the facts presented by the staff member with enthusiasm.) For example, if the conversation is lagging and you hand the class member the card that says, "Won a spelling bee," the class member might say, "Oh, and I understand that you are an excellent speller!" You can respond, "Yes, I am! I can even spell long words." This might lead to further conversation or even a spelling bee.

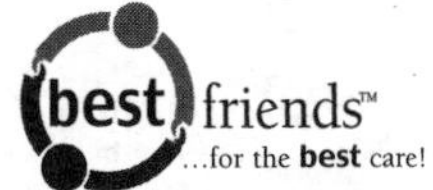

Tool 8.4 / Games for Learning
Nonverbal Role Plays

Here is another way to teach the importance of observation.

Ask selected staff members to act out one or more of the following behaviors that are sometimes observed in *persons* with Alzheimer's disease:

Pacing
Searching through a purse
Rummaging through a drawer
Undressing
Wringing hands
Reaching out for help
Hitting someone or something
Picking at things in the air
Tapping on the table
Frowning

Ask the class to describe what is going on. Name several reasons why the *person* is behaving this way. Should staff intervene? If so, in what way?

Variation: To make the point that we should also look for signs that the *person* is happy or content, act out positive expressions such as smiles, hugs, and laughter.

Tool 8.5 / Program Pointer

The Best Friends Approach to Communication

Post this list on bulletin boards, include it in newsletters, or distribute it as a handout to discuss with staff.

Check the environment

Remember the basics of good communication

Use the *person's* preferred name

Make a good first impression

Keep language simple

Ask questions using discretion

Employ good timing

Be conscious of nonverbal communication

Do not argue with or confront the *person*

Remember that behaviors communicate a message

Treat the *person* as an adult

Use the life story often

Maintain caregiving integrity

Respond to the *person's* emotional needs

Screen out troubling messages or news

Speak using positive language

Employ humor

Turn "no" into "yes"

Do most of the work

Tool 8.6 / Games for Learning
The Compliment Game

This fun game shows how the act of giving compliments can help a person *with dementia. Compliments are easy to give, cost no money, and take so little time. Staff also can be told that it is valuable to continue complimenting one another when good things happen.*

Choose somebody in the room and ask him or her to stand. Give the individual a compliment (e.g., on his or her appearance, job performance, personality, a recent achievement). Note the response—usually a blush, smile, or laugh. Ask the assembled group whether the individual looks downcast, depressed, or unhappy.

Make the point that compliments elevate us. They can disarm an agitated or unhappy individual and make all of us smile. Repeat the exercise by asking the staff member you chose to select another individual in the room to give a compliment to. Repeat the game four or five times.

Conclude the game by making the point that *persons* with Alzheimer's disease benefit from compliments. The compliments should never be forced or insincere. Hopefully there will always be some way to compliment a *person.*

Ask the class to think of compliments they can give *persons* in their care and list them on a board or butcher paper.

Variation: Ask the class to each give three compliments to fellow staff members or *persons* during their next shift. They should write down what they said on posterboard or butcher paper in a staff meeting room. Make every entry eligible for a raffle to be held later in the week. Review the compliments at the next staff meeting.

Variation: List the names of day center participants or residents on the board. Brainstorm compliments that staff could give to each *person.*

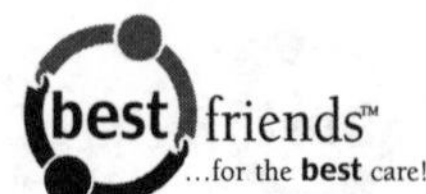

Tool 8.7 / Program Pointer
"Do's and Don'ts" for Communication

Post this list on bulletin boards, include it in newsletters, or distribute it as a handout to discuss with staff.

Do's for Communication

Listen carefully

Help a *person* fill in the blanks

Read facial expressions and body language and try to respond appropriately

Give compliments

Ask opinions

Ask open-ended questions

Give generous praise

Use common sense

Enjoy the *person* in every way possible

Take the blame and apologize

Be sincere

Use the *person's* life story regularly

Use positive language

Rely on humor

Keep language simple

Don'ts for Communication

Argue, confront, correct

Give orders, make demands

Talk down to a *person*

Talk about a *person* in his or her presence as if the *person* were not there

Ask questions that require remembering too many facts

Try to explain or prepare too far in advance

Take negative comments personally

Give too many choices

Take anything for granted

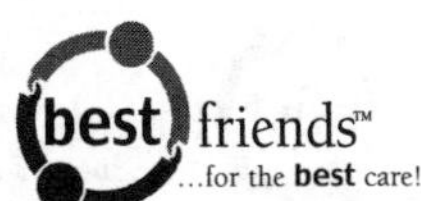

Tool 8.8 / Program Pointer

Making a Meal a Time for Conversation

For many *persons,* meals often are the highlight of a day. They should be treated as the important activities that they are. For a dependent *person,* a meal represents valuable time spent in one-to-one relationships in that it can be a social experience when the meal is shared. Meals should always be a pleasant sensory experience.

Jitka M. Zgola wrote in *Care That Works,*

"Every meal offers an opportunity for programming activities. It can be used to build relationships among participants, to offer occasion for reminiscence, and to reinforce old, and perhaps neglected, social skills. A meal can be a 'lunch bunch' or 'dinner at our place.' A wonderful thing happens when staff members participate, not as supervisors, servers, monitors, or feeders, but as people at the table enjoying a meal between staff and residents. This special touch goes a long way to building the trusting, respectful relationships that pay such dividends in the long run."

To make sure that meals are a pleasant experience for *persons,* use the following checklist for the dining table:

- ❑ Are the surroundings pleasant and uncluttered?
- ❑ Is the background music soft and instrumental (no vocals)?
- ❑ Is the table small enough for people to converse comfortably?
- ❑ Do the tablecloth, dinner plates, and even color of the food offer good contrast to one another?
- ❑ Is there a small arrangement of flowers on the table?
- ❑ Are the food, silverware, and plate appropriate for the functional level of the *person?*

The following list suggests ideas for the staff member's role as host or hostess:

- ✓ Do not leave the room or do paperwork; recognize that mealtime is a prime time for good communication.
- ✓ Float between tables and ask about the food; make appropriate introductions.
- ✓ Lead a prayer or a toast.
- ✓ Give compliments or ask opinions.
- ✓ Reminisce about past meals or favorite foods.
- ✓ Join residents or participants for lunch.

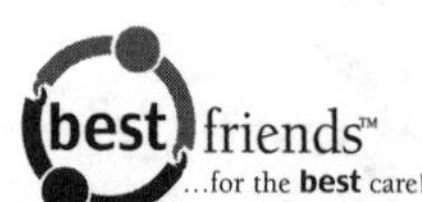

Tool 8.9 / Program Pointer
Question "Do's and Don'ts"

Post this list on bulletin boards, include it in newsletters, or distribute it as a handout to discuss with staff.

- ✓ Do provide cues and clues, such as, "How is your daughter, Marge, the viola player?"
- ✓ Do not ask for information that the *person* cannot recall (e.g., "How many children do you have and what are their names?").
- ✓ Do ask open-ended questions (e.g., "Did you enjoy your breakfast?" "Do you like chocolate?").
- ✓ Do exercise patience when you ask a question. Sometimes the *person* will answer; sometimes the *person* will not.
- ✓ Don't let a *person* hang out on a limb too long. If he or she really does not recall, then change the subject or answer the question yourself.
- ✓ Don't ask a *person* whether he or she wants to do a certain thing if there really is no choice.
- ✓ Do incorporate enough facts in the question to cue a *person* to respond.
- ✓ Do ask for a *person's* opinions.

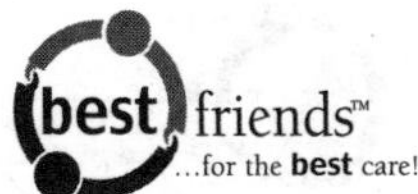

Tool 8.10

Turning No Knack into Knack

The purpose of this exercise is to show, with a dash of humor, the wrong way to do something. This is active learning that really sinks in, particularly when staff members themselves volunteer to take part in the role plays.

The following statements represent stereotypes or falsehoods about dementia. These examples of "no knack" can be used in a number of ways to explore staff attitudes and reinforce the lessons presented in this chapter. Draw them from a hat to discuss as a group or put them into role plays. Invite staff to comment on the mistakes. Then role-play or discuss the right way. The authors discuss the art of role plays in Tool 2.11. Use your creativity to have fun turning these examples of "no knack" into "knack."

I don't believe in watching my words. I just say it like it is. The residents won't remember it anyway.

I think it's nice to have the TV on all day because it gives the residents something to do.

Since you can't explain it to me, how can I know what you are feeling or what you want?

She's pacing and restless today. She's not her happy self. She must have gone into another stage of Alzheimer's last night.

She's always talking about going home, but when I show her the picture of where she lived for 60 years, she doesn't even recognize it as her home.

You only need to say things once, otherwise it might frustrate them.

This is not your coat. It's Mr. Garcia's. How many times do I have to explain it to you? Yours is blue and his is brown. Can't you see that?

Did you hear the news? A big storm is building up. It's going to be terrible out there.

No! Stop! You can't go that way! You are not allowed to go that way!

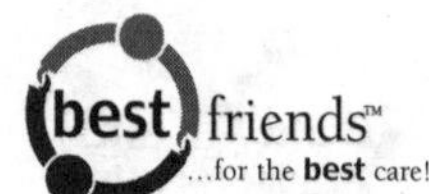

9

Being Together Using Best Friends Activities

What is friendship if it's not about playing together, working together, and being together? The Best Friends model has proven highly popular with activities professionals, who have found it an attractive framework for thinking about and implementing their programs. They like the model's philosophy that real friends do things together often—planned and spontaneous, simple and elaborate, short and long, fun and serious, physical and intellectual, spiritual and religious, vocational and avocational. Activities in dementia care should have the same flavor. They should include meaningful group programs but also allow the *person* with Alzheimer's disease to live between structured activities. Activities should reflect real life as much as possible. *Life is an activity!*

Virginia M. Sponsler, family life consultant in Portland, Oregon, supports this view with the following words that helped form the title for this chapter:

"Being together" is a term that can refer to activities. I like it because it refers to the relational part of the activity. It covers tasks, skill building, play, cooperative and parallel activities, doing, and "just being," the structured and the spontaneous.

Being together is part of good friendship. The following example demonstrates what can happen when staff and residents do not have this relationship:

> The building was beautiful. Platinum Palace Assisted Living had a grand entrance foyer, and the staff seemed friendly and supportive. As John and his wife Yvette toured the community as a potential home for Yvette's mother, they were impressed. "Wow, look at that chandelier," Yvette said to John. "I think I'd like to live here!"
>
> They both laughed as they walked the corridors. They had taken a formal tour last week, but decided to visit the place on their own for a second look. They came across a lovely bulletin board. On it was the activity calendar. Expecting to find a rich array of activities, they read it together. Listed for that day were bingo, crafts, and an ice cream social. They looked at the next day, hoping to find something

that would be of interest. Bingo, exercise, crafts, and a movie musical appeared. "Better, but shouldn't there be more, here at the Platinum Palace?" they wondered.

One class was going on in the activity area. John and Yvette both went in as an upbeat staff member led a crafts project. At first glance, it was hard for them to see what was going on, but then they understood. The residents were busy gluing sequins and decorations on fly swatters! They both walked away in silence, not sure whether to be shocked or amused by such a silly thing. "Mom certainly wouldn't give that the time of day," Yvette said.

They continued their tour and saw residents sitting around, some by themselves, doing nothing. The residents reached out to John and Yvette, wanting some human contact. John and Yvette both did their best to talk with them and touch and shake hands as they went down the hallway. "I'm feeling a bit sad right now," John said. "Me, too," replied Yvette.

They turned the corner and saw a lovely garden area. It was a beautiful day, and the flowers and fountains were inviting. "Where is everybody?" Yvette and John asked almost simultaneously. It seemed strange that the staff and residents were not using the gardens on such a nice day.

"Look—there's an exit," John said. "Let's get out of here. It's a beautiful place, but I think your mom would be bored here."

Feeling let down and frustrated, they decided to take a walk in the neighborhood and came across a small building. A sign said "Pretty Pennies Home." Curious, they walked through a door in a basement to find a simple, clean, well-lit space. It looked like the main residence was on the first and second floors with an activity room in the basement.

In the activity room, they found some sturdy chairs and folding tables. The activity calendar was posted on a dry-erase board that was hanging, a bit crooked, on the wall. There was too much on it to read at first glance.

There were about 15 residents in the room. "Look at that!" Yvette observed. To her left, one group was arranging flowers. They noticed another group had just set off for a walk, and a third group was looking at a collection of old photographs. A bulletin board showed off a project that apparently had been done the previous week—paper making and the creation of holiday greeting cards using the paper. A man who seemed to be a volunteer or family member was proudly playing with a golf putter, letting those present hold it one at a time. One resident was sweeping the floor.

Although some participants were sitting by themselves, John and Yvette could not help but notice that every few minutes a staff member would come up to the older adults, show them something, tell a funny story, or even just hold their hands for a little while. It seemed like nobody was lonely or sad. Yvette said, "John, let's stay here for awhile. It's not fancy, but I like this place. Maybe Mom should move in here!"

A dementia program can be put together with "platinum" or with "pennies." Obviously, resources can help build a more desirable, dementia-friendly environment, enhance marketing, attract staff with more experience and qualifications, and improve programming. Yet many adult day center programs thrive on fewer resources in church basements; good care can take place in a palace or in a modest home.

The Platinum Palace probably had well-intentioned, caring staff, yet more attention was put into the environment than into the programming. The activities listed on its calendar were, in general, not ones that mirrored everyday life. The crafts activity was suspect, even demeaning—would most families really be happy to see a decorated fly swatter or use it? There seemed to be little individualization. A wonderful garden space was underused. Residents who were desperate for one-to-one attention seemed to have their needs unmet.

The Pretty Pennies Home seemed to be getting things right. Individual attention was given, accompanied by fun and meaningful activities. The arts-and-crafts project (paper and card making) had a purpose. The residents were going outside. The resident who was sweeping was doing a meaningful chore. Pretty Pennies seemed to be a community of friends, enjoying their time together, being together.

An Activity Philosophy

The Best Friends program leader recognizes the importance of having a well-defined program philosophy underlying the activity program. The philosophy outlined in this chapter suggests that long-term care program activities should reflect everyday life as much as possible. Individualized activities are given as much attention as group activities. All staff participate in activities and are encouraged to bring their own interests to work. As stated at the beginning of this chapter, activities, like friendship, should be about playing together, working together, and being together.

Purpose of Activities

Activities are part of everyone's life. They serve a variety of purposes for all of us, but for *persons* with dementia, a rich and varied activity program can serve the following purposes:

- To socialize or to be with others—Most *persons* thrive on being with others in social settings, particularly in small groups and structured environments. If *persons* become isolated, then depression can easily occur; activities can prevent or diminish this sense of loneliness and despair.
- To be productive or to contribute—*Persons* need to feel that they are contributing something to the lives of the people around them. Good-quality dementia care programs may ask a homemaker to help set a table or ask a carpenter to help hang a painting. This helps the *person* to feel competent and useful.
- To experience success—Activities can help *persons* feel accomplished and successful. Even something as simple as successfully throwing a ball into a basket, passing out napkins, or tossing a ringer in a game of horseshoes helps *persons* feel good about themselves.
- To play—As children, play dominates our lives. After we become adults, however, many of us move away from this important and necessary part of life. *Persons* with Alzheimer's disease can experience joy in returning to simpler times.
- To build and retain skills—Activities can help *persons* practice and retain old, learned skills as long as possible, such as planting bulbs, playing musical instruments, playing simple card games, working puzzles, reading aloud, counting, and singing.
- To have a sense of control—Anger often stems from the loss of control that comes with developing dementia. Activities can help *persons* feel empowered and in charge of their world.

- To fill a religious or spiritual need—Activities should address the religious traditions and rituals of *persons* who are part of a faith community. Prayers, hymns, readings, and services all can support these religious beliefs. The arts, nature, music, and even volunteering to help others can fulfill spiritual needs.
- To experience growth and learning—Even though *persons* may not be able to retain most new information, they can enjoy the experience of being presented new material. This evokes in *persons* rituals of the schoolroom and provides intellectual stimulation and a sense of growth and accomplishment.

Let's look at the key concepts for Best Friends activities.

The Art of Activities Is Not in What Is Done; It Is in the Doing

Best Friends staff members understand that the process is always more important than the end result. When folding towels involves smiles, conversation, and friendly gossip, it should not matter whether the towels have perfect edges. For this reason, activity guides that contain detailed lists or steps on how to do even a simple activity such as singing ("hand out song books," then "open books," then "start singing") miss the point; any staff member who needs this level of detail in the instructions will surely fail. The following example demonstrates that the art of activities is in the doing:

One beautiful autumn day, participants and volunteers at the Helping Hand Day Center decided to take a walk while the changeable Kentucky weather was still cooperating. A volunteer walking with her Best Friend was hoping to get some exercise, but after only a few steps, the program participant stopped cold in his tracks to watch painters working on scaffolding along the walls of the church in which the Helping Hand program is located. A retired handyman, the participant watched the work in progress, fascinated by what the workmen were doing. He began counting the windows being painted, trying to estimate the cost and scope of the job. The volunteer was at first disappointed to miss their walk, but she enjoyed seeing her Best Friend count and recount the windows. The participant still got a workout, but it was mental instead of physical.

The volunteer recognized that the journey was more important than the final destination.

Activities Should Be Individualized and Tap into a *Person's* Past Interests and Skills

Best Friends staff members accept the challenge of individualizing care. With the creative use of volunteers and with staff's knowing each *person's* life story, individual attention can be given. Thus, artists should be encouraged to continue painting. Farmers can still tend gardens. An accountant can help balance figures. All of these activities can build self-esteem and promote high-quality care.

A participant at Toca das Horttensias is a retired plastic surgeon who was dedicated to helping poor children. He owned a farm where he grew vegetables and trees, and he often took children from the hospital to visit the farm. Now, when he gets sad, walks in the center's vegetable garden and among the mulberry trees, and visits from the children in the nearby social center cheer him up.

Staff used their knowledge of this participant's life story and personal values to evoke his memories of contributing to society and helping others (see Tool 9.4). They also knew that for this doctor, communing with nature and visiting with children renewed his spirit.

Hannah Herward, the administrator at Eden Pines, believes that individualized activities are particularly important for men. She developed specific programs that men traditionally enjoy, such as woodworking, talking about sports, visiting an antique car club, and discussing hunting and fishing.

Because many older men have not traditionally participated in group activities, Herward's individualized approach is especially effective.

Activities Should Be Adult in Nature

Best Friends staff members know that *persons* retain a sense of their past lives. Often, treating *persons* with Alzheimer's as children proves disastrous because it is perceived by them as demeaning. Some with Alzheimer's disease do respond to children's toys, such as dolls, but this should never be the starting point for programming. Here is a good example of an activity with a rewarding purpose:

The Riverside Adult Day Program has a partnership with the local Humane Society. The society brings pets to the facility to interact with the participants. The day program makes bone-shaped dog biscuits that are given as complimentary gifts when someone adopts a dog from the Humane Society. Everyone can participate in this project on some level, regardless of his or her functional ability. Some persons *can only poke holes in the biscuits, but even this is an important step in the process. They enjoy putting the finishing touches on the product.*

The idea of creating a product, having a *person's* work lead to a productive purpose, lends importance and a feeling of satisfaction to the biscuit-making activity. Sometimes the dogs come by the center to express their appreciation!

Activities Should Include Pets and Other Animals

Best Friends staff members recognize that pets can provide unconditional love. Although not every pet is appropriate for *persons* with dementia, especially animals that are overactive or aggressive, a gentle dog or an affectionate cat can bring joy to *persons* with dementia and can also be fun for staff (see Figure 9.1). They also can contribute to a more meaningful activity program by giving *persons* a sense of responsibility (e.g., brushing or walking a dog, feeding a cat or fish, watching for eggs to hatch in an aviary). Some problems must be acknowledged, including the cost of maintaining animals and that some *persons* may not like or be comfortable around animals.

A former movie star lives at Villa Bella Residential Alzheimer's Care, Santa Barbara, California. Cash, a cat, has acted in numerous movies and television commercials. Although he is rather independent, he is still a hit among most of the residents, who enjoy petting him and watching him strut around the campus. According to the administrator, Tom Henry, pets are welcome visitors, and many families will bring in their dogs to visit the residents.

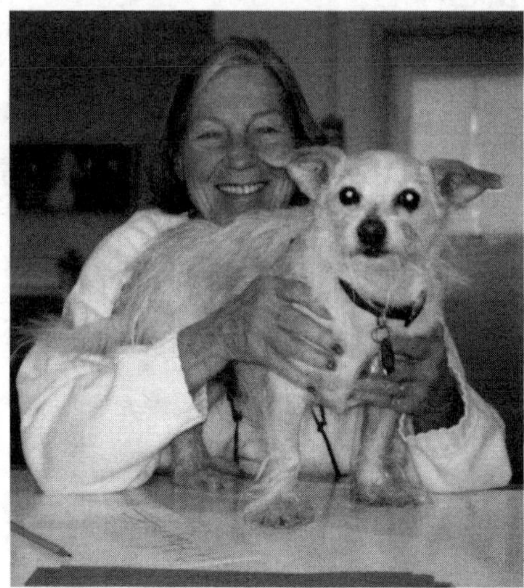

Figure 9.1. Volunteer Jane Owen with her dog, Henry, ready to interact with participants at the Helping Hand Day Center, Lexington, Kentucky.

Activities Should Recall a *Person's* Work-Related Past

Best Friends staff members recognize that most individuals with dementia are from a generation that shares a strong work ethic. Work-related activities are, in general, very successful and build pride and self-esteem. Activities also can be enhanced when the *person* feels that he or she serves some function or is helping others (e.g., getting a job or chores done, doing something for children or charity). Some day centers, for example, encourage families to tell their loved ones that they are going to class or to work; in a sense this is true in that effective day center programs have learning activities and "work" for participants.

At the Riverside Adult Day Program, residents wind a beautiful grandfather clock once a week, feed the goldfish, and take part in the care of plants in the garden. It makes the day program a caring, homey, "feel-good" place to be.

Doing chores around Riverside such as the ones described help participants believe that it is their home away from home. Staff can gently encourage a resident who is sad, for example, to "help around the house." Such an activity can change sadness to happiness.

Some programs show great flexibility in their willingness to accommodate family needs, as in the following case:

Vista del Monte Retirement Community in Santa Barbara, California, welcomed one resident's large executive desk when he was admitted to Pinegrove Special Care, its 10-bed special care residence. Although the desk fills much of the room, it gives the resident comfort when he is there.

Although the resident spends much of his time outside his room, the desk provides an endless source of ideas for activities, such as sorting mail and rolling coins. The staff encourage him to work on projects at his desk, just as he had for many years prior to joining the Pinegrove family.

Activities Should Stimulate the Five Senses

Best Friends staff members realize that stimulating *persons'* five senses (sight, hearing, taste, touch, and smell) keeps them connected to the physical world. Although age or infirmity diminishes some of the senses, many remain strong. For example, gardening can involve touching rich soil, seeing beautiful colors, smelling flowers, tasting vegetables or herbs, and hearing birds and insects.

The Fountains' Gourmet Club decided to make an apple pie. There was lots of laughter and conversation as they mixed the dough, peeled the apples, and measured the sugar. The feel of the dough, the color of the apples, the smell of the pie baking, and the taste of the warm apple pie stimulated all of the senses. As he enjoyed his slice of pie, one resident said, "This has been a happy day."

This activity produced rich rewards for all involved. If local licensing or health regulations discourage this kind of group cooking activity, then just the smell of a store-bought pie baking in the oven and the taste of the baked pie afterward can produce similar results.

Doing Nothing Is Actually Doing Something

Best Friends staff members know that good friends enjoy quiet times together. We do not always have to be busy or doing things. Just sitting outside on a bench in a garden or looking out a window watching the world go by can be an enjoyable activity for a *person*. Everyday life contains plenty of quiet moments, and long-term care should reflect this reality.

Cheri Taylor believes that holding a hand, touching a shoulder, or just sitting close is the most effective way to be a friend.

Being totally present for another *person* may be the best activity of all.

Leslie Congleton told the authors, "It is very important to provide quiet times of reflection in addition to outward socialization. So often professionals who are involved with providing activities for individuals with dementia focus on the outward, social, upbeat party times and neglect the thirst that each of us has for quiet inward times."

A good way to make this point with staff is to ask them how they spend their days off. Many will have spent time doing chores, sleeping, engaging in sports, shopping, visiting friends, or taking a trip, but many will say that their greatest pleasure stems from "doing nothing." Staff can be asked to talk about why doing the latter is sometimes just as important as doing the former.

Activities Should Tap into Remaining Physical Skills

Best Friends staff members encourage the *person* with dementia to remain physically robust. Activities that keep a *person* physically active should be encouraged, including those that stimulate eye–hand coordination and promote exercise. In this day of workouts and an obsession with fitness, the odds are high that many staff will enjoy taking walks and being physically active with a fit *person.*

The Memory Walk is a fund-raising event for Alzheimer's Association chapters throughout the United States. The Memory Walk coordinator in Santa Barbara, California, Dianne Timmerman, said that it is particularly meaningful to her that in addition to community members and caregivers, many persons *with Alzheimer's disease participate. "One man in Santa Barbara helps set up chairs and tables; another asks his Rotary Club for help. They all seem to get satisfaction from helping, as well as pleasure from being out-of-doors walking and enjoying the day."*

Even rather frail *persons* get caught up in the spirit of the day and do part or all of the Memory Walk. They also gain a sense of accomplishment and pride in helping a local charity continue its work.

Give staff permission to be creative.

—Joanne Rader, dementia care consultant and Associate Professor, Oregon Health Sciences University, School of Nursing, Portland, Oregon

We build our program around the gifts and talents of our staff.

—Rosemarie Harris, Program Director, Pinegrove Special Care, Vista del Monte retirement community, Santa Barbara, California

When the Omahanui Private Hospital began having trouble with sundowning, we thought of activities that might help reduce this problem. The problem seemed particularly acute among our male residents, who were harder to engage in meaningful activities late in the day. We decided to try using a stationary car and quickly found one with a sound body—no rust or sharp edges—and a tidy interior. A storage shed was

Activities Usually Are Initiated by Others

Best Friends staff members understand that *persons* with Alzheimer's disease may lose the ability to initiate activities. As one caregiver once told us, *persons* seem to have lost their "start button." They often need staff to model the activity or to show them the first step. An artist, for example, may still enjoy painting, but someone may have to hand him the brush and cue him about how to dip the brush in paint and stroke the canvas. Often, this extra push is all that is needed to make an activity a success.

The life story of a resident at The Fountains described how she loved to play the piano but had not done so for some time. When a staff member encouraged her to sit down at the piano, nothing happened at first. The staff member placed the person's *fingers on the keys and gently pressed down. Incredibly, the resident started playing again. A caregiver with knack helped her reclaim a favorite passion.*

Alzheimer's disease creates many paradoxes. In the case of the resident of The Fountains, she may not have been able to learn even a simple new song, but she could remember a complicated old one. Gentle cues brought back an old skill.

Activities Should Be Voluntary

Best Friends staff members know that most of us will rebel against things that we do not want to do. The same is true of *persons* with Alzheimer's disease, who will opt out of activities that do not interest them. Staff should always encourage participation in activities, however. Often if an activity is started in front of the *person*, or if a staff member asks for help, *persons* will join in.

Everyone Can Still Engage in Some Form of Activity

Best Friends staff members never exclude any *person* from the activity program. In her book *Care That Works*, Jitka M. Zgola provided an effective tool for reviewing this issue, which she calls "activity grading." She used the example of cookie baking and demonstrated that everyone can take part in similar activities. Some *persons* may be able to participate in all levels of the activity, what Zgola described as an "independent organizer-doer," a higher-level grading. Others who are more impaired may be at the lower level of grading, an "observer-critic" (tastes cookies) or "observer" (watches and listens). This inverted pyramid of activities drives home the point that all can participate. (See Tool 9.6 for more information about activity grading.)

The Helping Hand Day Center offers paper making as an activity. Some participants become deeply involved in the whole process, including cleaning, pounding, and brushing. Others are only able to dip the frames into the water solution. Some pat the moisture out. Everyone can see or touch the final product and feel a sense of pride.

This type of activity not only has meaning and purpose (creating a usable product) but also is one that everyone can enjoy.

built for it in our beautiful fenced back garden, with a workbench with cleaning cloths and buckets. The wipers, horns, lights, and indicators all work. The battery is regularly charged by our maintenance manager to ensure that this activity continues. Now our men get in the car, "drive" home to Omahanui from "work," and then sit down to enjoy the happy hour that we have every evening before dinner. The car is also a focal point for chores such as washing it and waxing it.

—Patricia Wesley, Administrator, Omahanui Private Hospital, New Plymouth, New Zealand

A wide range of music will promote a higher degree of involvement for a group of diverse persons with dementia.

—Leslie Congleton, Program Coordinator, Legacy Health Systems, Trinity Place Alzheimer's Day Respite Program, Portland, Oregon

I was soon to be married, and the other activity staff at Wellington Parc put together a surprise bridal shower for me as an activity. They provided each lady with a gift to wrap and to give to me at the shower. As I opened each gift, a few of the ladies could identify the gift they wrapped. I could tell they felt good about themselves and were excited to be at a bridal shower. Some said they had not been at one in years. I decided to send invitations to the ladies who I knew could attend my wedding. When the day came, the ushers seated them in the third row (after my attendants and parents). I remember being at the altar, looking out and seeing the ladies smiling and waving at me.

After the wedding, the photographer took our picture together. I gave them a picture to recall the special occasion which they were a part of for me. Upon returning to work, a few of the ladies remembered the wedding. They had kept the satin roses filled with birdseed. One resident called me by name and said she really enjoyed the wedding. Tears filled my eyes. When you work with

Intergenerational Activities Are Especially Desirable

Best Friends staff members encourage intergenerational activities. Children and high school and college students can add sparkle to a program and bring smiles to the faces of many *persons.* High school and college students also make excellent volunteers. They may not live close to their grandparents and thus may benefit from relationships with older *persons* and the unconditional love they give, as in the following example:

At the Haven Nursing Center in Columbia, Louisiana, the philosophy of Best Friends includes having children visit the facility. They come daily bringing pictures they have colored, take part in activities, and walk and even eat an occasional meal with the residents. The administrator, Jennifer Raeis, noted, "The residents have filled a void in the children's [lives] and the children in theirs."

When children work closely with *persons* in an activity, almost anything is possible. Many *persons* who would not normally engage in crafts, for example, will do them with children because the task seems more appropriate.

Activities that We Think Will Never Work Sometimes Do

Best Friends staff members recognize that risk is a part of life. Activities that are too conservative may end up being staid and boring. Trying new activities might lead to some misfires or disappointments, but usually the *person* and staff can recover quickly.

Staff at The Fountains asked a group of residents to help with the monthly newsletter of the Alzheimer's Association. "We did not know if this would work, but, to our surprise, they loved the drive to the office, folded and stapled hundreds of newsletters, and enjoyed a bag lunch with other volunteers and had a great time!" noted Diane Will.

This was rewarding for all concerned. Some staff thought it would not work, but the residents did a good job with the task. Other groups around the United States have involved *persons* with dementia in similar activities.

Participants at Legacy St. Aidan's Place Daycare, in Portland, Oregon, were busily examining seashells of various shapes and colors and reminiscing about the Oregon coast and seashore. Following a demonstration by the leader, the participants began making repeat pattern designs on colorful paper by tracing around the shells. Forty minutes later, a long time for such a formal activity, the group broke for a snack. Much to the amazement of the leader, some left the snack time early to return to their work.

Persons still have the capacity to try new things. Too often we make a decision for them that they would not be interested or that the activity would not work.

Activities Should Appeal to the Staff as Well as to the *Person*

Best Friends staff members are an integral part of the activity program. They understand that usually *persons* can sense whether the staff members are really challenged, excited, or satisfied doing an activity with them. Thus, program leaders should strive to develop activity programs that appeal to staff as well as to participants. They also should develop activity programs with variety; even a successful activity will become stale if repeated too often.

A volunteer and a participant in the Helping Hand Day Center have something in common: Both are authors. They talk at length about the joys and concerns of writing a book. They also look at each other's books and laugh and talk about the pictures and stories. Their friendship is strengthened by their common interests.

A volunteer Best Friend's enthusiasm and passion for writing is infectious. It brings out the best in the participant and the volunteer.

Personal Care Is an Activity

When Best Friends staff members redefine personal care as an activity, it can actually help complete these sometimes difficult tasks more easily. For example, staff with knack tell a funny story, ask the resident about his or her family, or sing a song to ease a *person's* anxiety before a bath.

Joanne Rader, associate professor, School of Nursing, Oregon Health Sciences University, Portland, is a pioneer in developing

persons with Alzheimer's disease, it's rare that someone can call you by name. It was then that I knew how special they felt being a part of my wedding and life.
—Stephanie K. Wilkerson, Medical Records Director, Wellington Parc of Owensboro, Owensboro, Kentucky

Structure is important, but the energy surrounding spontaneity is also important. We try to follow the Best Friends approach to activities by making everything an activity.
—Gayle Pennington, Program Director, Riverside Adult Day Program, Wilmington, Delaware

One joy scatters a hundred griefs.
—Chinese proverb

I'd rather one should walk with me than merely tell me the way.
—Edgar A. Guest

Actions speak louder than words.
—Old saying

I don't like the way you are feeding my Best Friend.
—One staff member to another, Serenity Nursing Home, Johannesburg, South Africa

more humane bathing programs and bathing philosophies. As a nurse working in long-term care, she arranged for CNAs to bathe her so that she could better understand how frightening and difficult an experience like this could be for a resident with dementia. She argues that a comfortable, homelike environment and caring staff can turn this daunting task into a more pleasant, successful experience:

"When it is suggested that staff arrange to be bathed in their own facility, they often refuse and are shocked, stating that it would be too embarrassing. Even thinking about that possibility helps them understand the need to change the focus of the bath from a task to do to someone to creating a pleasant activity to share with someone."

At Encore Senior Living Rediscovery™ Program, ADLs are listed on the activity calendar so that it reinforces their inclusion as part of each resident's life-enhancement program.

A Best Friends program embraces everyday personal care tasks as meaningful and productive activities (see Tool 9.7).

Activities Can Be Short in Duration

Best Friends staff realize that the *person's* attention span may be diminished as a result of his or her dementia. It can be difficult, therefore, for the *person* to participate in extended activities. Programs should embrace brief activities (see Tool 9.5) because these actions or tasks, repeated throughout the day, can accumulate to create a much larger impact, greatly enriching a *person's* life. Activities can be done in as little as 30 seconds; examples include showing a picture, smelling a fragrance, and applying hand lotion. One caregiver showed what can be done in 15 minutes:

Cindy Lynch, a dementia care consultant in New Concord, Kentucky, created a list of 15-minute Best Friends activities to do with her grandmother, who lives in a long-term care community. The list includes reading aloud, watching birds and squirrels outside the window, and visiting a wheelchair-accessible garden. (See Tool 9.2.)

Lynch cleverly posted the list for her grandmother's friends and family to see when they visit. This guidance makes their visit much more enjoyable and encourages return visits. One interesting aspect of Lynch's approach is that she asks staff and visitors to make a short note in a log about when they visited and what activity they did. She can now keep up with her grandmother's visitors and thank them for their attention and time.

Activities Can Happen Day or Night

Best Friends staff allow activities to happen at any time. Usually they take place during the daytime or early evening hours, but sometimes a *person* wants to get up and do something late at night. A good program accommodates this desire, and staff will make themselves available to the *person* when he or she needs them. One common problem in programs is the lack of after-dinner and evening activities.

Pinegrove Special Care at Vista del Monte has a full complement of evening and weekend activities for its residents, in addition to a full daytime program. Rosemarie Harris, program director, noted, "We want these times to look just like the weekday programs—active and alive!"

Some programs try to explain their lack of evening activities with the argument that *persons* "don't want this," or that they are "ready for bed." In fact, the reason why many are ready to sleep is boredom and lack of stimulation. Residents get up during the night because they went to bed too early. Pinegrove staff try to be flexible and support the residents' needs, not staff's convenience.

Activities Can Fill a Spiritual Need

Best Friends staff members recognize that every *person* with dementia has a spirit and that activities can nurture this spirit. When a *person* feels that he or she is helping another, this nourishes the spirit. When a *person* successfully completes a painting or poem, this nourishes the spirit. When staff members successfully share part of themselves with *persons,* this nourishes their spirits. When the *person* is part of a faith community, familiar religious traditions and rituals may be particularly helpful in meeting the *person's* need to be connected to God/a higher power, as in this example from Cheri Taylor, the executive director of Porterville Senior Day Care:

Spirituality is an important part of our program. Making get well and birthday cards for the local convalescent hospital fulfills a spiritual need of helping others. Familiar prayers, readings, and hymns of faith fulfill a spiritual need of connectedness for others who have been a part of a religious faith.

Activities can help *persons* feel connected to others and to their purpose for being part of this world.

Dorothy Seman, clinical coordinator of the Alzheimer's Family Care Center in Chicago, offers another example of activities filling a spiritual need:

When Anna, a vital member of a day center program, died suddenly at home, members of her group were surprised and struggled, as all of us might, to come to terms with her death. A staff member wondered whether we, as a group, would want to write a letter of condolence, reflecting the thoughts of Anna's friends. Some members of the group wrote their own message on the condolence card; others accepted the staff's offer to write their words and feelings as they were spoken. This beautiful tribute to Anna was given to her family by staff who attended her wake later that week. Anna's family was touched by the gesture as well as by the warm and genuine sentiments conveyed by those words.

Celebration of life and relationships and the expression of loss are felt along the full continuum of life. Sometimes one needs only to be asked to reveal what lies just below the surface.

Activities Are Everywhere

Best Friends staff can truly make something out of nothing. They can use items from a room, pictures from a magazine, even the weather for topics of discussion and doing things. Figure 9.2

20 Things to Do with a Colorful Scarf

1. Practice fly fishing.
2. Use it to substitute for a dance partner.
3. Talk about the color and design.
4. Practice nautical knots.
5. Turn it into a halter-top.
6. Try to figure out what country it's from.
7. Discuss how it could have been made.
8. Discuss and feel the fabric.
9. Try to name as many other fabrics as you can.
10. Cover your head to enter a sacred place.
11. Enjoy a risqué fan dance!
12. Model different ways to wear the scarf.
13. Use for S.O.S., flagging down a passing car.
14. Discuss the origin of the word *scarf.*
15. Guess its length.
16. Draw or paint a picture of it.
17. Imagine who might have bought it and worn it.
18. Guess how much it might have cost.
19. Use it as an arm sling.
20. Use it as a shawl to keep warm.

Figure 9.2.

lists activities that can be done with a simple scarf. Staff members do not need elaborate materials and supplies for an activity program.

One day a staff member at Legacy St. Aidan's Place Daycare asked the group to look at the chairs that they were sitting on. A wide-ranging discussion ensued about favorite chairs. One woman started talking about a chair that her father always sat in. She told the group with some humor, "No one else was ever allowed to sit in his chair." After much reminiscing, a game of musical chairs was enjoyed by all.

This staff member creatively looked around the room and made the most of what was there. Participants could not only reminisce but they also could take note of the texture of the chair fabric, the colors, and the overall comfort of the chairs. Finally, even music and play were involved in this fun, spontaneous activity. (See Tool 9.10 for Legacy St. Aidan's Place's list "Activities Are Everywhere.")

Conclusion

Staff with knack realize that there is no such thing as failure-free activities. If we did nothing, then we would never fail. Yet, in life it is hard to experience success without having also tasted failure. Success comes from innovating and taking chances. Best Friends programs realize this and are always innovative in the area of activities. Some activities will succeed beyond all hope; others will fail miserably. When failure occurs, what is important is how staff and volunteers deal with it. If they are relaxed and capable of joking when an elaborate pâpier maché sculpture collapses, then residents and participants will join in the laughter. Staff who become upset when cookies get burned or singing is off key do not belong in dementia care.

Best Friends program activities break the mold. The programs deemphasize a regular diet of games such as bingo and crafts without meaning (e.g., decorating a fly swatter) to make the program more reflective of daily life. They make activities out of ordinary chores and routines. They keep the *person* busy, challenged, and involved. They help reduce wandering and agitation and other challenging behaviors. They keep the *person* involved in life.

Best Friends programs also encourage staff to bring their interests, hobbies, and passions into the program (see Tool 9.9). When they do, staff seem to have as much fun as *persons*. When staff members can bring their interests to work, it helps change the culture of a workplace and builds a sense of community.

The ultimate question that the authors ask program administrators who are concerned about activities is this: If you were to break your ankle and you had to live in your facility for 1 month, would the activities keep you fully engaged? Hopefully, they would. If they would not, then it is time to embrace the Best Friends way.

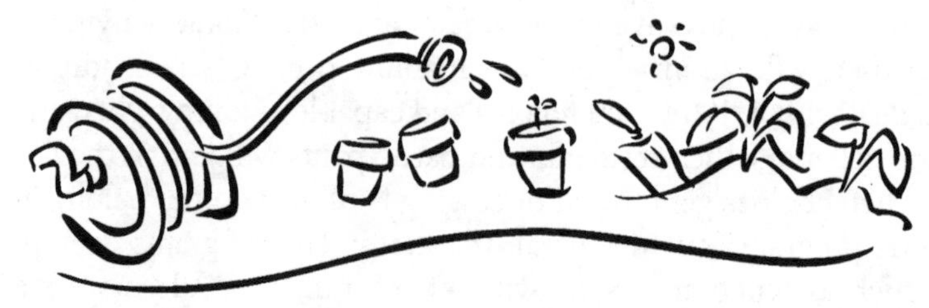

Training Tool Kit

Tool 9.0 / Warm-Up
The Best Friends Improv

Almost any item can be used for an activity. Activities are everywhere!

Take a look at various objects around your house, basement, attic, or office. Try to find 10–12 objects to bring to the staff meeting. They should include a few everyday items (e.g., coffee cups, hats) as well as some unusual items (e.g., cowbell, unusual seashell, belt buckle). Ideas include:

Old pictures	Postcards
Flat iron	Apples
Ugly necktie	Teapot
Road map	

At the meeting, ask the staff to break up into three or four groups. Give each group several items and ask them to come up with as many activity ideas as possible in 10 minutes.

After 10 minutes, use a board to list all of the ideas. Have fun in the process; let the staff act out or demonstrate ideas.

Variation: Invite a group of three or four staff members to sit at the front of the class and give them the objects, one at a time. Let them brainstorm or demonstrate potential activities.

Variation: Put items in a box, and ask a staff member to reach into the box and pull something out. Then ask him or her to brainstorm ideas for activities. The class can help. Ask the class how many of these activities could be done with residents or participants and whether they have items that could be brought in for use in activities.

Tool 9.1 / Games for Learning
Teaching Reminiscence

This exercise helps staff begin to learn and practice the technique of reminiscence. Reminiscence works well because Alzheimer's disease takes its toll on short-term memory, while leaving many longer-term memories intact. One way to get younger staff members interested in reminiscence is to practice it using people, items, and events from their immediate pasts (e.g., 1960s, 1970s, 1980s). Go to a thrift store for props or ask your friends to help.

Here are some ideas for you to consider for your staff:

Captain Kangaroo	*M*A*S*H* (television show)
The Beatles	Landing on the moon
Disco music	Ronald Reagan
Bell-bottom pants	Cabbage Patch dolls
Tie-dyed t-shirts	Nintendo games
John F. Kennedy	Martin Luther King

As you display or talk about these people, events, or items, ask staff what they remember about them. Did they ever own any of the items? What memories do they have about the events or people?

What similar objects or events would evoke memories for the *persons* for whom you care?

Variation: Ask staff what they remember about the decade that is common to most of them—ideally, when most staff were teenagers. List their memories on a chalkboard or flipchart, and have fun reminiscing.

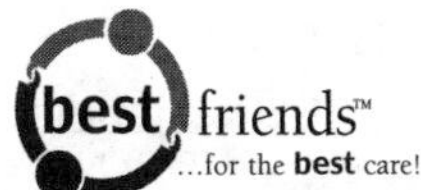

Tool 9.2 / Program Pointer
Activities for Grandmother

Cindy Lynch prepared the following list of 15-minute-long activities for her grandmother, who lives in a long-term care community. It is posted in her grandmother's room. Share this list with staff. Ask them to suggest other 15-minute activities for residents or participants in their programs.

Assign staff to engage in one 15-minute activity each day with a resident or participant. See how this Best Friends approach adds richness to your program's day.

Wanted: Best Friends Who Will Spend 15 Minutes to Help Me Enjoy . . .

Rocking in my rocking chair
Reading aloud
Combing my hair or polishing my nails
Sharing dessert and a cup of coffee
Watching birds and squirrels that live outside my window
Watching and helping someone do chores like dusting or mending a sweater
Visiting a wheelchair-accessible garden
Looking closely at an indoor garden
Looking at the pretty fish in an aquarium
Listening to my favorite music or nature sounds on the tape player
Providing an update on my favorite sports team or happenings around town
Experimenting with art materials
Making cookies or brownies from a mix
Looking at family pictures and postcards in my photo album
Visiting with pets
Watching the sky at sunset
Choosing fabric for specially adapted clothing or for slipcovers for my bedrail cushions
Watching an old TV show, a movie, or a cartoon
Looking at beautiful photographs of nature and of people's faces

Cindy Lynch is a dementia care consultant and researcher in New Concord, Kentucky.

Tool 9.3 / Program Pointer
Worksheet for Activity Ideas and Planning

Ask staff to complete this worksheet in a class setting or care plan meeting.

How would you help *persons* to:

Feel more productive or independent?

Feel that they have more choices?

Maintain abilities, skills, or memories?

Share feelings and express emotions (laughter, sadness, joy, frustration, anger)?

Keep physically active?

Use their senses (touch, sight, movement, hearing, taste, smell)?

Feel connected to the larger community (family, friends, current events)?

Express their spirituality (through ritual, nature, religious, and nonreligious traditions)?

Adapted from a form created by Leslie Congleton, Program Coodinator, Legacy Health Systems, Trinity Place Alzheimer's Day Respite Program, Portland, Oregon.

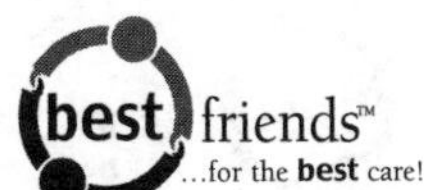

Tool 9.4 / Games for Learning
Make a Connection

This valuable exercise helps staff make the connection between the life story and activities.

Take facts from a sample life story from your facility or write a life story. You can use the sample facts below as well. Give them to staff and ask them (as a large group or in smaller groups) to brainstorm activity ideas that flow from this *person's* life story. Are there some that should be avoided? Is there an obvious source of potential volunteers who might consider being a Best Friend to this *person?*

Sample Facts from a Life Story: Virginia Smith

Dislikes busy work, things that are too silly

Volunteered during World War II as a USO entertainer

Lived in New York City all of her life

Is serious and full of strong opinions

Is Catholic and still attends Mass

Is artistic

Was married to a famous jazz musician

Speaks fluent French

Loves almost every kind of food but hates vegetables

Doesn't like children (did not have any) but loves animals

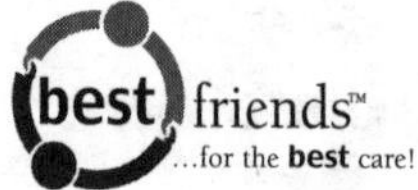

Tool 9.5 / Program Pointer

30 More Things to Do in 30 Seconds or Less*

Post this list on bulletin boards, include it in newsletters, or distribute it as a handout to discuss with staff. Note that an activity need not take a lot of time.

1. Whistle
2. Comb someone's hair
3. Give a comforting hug
4. Show a funny toy
5. Hum a tune
6. Feel a flower petal
7. Blow a kiss
8. Smell a fragrance together
9. Look at clouds in the sky
10. Demonstrate a jumping jack
11. Hold hands
12. Address someone by his or her full name
13. Make up a funny rhyme
14. Yodel
15. Spell someone's name
16. Give a compliment about someone's dress/appearance
17. Plant a kiss on the forehead
18. Show a funny drawing or cartoon
19. Sit next to someone for 30 seconds
20. Make a funny face
21. Wave to the *person,* or together wave at someone passing by
22. Comment on a piece of jewelry
23. Compare neckties
24. Ask for an opinion: "Do my shoes need shining?"
25. Blow a bubble with bubble gum
26. Straighten out a crooked picture on the wall
27. Play a tune on a mouth harp
28. Recite a poem
29. Show pictures of your children or pets
30. Taste a piece of fruit or candy

Variation: Work in small groups and ask staff to come up with their own lists of 30 activities to do in 30 seconds.

---

*The original "30 Things to Do in 30 Seconds or Less" appeared in *The Best Friends Approach to Alzheimer's Care.*

Tool 9.6 / Program Pointer
Activity Grading—Baking Cookies

Activity grading is the process of breaking down an activity to accommodate the abilities of any individual who is interested in participating. Discuss this valuable tool at your care planning meetings. This chart can be used to match persons with Alzheimer's disease to appropriate activities. It is not meant to be a rigid scoring system. Instead, it is designed to encourage programs always to find a way to involve persons in activities. Whether they are at the top or the bottom of the scale, there is always a way to include persons with Alzheimer's disease in an activity.

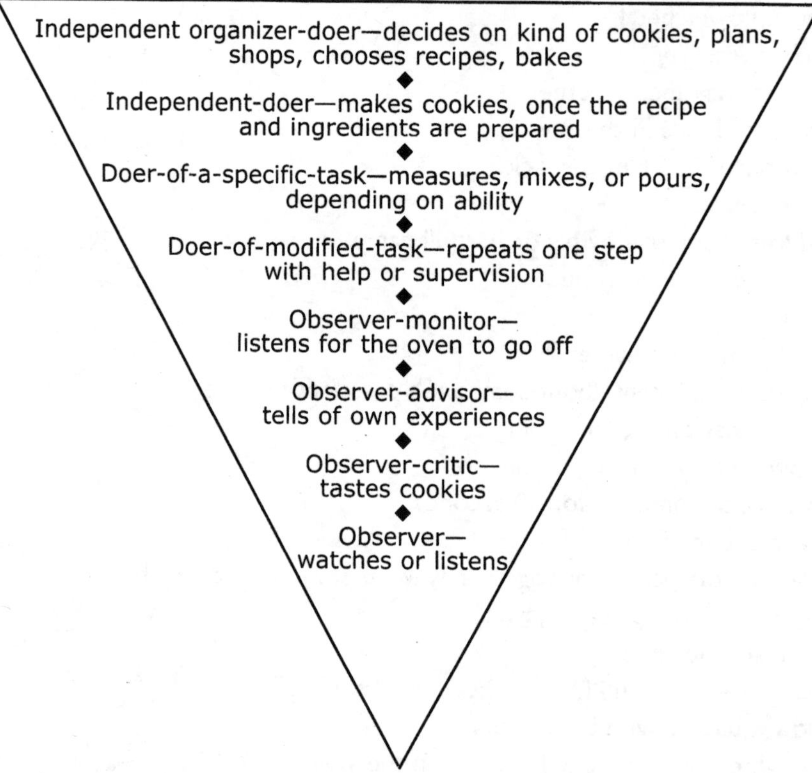

From Zgola, J.M. (1999). Care that works: A relationship approach to persons with dementia *(p. 177). Baltimore: The Johns Hopkins University Press; reprinted by permission.*

Tool 9.7 / Program Pointer
Personal Care as an Activity

This activity can help staff be less task oriented and more person *oriented.*

Ask staff to break into small groups and use this list to come up with as many ideas as possible on how to turn each personal care task or daily activity into a Best Friends activity. Cue them about the Best Friends model (i.e., are we here just to complete the task or to help the person?).

Dressing can be: ______________________________

Brushing teeth can be: ______________________________

Combing hair can be: ______________________________

Even toileting can be: ______________________________

Applying makeup can be: ______________________________

Getting a manicure can be: ______________________________

Getting a massage can be: ______________________________

Eating a meal can be: ______________________________

Going to bed can be: ______________________________

Taking a bath can be: ______________________________

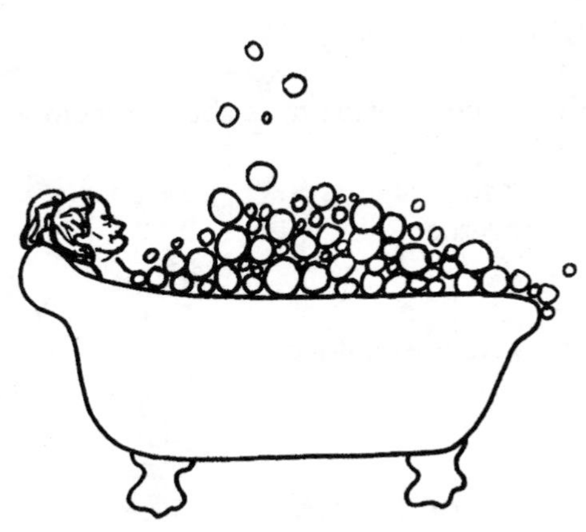

Tool 9.8 / Program Pointer
101 Things to Do

1. Clip coupons
2. Sort poker chips
3. Count tickets
4. Rake leaves
5. Vacuum
6. Look up names in a phone book
7. Bake cookies
8. Read the daily paper aloud
9. Ask a friend with a baby or a young child to visit
10. Read a relative's letter aloud
11. Listen to relaxing or favorite music
12. Plant seeds
13. Look at family photos
14. Toss a ball
15. Color pictures
16. Make fresh lemonade
17. Wipe off the table
18. Weed the flower bed
19. Make cream cheese mints (2 pounds of powdered sugar, 8 ounces of cream cheese, 2 drops of peppermint extract; knead and press into shapes)
20. Have a spelling bee
21. Read from *Reader's Digest*
22. Fold clothes
23. Arrange a visit with a calm pet
24. Cut out pictures from old greeting cards
25. Wash silverware
26. Bake homemade bread
27. Sort objects (e.g., beads) by color
28. Sing Christmas carols
29. Say "Tell me more" when a *person* talks about a memory
30. Put silverware away
31. Make a Valentine collage
32. Sing favorite songs together
33. Take a ride
34. Make a cherry pie
35. Read a favorite story or poem aloud
36. Dye Easter eggs
37. Sort a basket of socks
38. Take a walk
39. Reminisce about the first day of school
40. String Cheerios to hang outside for the birds
41. Make a fresh fruit salad
42. Sweep the patio
43. Color paper shamrocks with green crayon or markers

(continued)

Tool 9.8. 101 Things to Do *(continued)*

44. Roll coins
45. Have afternoon tea
46. Remember great inventions
47. Play a favorite game (e.g., Pictionary)
48. Paint a sheet
49. Cut out paper dolls
50. Identify states and their capitals
51. Make a family tree poster
52. Color a picture of the American flag
53. Cook hot dogs outside
54. Grow Magic Rocks
55. Water houseplants
56. Reminisce about a first kiss
57. Play horseshoes
58. Dance
59. Sing favorite hymns
60. Make homemade ice cream
61. Force bulbs for winter blooms
62. Make Christmas cards
63. Sort playing cards by suit or color
64. Write a letter to a family member
65. Dress in favorite team's colors for Sunday or Monday night football
66. Pop popcorn
67. Name the U.S. presidents
68. Give a manicure or pedicure
69. Make paper butterflies
70. Plant a tree
71. Make a May basket
72. Make homemade applesauce
73. Finish famous sayings
74. Feed ducks
75. Make shapes out of Play-Doh
76. Look at photos in *National Geographic*
77. Put a simple puzzle together
78. Sand wood
79. Rub in a pleasantly scented hand lotion
80. Decorate paper placemats
81. Arrange fresh flowers
82. Remember famous people
83. Straighten underwear/lingerie drawers
84. Finish nursery rhymes
85. Wipe off patio furniture
86. Make peanut butter sandwiches
87. Cut up paper for scratch pads
88. Take care of a fish tank
89. Trace and cut out leaves
90. Ask simple trivia questions

(continued)

Tool 9.8. 101 Things to Do *(continued)*

91. Finish Bible verses
92. Paint using a string
93. Cut out pictures from magazines
94. Read classic short stories
95. Put coins in a jar
96. Sew "sewing" cards
97. Put birdseed in bird feeders
98. Carve a pumpkin
99. Roll yarn into a ball
100. Reminisce about a favorite summer vacation
101. Make a birthday cake

From Susan Lonn, Director of Community Services, Madonna Rehabilitation Hospital, Lincoln, Nebraska; reprinted by permission.

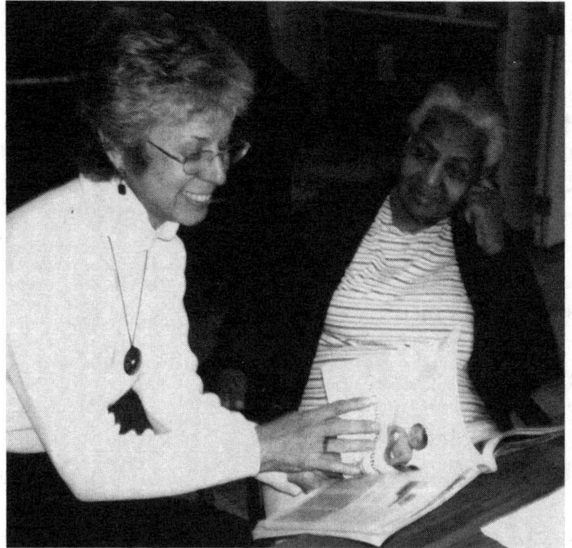

Aileen Wiglesworth (left), a Ph.D. student, reminisces with Helping Hand Day Center participant Lucy King using a variation on #93.

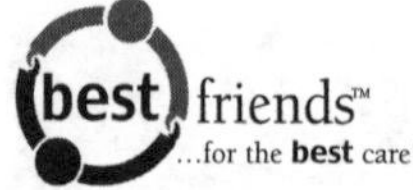

Tool 9.9 / Program Pointer
We Want You!

Copy and circulate the list below. Ask staff to sign up if they have a special interest or hobby and would be willing to demonstrate it in your program.

We Want You—To Be Part of Our Growing and Changing Activity Program
Would you consider sharing a special hobby or talent with our residents (or day center participants)?

Hobbies/Skills/Talents

- ❑ Tool collection
- ❑ Weddings
- ❑ Pets
- ❑ Sewing
- ❑ Music (singing or instruments)
- ❑ Cooking
- ❑ Weaving or handwork
- ❑ Woodworking
- ❑ Camping/outdoors
- ❑ Hats
- ❑ Bird watching
- ❑ Doll collection
- ❑ Quilts
- ❑ Collecting old toys/antiques
- ❑ Reading
- ❑ Writing
- ❑ Sports (please list)
- ❑ Others (please list)

____

____

____

____

________________________ __________________

Staff Member's Name Phone/Extension

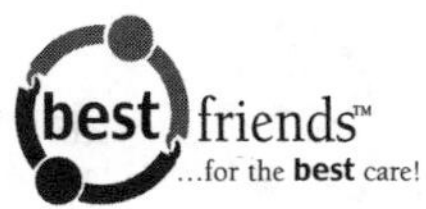

Tool 9.10 / Program Pointer
Activities Are Everywhere

Everyday items or situations can be used to create activities. Try it in your day center or dementia program.

There is always a conversation or activity waiting to happen if we just look around. At St. Aidan's Place we have had so much fun with items that are in the room.

A landscape painting—One day we took a landscape painting down from the wall and said to *persons,* "Let's go where this picture is taking us. How should we go? Should we walk, ride a horse, ride a bike, or take a train? Do we go this way, or that way (pointing in directions)? What will we do when we get there; have a picnic, or a party? Is it hot or cold there?" Each *person* gave his or her own answer—we created a picture within a picture. Ask a staff member to write the answers so they can be put into a story or poem. Then read the story or poem to the group to enjoy the adventure all over again.

Jewelry—There is always at least one person wearing jewelry, and it remains a fascinating topic. Let everyone admire the piece and ask for his or her favorite stone shape or color. Tell them their birthstones (information from the life story). If you do not have pictures of the gems, point to objects around the room that are the same color. Bring in costume jewelry for participants to wear and enjoy. Ask the men why they do not want to wear jewelry. Make some simple jewelry as an art project or talk about mining (one of our participants actually had been a miner).

Meals—One day when a group was sitting around a table we were told that we looked like a big family ready to eat dinner. This started a wonderful conversation about what everyone ate at dinner time, what dinner table rules were (napkins on lap, do not talk with your mouth full), and who was supposed to wash and dry the dishes.

Curtains—Looking at and then feeling the curtains at the day center started a delightful conversation about sewing, material, patterns, flower sacks used to make dresses, and swimsuits made out of wool.

Courtesy of Terrye Alexander, Director, Legacy St. Aidan's Place Daycare, Portland, Oregon.

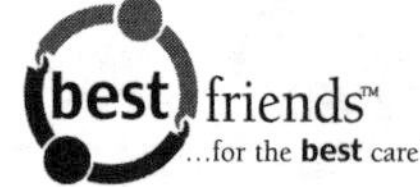

Tool 9.11

Turning No Knack into Knack

The purpose of this exercise is to show, with a dash of humor, the wrong way to do something. This is active learning that really sinks in, particularly when staff members themselves volunteer to take part in the role plays.

The following statements represent stereotypes or falsehoods about dementia. These examples of "no knack" can be used in a number of ways to explore staff attitudes and reinforce the lessons presented in this chapter. Draw them from a hat to discuss as a group or put them into role plays. Invite staff to comment on the mistakes. Then role-play or discuss the right way. The authors discuss the art of role plays in Tool 2.11. Use your creativity to have fun turning these examples of "no knack" into "knack."

We have a deadline to get these pictures painted for the art show!

Stay inside the lines. Remember how you used to color in your coloring books.

Don't try individual activities. They've forgotten what they want to do.

Persons with Alzheimer's disease don't enjoy work any more. They are tired of working.

Activities should not be stimulating. A *person* with Alzheimer's disease can't deal with being stimulated.

If someone wants to do something, the *person* can do it on his or her own.

Children don't mix with Alzheimer's *persons.*

We don't have the money for a good activities program. Those materials cost too much.

A 1000-piece puzzle should keep the restless ones busy for awhile.

Let's learn some new card games.

Everyone likes bingo.

Television is the best group activity!

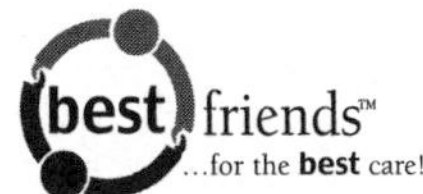

10

Caregivers as Members of the Best Friends Team

Alzheimer's disease can bring families together or tear them apart. Staff members in day centers or residential communities often witness this family dynamic. Staff can be present to educate and inform, suggest options, mediate, and offer support. Unfortunately, staff without experience or proper training can be part of the problem, not part of the solution, ending up inappropriately taking sides, being judgmental, or giving unsolicited and inappropriate advice. They can become embroiled in a familial civil war.

Best Friends staff members are taught that caregivers are an important part of a dementia care program, key players that we want to encourage to be part of the Best Friends team. They can be partners in providing excellent care, be somewhat detached, or work against staff efforts; the job of the Best Friends staff is to encourage the first option. This does not always happen, as seen in the following example.

The No-Clue Day Center

It had been a pretty good day at the No-Clue Day Center. The participants had enjoyed themselves, and several new ones were adjusting to the program well. Maggy, the program director, noticed that the activities assistant, Lulu, was walking out to the parking lot with one participant, Mike, and his wife.

"So just remember what I told you," Lulu said to the family member. "Have him on at least five of those Ginkgo pills a day and lots of carrots. I read that may stop Alzheimer's. I also think Mike should only come half-days; he gets pretty tired after lunch."

Meanwhile, Maggy left her office and was speaking to another family member who had come to pick up her father. He was fairly new to the center and was thriving, but his daughter looked frazzled. Maggy thought it would be helpful to give her some good news. "Your dad is so great. He is terrific. You can't believe the help he is here at the center. Whatever we ask him to do, he does." Maggy was sure that she would be happy with this great report card, but she noticed that the more she said, the more disgruntled the daughter looked.

"He doesn't do any of that for me," she snapped. "Maybe he should move in with you!" With that she stomped away, leaving her dad looking a bit worried and Maggy completely puzzled.

Lulu helped another participant walk outside. The woman's daughter greeted her: "I tell you, Lulu, that family of mine is just no good. I'm the only one who cares." Lulu replied, "I know! I just can't believe your brother won't do more for his mom. Like you said, I guess he just doesn't care."

The following Monday, Maggy walked into her office after a pleasant weekend. She immediately noticed two messages on her voice mail. Mike's wife left a message saying that he would be coming just once a week now instead of three times a week. Another client said he would not be coming back to the center at all. Stunned, Maggy wondered what had happened.

Just then the phone rang. "Who is it?" Maggy asked her secretary. "I didn't quite get his name," her secretary said, "but he's pretty angry. He said someone at our center has been saying bad things about him and getting involved in his family problems." "Oh, boy," said Maggy. "This week is getting off to a bad start."

Like most people who choose to work in long-term care, Maggy and Lulu are probably doing their best. They may, in fact, have a good program that has much to offer participants, but they have no insight into the family dynamics surrounding Alzheimer's disease. Both made a lot of mistakes, including giving unsolicited advice and erroneous information (recommendations about unproven therapies/treatments), allowing multiple "spokespeople" (program director and activities assistant) to deal with family members, involving themselves in family disputes (the brother and sister dispute), and overpraising a participant's achievements (Maggy inadvertently making the adult daughter feel inadequate about her relationship with her father).

The staff at the No-Clue Day Center certainly lived up to the program's name.

THE BEST FRIENDS WAY

The Best Friends staff are never clueless. Their goal is to model excellent care for caregivers in every setting. Best Friends staff members also make an effort to know caregivers well. They show an interest by learning names and understanding the family situation. They greet family members with respect and appreciate their involvement. They bring families into the caring community that a Best Friends staff tries to create.

The following are important concepts that staff should learn about caregivers and their impact on long-term care programs. Learning these concepts will increase the likelihood that families will become part of the Best Friends team.

UNDERSTAND THAT THE DEFINITION OF "FAMILY" IS CHANGING

Best Friends staff members understand that traditional nuclear families are no longer the norm. A national poll found that most Americans conceive of family as "a group of people who love and care for each other." These families include traditional families with a wage-earning father and homemaker mother; reversed-role families with a homemaking father; families headed by a dual-career mother and father; families in which grandparents are raising grandchildren as a result of parental incapacity or death; families with stepchildren; single-parent families created by abandonment, divorce, death, unplanned pregnancies, or choice; gay and lesbian households; families that postpone childbirth past traditional child-bearing age; "sandwich generation" families, in which parents care for their own children and older family members at the same time; multi-, even four-generation households; unmarried domestic partners; and many examples of older adults living together who may not marry.

The consequence of this change in what constitutes the family is that program leaders must talk to staff about each *person's* caregiving situation. They should be reminded that a Best Friends program respects diversity and supports the *person's* family situation—whatever it is. Marie B. Smart, Alzheimer's care specialist at The Breckinridge in Lexington, Kentucky, supports this view:

In a decade spent as family counselor at the University of Kentucky Alzheimer's Disease Research Center Memory Disorders Clinic, I worked with every possible family combination. I can attest to the fact that traditional and nontraditional families can be equally caring and sensitive.

This is an important point that staff will learn for themselves, as they work with more and more families during their careers.

Remember that Each Family's Response to Alzheimer's Disease Is Unique

Best Friends staff members appreciate the fact that families will differ in their ability or desire to be involved in care. Most families have a desire to give care themselves as long as possible; however, resources, abilities, and situations differ. Some families seem to muster the resources to care effectively for a loved one for a long time in a home setting, even when the *person's* behavior is quite challenging. Others do not.

Once a placement has been made, some families visit often and are very involved, whereas others visit infrequently. The fact that family members do not visit does not mean that they no longer care. Many families live far away from the *person*. Some caregivers are themselves old and frail. Still others might find it too painful to visit frequently with a loved one in a residential program.

Lisa Gwyther, director of the Duke University Medical Center's Alzheimer's Family Support Program, Durham, North Carolina, said, "Almost all families struggle with placement decisions, even those that seem like they do not care." She encourages staff to treat each family as unique: "When you've met one family coping with Alzheimer's disease, you've met just one family" (see Tool 10.5).

Staff must learn to be as caring and concerned about families as they are about the *persons* for whom they care.

Realize that Placement Does Not Always Make Things Easier, Only Different

Best Friends staff members recognize that a caregiver's worry, stress, and anxiety do not necessarily end with placement. The caregiver may no longer have the heavy physical care of the *person* as a responsibility and may be getting more sleep, but new worries develop: Will the facility keep my loved one? Will the facility be safe? Will my loved one adjust? What am I going to do with myself now that I have more time? Did I do the right thing? Could I have tried harder? Robin Hamon Kern, family support coordinator, Alzheimer's Disease Research Center Memory Disorders Clinic, Sanders-Brown Center on Aging, University of Kentucky, noted:

At times, caregivers don't know what to expect after a placement has been made. Often, they fear that they won't have any say any more. I tell them that although their role will change, it does not mean that they aren't needed. Their loved one still needs them to be involved.

The Best Friends staff recognize this, and they remind family members that many *persons* with Alzheimer's disease do well in residential care. A social milieu can bring out the best in them, they respond to a routine that can be difficult to create in a home setting, and trained staff often can do a better job with personal care. Families should be reminded that *caring* does not stop once a *person* moves to a residential program. Instead, responsibilities change and the burden of heavy, physical care actually can create less stress and allow for more "quality time" for the *person* and his or her caregivers.

Family participation is an important part of our program. They bake goodies for our parties, send in personal stories, picture albums, and special items to share with the group.

—*Cheryl T. Weidemeyer, Director, Christiana Care/Visiting Nurse Association, Evergreen Center I, Alzheimer's Day Treatment Program, Wilmington, Delaware*

I think it's very important for a program to share its admission and discharge criteria with the family early on. If a program works to allow *persons* to age in place, this is important for families to understand. If a program often discharges more challenging *persons* or moves them to a different setting, families should be told that this is a possibility early, rather than facing an unpleasant surprise.

—*Tonya M. Tincher, Chapter Programs Director, Lexington/Bluegrass Alzheimer's Association, Lexington, Kentucky*

Share a Defined Philosophy of Care with Families

Best Friends staff members communicate their philosophy of care and goals with families on a regular basis. Programs may wish to develop their own statement of philosophy or mission statement (the Alzheimer's Disease Bill of Rights [see Chapter 1] can be helpful in doing this), or the program can adopt the Best Friends philosophy that "what people with Alzheimer's disease need most of all is a good friend, a Best Friend."

Villa Alamar's philosophy reflects the residents' world of Alzheimer's disease, instead of asking them to conform with our world. For example, families are told that if residents are wearing each other's robes or hats, then the staff will not make a change unless it is upsetting to the person *to whom the garment actually belongs.*

Villa Alamar's decision had a great impact on staff and families, even in some seemingly simple areas. Regarding clothing, the administrator, Jackie Marston, commented that this philosophy has saved staff hours of time and lots of frustration trying to retrieve and return misplaced clothing to the original owners. Several families were quite upset when clothes that they had purchased for their loved ones ended up being worn by another resident. Jackie and her staff quietly repeated their philosophy and rationale, noting that this would happen in any dementia care unit. One very angry caregiver finally took this message to heart. Now, when he sees another woman wearing his wife's robe, he says, "My, you look nice today. Someone with very good taste must have given that to you!"

Villa Alamar's philosophy has not only made staff members' jobs easier but it also has helped them defend other decisions, such as letting residents sleep later in the day and wear clothes that they prefer. Most important, it has helped families better accept their loved one's diagnosis.

Professionals cannot force families to use services or not to use services. Families have their own schedule. Many families considering residential placement will reach out fleetingly, drop their efforts, and then come back again. Staff need to be aware of this and keep in regular contact with families considering their programs.
—*Lisa Gwyther, Director, Duke University Medical Center's Alzheimer's Family Support Program, Durham, North Carolina*

Believe that Most Families Are on Your Side

Best Friends staff members recognize that most families show appreciation, give compliments, and support the efforts of a program to give good care. Unfortunately, having even one or two difficult and challenging families can make a staff feel that "everyone is against you."

Lisa Gwyther pointed out that one way to improve relationships with families is to recognize that families will choose favorites among staff, often for idiosyncratic reasons: "This is not a bad thing. Programs should take advantage of this to encourage this staff member or staff members to play a greater role with that family."

Because each family is different, each will respond differently to the same staff member. In some cases, a staff member's folksy personality will be very appealing. Other family members may relate better to a staff member who gets right to the point or is very businesslike. When programs understand and accept these differences, they may find just the right "ambassador" to work with a challenging family.

Create a Care Plan for Families

Best Friends staff members have put strategies in place to help families cope with frustration and loss (see Tool 10.1). A good long-term care program sponsors its own support group and has links to local services, including the Alzheimer's Association. It is important to connect families to services that will help them cope better with their situation.

By linking families to community-based services, a program takes some pressure off itself to be the total support system for families. It can be healthier for families to meet other families that have similar issues and concerns but whose loved ones are in different settings or programs.

Grief is not an event, it is the process of healing.

—Linda Blair, grief and bereavement counselor, Frankfort, Kentucky

Leena's Home, in Helsinki, Finland, a special care unit for persons *with dementia, makes available 20 beds for 2- to 4-week-long respite periods. The goal of the program is twofold: to maintain the functional level of the family member and to support families that are trying to keep loved ones at home. Home visits from staff are routine, as is telephone support. One family member wrote, "It's really important to me that I'm not left alone when I'm taking care of him at home. I can always call the primary nurse and she will help support me. I'm very thankful for these discussions with her. Many times they help me make it through the day."*

We also feel a responsibility for the families of our patients. We encourage our families to visit and spend time—as if they were still visiting in their own home.

—Patricia Wesley, Administrator, Omahanui Private Hospital, New Plymouth, New Zealand

When families know that a program will back them up, it takes a huge weight off their shoulders.

Never Give Advice

Best Friends staff members recognize that their job is to give good information and trust families to make good decisions. When staff take on the decision-making role, it inhibits caregiver growth and learning. A caring staff works to empower caregivers to make their own decisions.

Your staff brought back Izzy's joy of music. I know how much pleasure it brought to her and the staff and the other residents as well. She regained self-confidence and the attention she received brought joy to her heart and to ours, too. Be sure of that!

—Pat and Ian Crow (Izzy's daughter and son-in-law, in a letter to Villa Alamar)

Deborah Dunn, director of patient and family services for the Santa Barbara (California) chapter of the Alzheimer's Association, believes that this area is quite important for professional staff to understand well: "It is very risky to put yourself in a position of knowing it all. In dementia care, there is often not a right or wrong answer or decision. My goal as a family counselor is to empower families to make a good decision. I don't ever fall into the trap of deciding for them."

Families under stress and strain often ask professionals to become the decision makers; staff can be taught appropriate boundaries so as not to overstep their roles.

Involve Families in Care Decisions and in the Program

Best Friends staff members encourage families to come to care planning meetings and to attend the facility's educational programs. There are many other creative ways to encourage involvement, such as asking families to write a memory book or create a scrapbook, design a bulletin board, write a letter to the editor of the in-house newsletter or the local newspaper, help with outings, support fundraisers, or speak at a staff meeting (see Tool 10.6). According to Marie B. Smart:

Families need to be coached on the most effective ways to be involved at a long-term care residence. Good programs put out the welcome mat and give families tips about how to be part of the community.

These suggestions can include encouraging shorter, more frequent visits. Families also can be encouraged to bring their own interests with them. Perhaps a caregiver can read a good book while simply sitting next to a loved one, holding hands now and then.

Staff sometimes express frustration or disappointment that, despite these efforts, families do not seem to get involved. The Best Friends staff keep trying. Also, the Best Friends staff learn to be specific. "I know your daughter and her school art class are looking for projects. Could you take on our June bulletin board?" "We're taking the residents to the Alzheimer's Association Memory Walk. Can we count on you to come Saturday morning for 2 hours to lend a hand and support a great cause?"

Develop Honest, Effective Dialogue

Best Friends staff members have honest dialogues with family members. They encourage family members to express concerns and let family members know that the program also will conduct an honest dialogue with them.

As in the earlier example from the No-Clue Day Center, it is important for staff to be "on the same page," deliv-

I call my case managers "Best Friends." This is less threatening and more friendly for families.
—Meredith Gresham, writer and consultant, Avon, Connecticut

Robert Barrett regularly visited his wife Jean at Villa Bella in Santa Barbara, California. He became friendly with many staff members. A retired college professor, he encouraged them to continue their education and think about their futures. For Christmas, he offered one CNA the choice of a gift certificate at a local department store or a book on Alzheimer's care. He was delighted when she chose the book: "I believe that many line staff have a keen desire to learn. I think they really appreciate family members' taking an interest in them and being encouraging."

ering the same message. There is a chain of command in dementia care programs, so, for example, CNAs should not discuss frequency of day center visits with families. Likewise, families should be told to whom to address complaints and concerns. Robin Hamon Kern suggested:

Family members should be encouraged by staff to ask for meetings with the appropriate parties early, before the problems grow too big, and to keep the lines of communication open.

It is important for staff to feel that they can give feedback to families when problems occur. If a family member, for example, is speaking inappropriately about the *person* in his or her presence (e.g., "Does Mother need to go to the bathroom now?"), then staff members should model the Best Friends way (by leaving the room when talking about him or her). They also can give the caregiver some careful feedback (e.g., "Margie, one of the things we try so hard to do here is never talk about someone in their presence. It's hard for me to remember this sometimes. Would you mind helping me stay on track? Let's go into the hallway if we're going to talk about your mom."). The latter example shows great sensitivity and tact.

Handle Conflict Appropriately

Best Friends staff members accept that conflicts with families are inevitable. In fact, conflict can be very positive. It can bring issues out in the open and start the process to find solutions.

Conflict can occur with regard to failed expectations or promises that go undelivered. For example, if a family is concerned about staff turnover, then a thoughtful program leader will talk to the family about the steps that the program is taking to improve the situation (assuming that this truly is the case). However, it would be foolish to make promises ("Your mother will have the same staff take care of her from now on") that cannot be delivered on.

Often, family members are not expecting immediate solutions. They are expecting to be heard. A good program leader is a good listener. He or she may ask the family member, "What ideas do you have to solve the problem?" Such a question shows respect and that the program values the family member's opinion.

Deborah Dunn notes that sometimes you can be right but still have to be wrong. She comments:

There are times when a program leader must "fall on the sword" for a family member. Even if the program is "right" and the family "wrong," it can sometimes be wiser not to argue, make a simple apology for any misunderstanding, and say, "I'm so sorry you feel that way." However, staff members do not need to take abuse from family members. When this happens, staff should be encouraged to refer the person to the supervisor, or take other steps to defuse the situation.

The program pointer in Tool 10.2 targets working with challenging family members who seemingly may never be happy with the quality of your program.

Encourage Use of Services

The Best Friends staff encourage families to take advantage of community-based services and the continuum of care offered in many communities. One effective approach for encouraging the use of day services and eventually residential care is to stress the benefits to the *person* instead of to the caregiver. By saying, "Your mother (with Alzheimer's disease) would really benefit from being with others at our day program," rather than, "If you don't take a break, you'll collapse," a staff member is stressing the positive outcomes for the *person* instead of potentially evoking feelings of inadequacy in the caregiver.

Tonya M. Tincher, chapter programs director, Lexington/Bluegrass Alzheimer's Association (Kentucky), told us about some of her experiences in trying to get families to use adult day center care:

I struggle to understand why families are often so reluctant to use adult day care services. Then I remember that they are doubtful their loved one will come; families are under stress, fearful about the future, and guilty about letting go. The solution, I think, is to stay in regular touch with these caregivers, encouraging them to drop in for a special lunch, and letting them know that most of our participants in the Helping Hand Day Center have families who shared the same feelings. I like to tell them that about 90% of our families initially think day services will never work. Later they are calling asking if Mother or Father can't attend more days a week!

Encouraging caregivers to try services involves gentle persuasion and repeated contact. Without such encouragement, most dementia programs—no matter how good—will struggle to build and maintain their censuses (see Tool 10.8).

Help Families Recast Relationships

Best Friends staff members help families accept the changes that come with Alzheimer's disease. Staff members make a shift in their roles from workers to friends. Families can be encouraged to similarly recast their relationships.

After a visit to The Fountains, one daughter expressed sadness that her mother no longer recognized her. She said that it was increasingly hard to visit her mother. Diane Will, to whom she expressed these feelings, noticed that the visit actually seemed to include smiles and animated conversation. She said to the daughter, "Isn't it nice to know that your mother still seems to respond to you in such a warm, friendly way? You've graduated from daughter to friend."

Diane's thoughtful and kind remark helped the daughter recast her relationship. The daughter feels better about her visits and more accepting of her mother's Alzheimer's disease.

The idea of recasting relationships is jarring at first to some family members, but a common experience of Alzheimer's disease is that the *person* begins to forget or mistake identities. For example, the *person* may now see his wife as his mother, his sister, or his daughter or even as someone else. Understandably, this is very upsetting to family members.

Best Friends staff are there to remind families that this confusion of identity is common. The family member may physically resemble another family member. The *person* may think that he or she is 30 or 40 years younger than his or her real age, adding to the confusion. Language can be affected. The brain may no longer be able to process the visual image and retrieve the memory of the name.

The suggestion that families recast relationships does not negate the past. It helps families seize control of the situation and turn a negative situation into a positive one. We may no longer be remembered as a daughter or spouse, but we can be remembered as a friend, a Best Friend.

Conclusion

Often, Best Friends staff have the opportunity to get to know families as well as they know the *persons* in their care. Best Friends staff exhibit knack with family caregivers, treating them with love, good humor, and respect. Best Friends staff members provide good information and support and encourage the use of services to help family members work through denial and develop an effective plan of care for their loved ones as well as for themselves:

Natasha Land's grandmother had been an especially beloved figure for her, in part because the grandmother got her involved in dance—now Natasha's passion—as a young girl. Here are her words excerpted from a letter to her grandfather, Berdine Erickson, of Rochester, Minnesota, a dedicated caregiver for his wife for many years:

Grandma doesn't know me any more ... but most important is that I carry a big piece of her in my heart. I will not forget her. She encouraged my parents to give me dance lessons. That has given me so much joy, continually, all through my life. Alzheimer's disease cannot take away what has already been. It only transfers the responsibility of remembering to those who love the one that is afflicted. It is with great joy that I accept this, as do all, I hope, that love and cherish Grandma.

In the same letter, Natasha praises her grandfather: "It seems to me that you have become even more sensitive, loving and gracious . . . you are not swallowed up by your pain." Staff members' spirits are renewed when they see families travel a path from despair to hope, from darkness to light.

In the 1970s and 1980s, much of the literature and research surrounding caregiving issues painted a bleak picture of stress, strain, and burden. It seemed true that the caregiver often would be at greater risk for premature death and disability than the *person*.

The sadness, losses, and challenges associated with Alzheimer's disease remain the same. Yet Best Friends staff understand that when they do their jobs well, caregivers will come out on the other side of the illness intact, sometimes even stronger for having faced the challenge. Just as Natasha's grandmother gave her the gift of dance, Best Friends staff members can give families the gift of good-quality care and love.

Working with families in a caring and empathetic way also can help staff members review their own family situations and develop new skills and confidence to address problems and conflicts. One CNA was able to leave an abusive relationship with the support of coworkers. Another CNA in a Best Friends program addressed his family situation this way: "I'm trying now to be a Best Friend to my own family, to be less judgmental, to lighten up and have more fun with them. At the same time, I want them to be a Best Friend to me—to give me more respect for the person I am and the hard work I take on to help all of us." His workplace was a good environment for him to learn and practice caring for others and for himself.

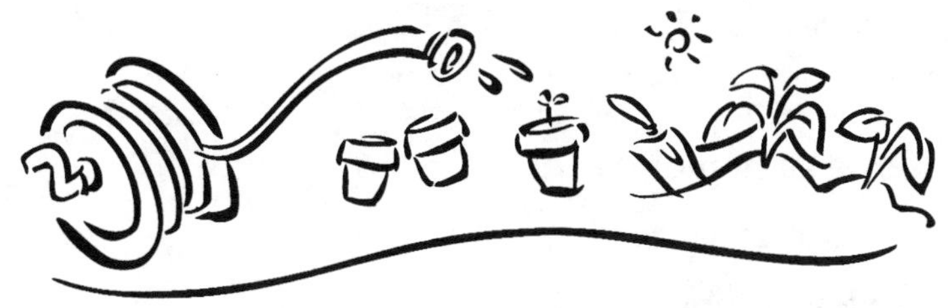

Training Tool Kit

Tool 10.0 / Warm-Up

One Face Seen Three Ways

Display this picture as an overhead or on a handout. Ask staff what they see. Challenge them to find the three images in the picture. Make the point that we can often look at one thing in many different ways.

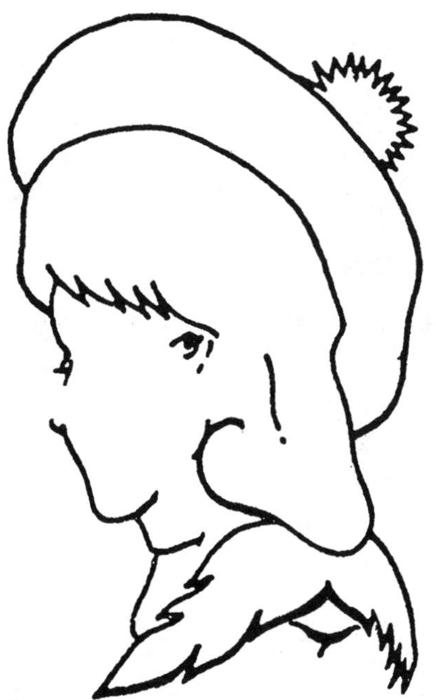

Mother, father and daughter

Suggested by Kathy Laurenhue, President, Better Directions, San Diego, California.

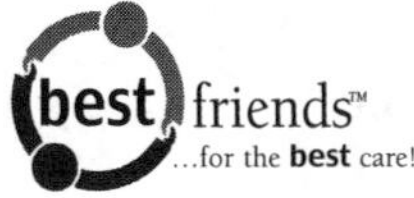

Tool 10.1 / Program Pointer
Tips for Helping Families Cope with Stress

Use this list as a handout for staff or families.

Maintain a sense of humor.

Seek out someone to confide in.

Set realistic expectations.

Practice assertiveness.

Develop strategies for handling unhelpful advice.

Keep in contact with the outside world.

Stay in touch with your faith community (if one has been a part of your life).

Modify or change your living environment when appropriate.

Fulfill creative impulses.

Listen to your body.

Be good to yourself.

Plan ahead.

Forgive others and yourself.

Keep a diary or notes of caregiving experiences.

Use services early rather than late.

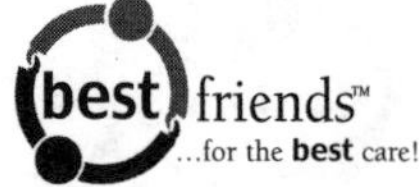

Tool 10.2 / Program Pointer

Suggestions for Working with Challenging Families

For families that cannot overcome denial

Recognize that denial can be a healthy response if it does not go on too long.
Educate in small doses; supply a few brochures at a time or take the family to a workshop.
Encourage support group attendance.
Do not push too hard; give them time to adjust.

For families that have trouble accepting change

Acknowledge their skepticism up front.
Ask them to listen carefully to a suggestion.
Ask them to think about why an idea might work.
Ask another family member to be a mentor.

For families that are uninformed

Take them to a conference or workshop.
Go through printed materials with them, making points one at a time.
Offer lectures or workshops at your program.
Use the Internet and e-mail appropriately.

For families with unrealistic expectations

Use a visualization exercise such as "Imagine Walking a Mile in the Shoes of . . ."
Invite them to a care planning meeting.
Let them know the consequences of expecting too much from the *person.*
Describe staff goals and expectations.

For families that are overly critical of/angry with/can never be pleased or happy with staff

Be certain that you are listening to and acting on legitimate concerns.
Ask them to write out a list of what is wrong and what is working well.
Appoint one spokesperson from staff or ask a third party to mediate.
Make your care philosophy and plan very clear to family members.
Give them feedback on how their criticism is received by staff.

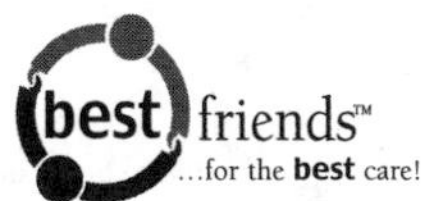

Tool 10.3 / Games for Learning
Role Plays

Role play is one of the best techniques for teaching staff to work with families because it helps staff members better understand what works and what does not. Here is one role play scripted out. Use the examples in Tool 10.9 to write more.

Topic: Staff Griping About One Another (Unprofessional Behavior)

Scene: A staff member talking to a family member

The Wrong Way

FAMILY MEMBER: Do you know Calvin, the aide who takes care of my Charlie on the day shift?
STAFF MEMBER: I've met him.
FAMILY MEMBER: Well, he's just the worst. I've told him over and over again that Charlie likes to get dressed right after getting up. Today, I found him in his pajamas.
STAFF MEMBER: You said it! Just between us, he doesn't care. He gets by with as little work as possible. He's a disgrace!

Discuss this situation with the class, noting the result when staff do not respect one another. Ask whether this approach helped the family member get his or her concerns heard.

The Right Way

FAMILY MEMBER: Do you know Calvin, the aide who takes care of my Charlie on the day shift?
STAFF MEMBER: Yes, I do.
FAMILY MEMBER: Well, he's just the worst. I've told him over and over again that Charlie likes to get dressed right after getting up. Today, I found him in his pajamas.
STAFF MEMBER: It's possible that Charlie didn't want to get dressed. All of us work hard to take family wishes seriously, but we don't like to force Charlie.
FAMILY MEMBER: Well, I think you should get the job done.
STAFF MEMBER: I hear your concerns. I really encourage you to talk to the administrator, or maybe we can sit down with the rest of the staff to think of some ways to keep you and Charlie happy.

Discuss the positives with the group—the family member felt heard, staff respected one another, simple explanations were given without argument, the suggestion was made to bring in the administrator, and the staff member did not put herself between a family and another staff member.

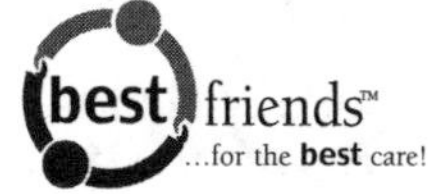

Tool 10.4 / Games for Learning
Whose Job Is It When Families . . . ?

Use this game to talk about what staff should do in certain situations with families. It also can be a good way to reinforce roles and teach staff where they can turn for help.

Write the following items on slips of paper, put them in a hat, and ask staff to draw a slip of paper, read the item aloud, and then discuss it as a group. Make the point that it is everyone's job to be helpful and courteous but that some situations can be handled on the spot and others need to be referred to another staff member.

Whose job is it when families . . .

Ask how Mother is doing today?

Ask what activities are scheduled or what the afternoon schedule looks like?

Need fresh bed linens?

Need a wheelchair to take Mother out in the garden?

Ask for help taking Father out to the car for an afternoon drive?

Say they are really feeling down and depressed today and could use some love?

Are angry that Mother is being moved to another level of care and begin asking questions?

Are angry that clothes are being lost and demand an immediate search for slippers?

Have a bunch of new ideas for recruiting volunteers?

Have questions about a medical problem?

Ask what happened to a staff member who was fired?

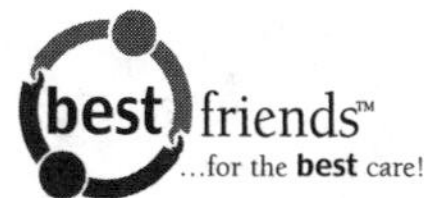

Tool 10.5 / Games for Learning
Putting the Pieces Together

This exercise helps staff understand the impact of dementia on families.

Prior to the training session, cut art foam board into puzzle pieces and attach a strip of Velcro to each piece. On a slip of paper, write the terms that you have decided to use from the possibilities listed below. Cut out each term and stick one term on each of the puzzle pieces. Divide the class into groups and give each group one or more pieces. Ask them to discuss the content of the piece and how it relates to the impact of Alzheimer's disease on caregivers. At the end of the session, ask a volunteer to come to the front of the room and put each group's piece back into the puzzle (you can create a master outline to lay on the tabletop).

Sometimes in denial
Angry
Sad
Tired
Still want to provide care themselves
Embarrassed
Worried about confidentiality
Appreciative
Caring
Need more information/education
Gave care by themselves for a long time
Financial pressures
Helped by using services

Variation: Use the terms for general discussion. Ask staff to draw slips of paper from a hat and discuss the term. Discuss real family situations that they have encountered, and talk about possible solutions.

Note: Make the point that all families are different, but we should try to empathize with their situations.

Adapted from Putting the Pieces Together, *by Susan D. Berry, Alzheimer's consultant and trainer, Warsaw, Indiana.*

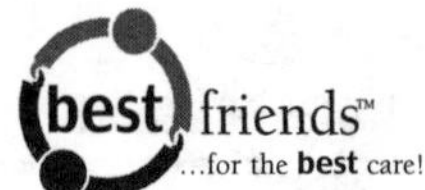

Tool 10.6 / Program Pointer

25 Ways to Get Families More Involved in Your Program

1. Ask them to come to care planning meetings.
2. Create a family council or advisory board.
3. Match them with *persons* for one-to-one activities.
4. Be a guest chef.
5. Invite them to theme and holiday parties/meals.
6. Ask them to help with field trips.
7. Form a team at a community walk or fund-raiser.
8. Ask them to share a hobby or special skill for show-and-tell.
9. Give a concert on a musical instrument or play piano for a sing-along.
10. Share a family member's life story at a staff meeting.
11. Ask them to help plant a vegetable or flower garden.
12. Invite them to participate in art classes or activities.
13. Ask them to mentor a new family.
14. Ask them to read aloud to a *person.*
15. Invite them to participate in a barbecue or dessert party.
16. Host an afternoon tea or after-work "happy hour."
17. Ask them to get their service club involved in a project.
18. Have a "poodle parade" or a "bring your pet day."
19. Host meetings or community rehearsals in the building.
20. Ask them to help with publicity or be on a speaker's bureau.
21. Have a carnival or circus or special event for staff and family members' children.
22. Ask them to be involved in birthday celebrations for staff, not only *persons.*
23. Invite them to exercise or work out with fit residents.
24. Ask them to be a translator for a *person* who speaks the same language.
25. Ask them to be teachers in your educational programs.

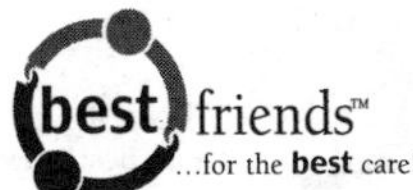

Tool 10.7 / Program Pointer

Creating a Resource Center or Shelf for Families and Staff

Use this list to create a resource center or shelf for families and staff.

A resource center or shelf for families (and staff) can contain the following items:

Basic brochures and fact sheets about dementia

List of local support groups

List of local geriatricians or other physicians

Alzheimer's Association newsletters and telephone numbers

Autopsy information

Books to borrow or buy

Calendar of upcoming education events/workshops

List of dementia-friendly dentists, dental services

List of homemaker and visiting nurse services

Information about legal services or powers of attorney, conservatorships, living wills

List of nearby university clinics or research centers

List of possible in-home sitters or in-home workers

Telephone numbers of older adult nutrition services/Meals on Wheels

List of senior centers

List of older adult peer counselors or other mental health services

Ombudsman telephone numbers

Area Agency on Aging telephone number

Telephone number of adult protective services

List of church and interfaith volunteer programs

Senior or community hotline/helpline telephone numbers

Tool 10.8 / Program Pointer

Tips for Getting Families to Use Services

Families often wait a long time to use services. Here are some tips to ensure that your Best Friends program is doing its best to reach out to families in need and to encourage them to use in-home services or adult day center care or to consider resident placement.

Assess Your Program

If you were a caregiver needing help, would your program be useful?
Are the hours appropriate (e.g., is the day center open only 4 hours a day, thus excluding many working caregivers)?
Is your location good?
Have you considered weekend or evening hours?
Have you addressed any other barriers to use?

Assess Your Activities

Is the activity program appealing to visitors?
Is the activity program something that staff would enjoy doing themselves?

Assess Your Print Materials

Are they clear?
Are they sensitive to multicultural/aging issues?
Is the language too advanced or filled with jargon?

Assess How Potential Clients Are Greeted in Person or on the Telephone

Are they made to feel welcome?
Does the mention of the word "waiting list" scare off prospective clients?

Assess Follow-Up

Do you have a system in place to follow up regularly with clients interested in your program?

Assess Benefits

Do you stress the benefits of the program to the *person*? Mentioning respite care also is valuable but should be secondary.

Assess Policy on Confidentiality

Do potential clients believe that confidentiality will be respected?

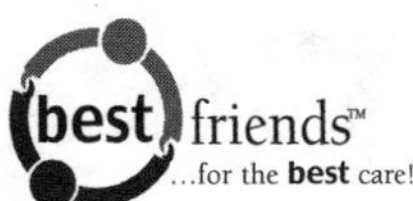

Tool 10.9

Turning No Knack into Knack

The purpose of this exercise is to show, with a dash of humor, the wrong way to do something. This is active learning that really sinks in, particularly when staff members themselves volunteer to take part in the role plays.

The following statements represent stereotypes or falsehoods about dementia. These examples of "no knack" can be used in a number of ways to explore staff attitudes and reinforce the lessons presented in this chapter. Draw them from a hat to discuss as a group or put them into role plays. Invite staff to comment on the mistakes. Then role-play or discuss the right way. The authors discuss the art of role plays in Tool 2.11. Use your creativity to have fun turning these examples of "no knack" into "knack."

Family to Staff

Can you promise me that you'll bathe and dress my husband first?

What is the story with Mr. Giordello's family? Why don't they ever visit?

Do you really think George should be working here? I don't think he does a very good job.

Who do you think is stealing Mother's socks? I can't believe that you'd allow this to happen!

Mother tells me that you haven't given her any food today.

Staff to Family

I can promise you that your dad will get that new room. I'll talk to the administrator.

He never wants to go to physical therapy. I don't think it's worth it.

When I look at Harry, I'm so glad that I gave up drinking before that alcohol-related dementia hit me.

If you'd like to keep your mother coming to the day center, I could give you some extra hours at home on the side.

In all the time she's been here, I never knew she was a nurse. I guess it doesn't matter anyway, now that she's got Alzheimer's.

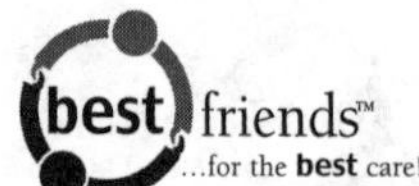

Conclusion

A Best Friends program is not possible without a Best Friends staff. The important message of this book is that programming and staffing are invariably linked. Yet in the literature of long-term care, it seems that there is a single effort under way to improve programming and another, separate effort to enhance staffing.

When these efforts are linked to support *persons* and staff, a caring community that brings out the best in all of its citizens can be created. This culture change can be created by following some simple guidelines:

- Invest in staff
- Treat staff with the same respect that good programs give to their residents or participants
- Recognize that staff have a desire to be part of a caring community
- Give staff the tools that they need to build effective job and life skills
- Involve staff in decision making
- Recognize that leadership is vital to a program's success
- Encourage staff to be involved with residents and participants through group and individual activities
- Assign a Best Friend to each staff member

Invest in Staff

If there is a silver lining to the current staffing crisis, it is that line staff wages have risen. Although this improvement has challenged the bottom line of many businesses, we believe that these staff members deserve to earn a living wage. Many long-term care communities are rising to the challenge, offering health insurance, child care, transportation, and employee assistance programs. The Santa Barbara (California) chapter of the Alzheimer's Association has even started a club for long-term care line staff that provides social and professional support. Career ladders for CNAs are also under discussion. Groups such as the Pioneer Movement are devising ways to reward outstanding staff members and to encourage them to stay in the field of long-term care. It is our hope that good people remain hands-on workers but that many of today's Best Friends CNAs will be tomorrow's administrators, even owners, as they grow personally and professionally.

Treat Staff with the Same Respect that Good Programs Give Their Residents or Participants

Best Friends program leaders understand that they cannot treat staff badly and then expect staff to treat the residents or participants well. The message that staff are important must come from top management and work its way down through the ranks. The authors endorse the ideas of Patricia Wesley, administrator of Omahanui Private Hospital, who confirms this view: "I treat my staff as I expect them to treat the residents—I can do no less for them, and they make me very proud."

Recognize that Staff Have a Desire to Be Part of a Caring Community

Many people are attracted to long-term care settings for more than the often-limited financial rewards. They are attracted to this line of work because their relationships to residents and participants build self-esteem and pride. The caring community of a Best Friends program can be a "shelter in the storm," a place to find success for some staff members with difficult personal lives. Cynthia Belle, a dementia care consultant and trainer, thanks staff often for their contribution to caring communities: "Realize that, through your caregiving, you hold the key to the success of the *person's* journey through this disease, and because of this you are a rare and special individual."

Give Staff the Tools that They Need to Build Effective Job and Life Skills

Best Friends staff members need to learn information about Alzheimer's disease, but, even more important, they need to learn and develop skills. A Best Friends program helps staff members grow and develop as people and professionals. It teaches staff the basics of dementia care and ways to be a Best Friend to *persons* in their care. It also teaches practical life skills, including assertiveness, conflict resolution, and money management.

Involve Staff in Decision Making

Best Friends staff members believe that they have a stake in their community and in decisions involving their work experience and *persons* for whom they care. When staff have heavy responsibilities but little or no control, stress and burnout are inevitable. When the voice of a staff member is heard, it not only improves morale but it also ensures that good ideas about care planning and execution are not lost. Yvonne Smalls Prosper, the care plan coordinator of The Fountainview Center, wrote, "Since our CNAs have been coming to our care plan meetings, I have seen a more widespread use of hugging, talking, and smiling with our residents. Because staff now feel more informed and more involved, they also can make a greater connection with the residents."

Recognize that Leadership Is Vital to a Program's Success

Best Friends staff members benefit from strong, effective leadership. When top management embraces quality improvement and has the vision to create a caring community, it elevates everyone. It inspires staff to do more than the minimum required in their daily routine. When St. Basil's Homes implemented a quality improvement program across its sites and services, the process involved staff members, families, even board of directors' members. This process revealed that it was critical to have strong leadership at the top to have an impact on direct care staff.

Encourage Staff to Be Involved with Residents and Participants Through Group and Individual Activities

Best Friends staff members take part in activities with residents and participants. This involvement is an essential part of living in a community—making a contribution and being involved with friends and neighbors. This concept is critical for programs to understand and embrace. Some managers might rebel at the thought of a housekeeper, gardener, or bookkeeper being given time to spend with the participants or residents away from their usual duties, but it is, in fact, *why* they are there—to build programs that benefit *persons* and their caregivers. Giving nondirect care staff a chance to participate enriches their lives. It is bound to have a positive effect on morale.

Assign a Best Friend to Each Staff Member

Best Friends staff give good care to all *persons*. Programs should build on this commitment by encouraging staff to "adopt" a specific individual. This can immeasurably improve the quality of care. It is also easy and costs virtually nothing to implement. Karen Wyan, assistant administrator at Laurel Heights Home for the Elderly, wrote to the authors that all of her staff have chosen a resident to be a Best Friend: "It is such a nice experience that we are not limiting it to just residents with Alzheimer's disease. Every resident needs a Best Friend."

The Best Friends Model as a Tool for Change

The Best Friends approach was developed as a model or philosophy of dementia care. The goal of the model is to develop family and professional caregivers with knack and to move the *person* away from the feelings that are listed on the left side of Figure 1 to the ones that are listed on the right. The shift may only be momentary, but person-centered care suggests that when we link these moments together, challenging behaviors are reduced and the quality of life is improved for the *person* with Alzheimer's disease.

The Best Friends staff training and development philosophy as outlined in this book can have a similar impact on staff. Not every staff member will experience the feelings noted on the left side of Figure 2, but those who do will find that this caring community can help them move toward the feelings noted on the right side of the figure.

Loss	→	Fulfillment
Loneliness	→	Connectedness
Sadness	→	Cheerfulness
Confusion	→	Orientation
Worry/anxiety	→	Contentment
Frustration	→	Peacefulness
Fear	→	Security
Paranoia	→	Trust
Anger	→	Calm
Embarrassment	→	Confidence

Figure 1. Changes for persons *that result from the use of the Best Friends model of care.*

The Best Friends philosophy can help staff members move from failure to success. Unlike the changes in Figure 1, those that are listed in Figure 2 can be long-lasting. When a program leader gives his or her attention to a staff member, not just to the *person,* it can bring out the best in that staff member. It can elevate staff and help them grow personally and professionally. It can improve job performance and the quality of care. Special attention can move staff to a place of fulfillment, connectedness, purpose, clarity, and success.

Looking back on the interviews with the CNAs in Chapter 2, the authors noted that many had experienced tough times in their lives. Conventional wisdom suggests that these individuals would not be good long-term care employees. The Best Friends approach to staff development, however, can give these individuals an opportunity to learn new skills and join a caring community. It can help these individuals be more effective and successful employees. It can help them develop a career instead of just have a job. It can help them grow as people and thus have more to give to the *persons* for whom they care.

For other staff, including program leaders, a Best Friends model can vastly improve morale and provide a workable philosophy for implementing almost any program. Developing a Best Friends staffing model also can improve staff recruitment and retention in a very challenging employment market. Michael Livni, the administrator of Serenity Nursing Home, acknowledges this. Clearly, the Best Friends philosophy has affected and supported him personally and professionally as much as it has his staff. The approach moves not only people but also programs toward success.

Barbara Susan Dicker, the team facilitator of a dementia care unit at Carinya Village, Church of Christ Homes, Inc., Mt. Lawley, Western Australia, wrote to the authors about the impact of the Best Friends approach on her program:

Loss	→	Fulfillment
Isolation	→	Connectedness
Sadness	→	Cheerfulness
Drifting	→	Purpose
Restlessness	→	Contentment
Frustration	→	Satisfaction
Low self-esteem	→	Pride
Fear	→	Confidence
Uncertainty	→	Clarity
Failure	→	Success

Figure 2. Changes for staff that result from the use of the Best Friends approach.

The most gratifying aspect of the Best Friends model is that the team truly owns the project and it appears to be working well for us and our residents. If we make mistakes along the way, that's all right, too, as we have the ability to analyze what we are doing, make changes, and try new strategies. In this way, we hope to continue to transform our unit from the nursing wing it once was into a truly caring community of friends.

Here is another example:

At Karrington Cottages, one young CNA accompanied a resident to her room to help her get ready for bed. As they walked to the resident's room, the woman insisted that she wanted to help the CNA get to bed. She said she had to do this before she could go to bed herself. Thinking on her feet, the CNA went to an empty room, slid under the covers of a bed, and allowed the resident to tuck her in for the night. The person *then went to her own room and another staff member helped her get to bed.*

This CNA with knack was truly being a Best Friend to the resident by letting her recall the comforts of home, the time when she would tuck in her own children, and the kiss that she would plant on their foreheads. A Best Friends program and new culture of care can begin this way, with just one staff member, taking one small step, changing his or her way of doing things.

Notes and References

Introduction

Fagan, R.M., Williams, C.C., & Burger, S.G., Meeting of Pioneers in Nursing Home Culture Change, Final report, Rochester, NY, 1997.

Chapter 1

Kitwood, T., & Breden, K. (1992). *Person to person: A guide to the care of those with failing mental powers.* Loughton, England: Gale Centre Publications.

The concept of "knack" has proven very popular in the field of long-term care. An expanded discussion of knack can be found in *The Best Friends Approach to Alzheimer's Care.* Baltimore: Health Professions Press, 1997.

Zgola, J.M. (1999). *Care that works. A relationships approach to persons with dementia* (p. 170). Baltimore: The Johns Hopkins University Press.

Chapter 2

"Nursing assistant shortage hits hard: Area suffers as nursing home beds go empty." *Rochester (MN) Post Bulletin,* December 15, 1998.

Hellen, C.R. (1998). *Alzheimer's disease: Activity-focused care* (2nd ed., p. 49). Woburn, MA: Butterworth-Heinemann.

Hellen, p. 47.

Bell, V., & Troxel, D. (1997). *The best friends approach to Alzheimer's care* (pp. 91–112). Baltimore: Health Professions Press.

Hellen, p. 41.

My Challenge with Alzheimer's Disease. (1996). [Video]. (Distributed by Terra Nova Films, 9848 S. Winchester Avenue, Chicago, IL 60643.)

Chapter 3

Alzheimer's Association. (1997). *An overview of Alzheimer's disease and related dementias.* (Publication No. ED205Z). Chicago: Author. Used by permission.

Chapter 5

Hellen, C.R. (1998). *Alzheimer's disease: Activity-focused care* (2nd ed., p. 164). Woburn, MA: Butterworth-Heinemann.

Chapter 6

Helping Hand Day Center. (1997). [Video]. *Best friends.* (Distributed by Health Professions Press, 888-337-8808. www.healthpropress.com.)

Quotations in Tool 6.5 from Berman, K. (Ed.). (1996). *Friendship.* Kansas City, MO: Ariel Books/Andrews-McMeel; reprinted by permission.

Chapter 7

Tool 7.9 was adapted by Susan Maxwell Jones from Bell, V., & Troxel, D. (1997). *The Best Friends approach to Alzheimer's care.* Baltimore: Health Professions Press; and Beedle, J. (1990). *The care book: A workbook for caregiver peace of mind.* Portland, OR: Lady Bug Press.

Chapter 8

Zgola, J.M. (1999). *Care that works. A relationships approach to persons with dementia* (p. 170). Baltimore: The Johns Hopkins University Press.

Chapter 10

Massachusettes Mutual Insurance Company survey. (1990, Winter/Spring). *Newsweek* Special Edition.

Bell, V., & Troxel, D. (1997). *The best friends approach to Alzheimer's care* (pp. 147–148). Baltimore: Health Professions Press.

Conclusion

Bell, V., & Troxel, D. (1999, January/February). Another face of Alzheimer's disease. *American Journal of Alzheimer's Disease, 14*(1) 60–64.

Appendix A

Programs Featured in *The Best Friends Staff*[1]

The following adult day and residential dementia programs contributed stories to *The Best Friends Staff*. Each story or quotation reflects the Best Friends philosophy at its best. The authors thank them for their contributions to this book.

ADCare, LifeSpan Services Network, Inc., San Luis Obispo County, California
ADCare offers adult day services to adults with dementia and other conditions at three centers. It is a program of LifeSpan Services Network, Inc., a private, nonprofit umbrella organization offering a variety of programs in San Luis Obispo County and the Santa Maria Valley. ADCare has provided adult day services since 1985 and holds a prestigious Alzheimer's Day Care Resource Center grant from the state of California. All of its centers incorporate intergenerational activities, including volunteer opportunities for local college and university students.

Alzheimer's Care at Aspen Ridge, Bend, Oregon
Part of a full-service campus, Alzheimer's Care at Aspen Ridge offers 42 units of specialized dementia care. The facility's philosophy is to provide compassionate, individualized care to *persons* with Alzheimer's disease or a related dementia. The life story is central to living that philosophy, providing staff with an opportunity to learn each resident's habits, traditions, and facts about his or her life. The community is divided into three neighborhoods, each complete with a "mom's"-style kitchen and comfortable living spaces. This arrangement helps decrease stressful encounters and facilitates the creation of a personal approach to care.

Alzheimer's Four Seasons, Santa Barbara, California
Alzheimer's Four Seasons is a six-bed dementia-specific facility that was licensed in 1996. The home specializes in making connections with its residents. Massage therapy gives the staff a wonderful way to connect and create bonds not previously observed in residents and staff. Another connection is with a nearby elementary school through a program called "Adopt a Grandparent." The residents go to the school for sing-alongs, plays, and puppet shows. The children come to Four Seasons for games, reading to residents, a ride on the antique fire en-

[1]The program summaries were submitted by the programs themselves and edited by the authors for length. The inclusion of these programs does not reflect an endorsement of either party to the other.

gine, or birthday celebrations. "The goal of our program is to give moms and dads a soft pillow to land on in their dementia days," Dana E. Newquist, owner and administrator, explained.

The Breckinridge, Lexington, Kentucky
The Breckinridge, a licensed personal care facility for *persons* with Alzheimer's disease or a related disorder, is located on a wooded, three-acre lot in a quiet residential neighborhood. One acre is enclosed by a security fence and provides opportunity for walking, gardening, birdwatching, star-gazing, and other outdoor activities. The staff of The Breckinridge think of it as the residents' home, where staff are visitors. Although the facility is proud of the professional credentials of its staff and advisors, the primary qualification for being on staff is having the kind of heart that allows each to be friend, caregiver, and encourager to people who are losing their ability to remember and function independently.

Care Club of Collier County, Inc., Naples, Florida
Care Club was founded in 1991 to provide high-quality day services for *persons* with Alzheimer's disease and other forms of dementia, regardless of their ability to pay. The center is a social-model day program that serves 41 participants 6 days a week. It provides a homelike setting in a safe and stimulating environment. One of the center's goals is to have fun throughout the day. Family caregivers get peace of mind, knowing that their loved ones are safe and well cared for. The beautiful weather in Naples, which is situated on the southwest coast of Florida, makes outdoor activities popular throughout the year, and the abundance of flowers year-round bring joy to all of the residents.

Carilion Adult Day Center, Bedford, Virginia
Carilion Adult Day Center was founded in 1993 with the mission of preventing isolation, maintaining functional and cognitive abilities, and enhancing a sense of well-being for a diverse group of participants, including *persons* with Alzheimer's disease. The center is licensed for 25 participants and averages 14 participants a day. The center takes pride in its high participant and caregiver satisfaction ratings. This rural setting provides an impressive view of the Peaks of Otter, part of the Blue Ridge Mountains.

Carinya Village Nursing Home, Churches of Christ Homes and Community Services, Inc., Perth, Western Australia
Carinya Village Nursing Home is a 44-bed traditional nursing facility. In 1997, an 18-bed dementia-specific unit was established to cater to both ambulatory dementia residents and residents with challenging behaviors. The project aimed to develop a high-quality lifestyle for its residents within a caring community while providing caregivers with the knowledge, skills, and resources required to provide optimum care for *persons* with dementia. An Action Learning Model was employed to encourage ownership of the project by team members. In 1998, the Best Friends approach to Alzheimer's care was adopted as the team's method of care delivery because it seemed to be the most compatible with the team's vision for the unit. The result has been happier, more secure residents and families and greater job satisfaction for staff.

Christian Health Center, Christian Church Homes of Kentucky, Lexington, Kentucky
The Christian Health Center is a 150-bed approved residence offering nursing and skilled care. Private and semiprivate rooms await new residents, and they are encouraged to bring decorative items to personalize their environment. In celebration of each person's gifts, talents, and life, opportunities are provided that promote independence, encourage self-fulfillment,

and maintain personal dignity. A unique feature is a live-in rabbit, which provides many hours of stroking, holding, and caregiving opportunities. The most fun of all is looking for him when he is hiding, probably escaping for a moment of respite.

Christiana Care/Visiting Nurse Association, Evergreen Center I, Alzheimer's Day Treatment Program, Wilmington, Delaware

Evergreen Center began in 1987 in response to the community's need for care for *persons* who have received a diagnosis of Alzheimer's disease or a related dementia. The center serves 24 participants each day. The center provides music therapy, art therapy, sensory stimulation, physical exercise, reminiscence, and a variety of games. "Our specialty revolves around learning the most possible about better ways of relating and communicating with *persons* with failing memories. Friendships are formed as we work and play together, and there is little turnover in staff due in large part to the fun, rewarding days that we all experience together," according to Cheryl T. Weidemeyer, director.

Eden Pines, Lynchburg, Virginia

Eden Pines, which opened in 1999, is an assisted living community with a capacity for 55 residents. It offers a safe and secure place to live and a respite program for families who are caring for *persons* with Alzheimer's disease at home. The caregiving goal at Eden Pines is to keep residents as independent as possible for as long as possible. For residents who require a higher level of care, the community has an extended care wing. Each wing has its own wandering garden that allows the residents to walk freely and safely outdoors and enjoy the flowers, gardening, or just sitting and relaxing.

Encore Senior Living Rediscovery™ Program, Portland, Oregon

Encore Senior Living Rediscovery™ provides three options for residency: congregate with assisted living, traditional assisted living, and assisted living specializing in Alzheimer's care. The last program is known as the Rediscovery Program. Rediscovery trains care specialists to help residents live comfortably with dignity within their own perception of reality. This approach bolsters *persons'* self-worth and creates for them a less frustrating world. Care specialists use redirection, coaching, cueing, and task breakdown methods to maintain *persons'* levels of independence for as long as possible. Noted Delores M. Moyer, senior vice president, "We try to create small victories, one success at a time, through love, empathy, and innovation."

The Fountains Continuum of Care, Inc., Tucson, Arizona

The Fountains, a privately held company based in Arizona, developed and trademarked "The Gardens," a residential-social model of care, including high staff–resident ratios, specialized training programs, and activity-focused care, a departure from the traditional medical model for Alzheimer's care. The Fountains operates The Gardens in nine states. Licensure, as applicable, falls under assisted living guidelines. The main goal is to preserve the dignity of each *person* with dementia while building on their remaining strengths. True to its name, The Gardens features gardening as a therapeutic focal point, including butterfly and vegetable gardens to engage residents in the joys of nurturing and nature.

The Fountainview Center for Alzheimer's Disease, Atlanta, Georgia

The Fountainview Center, Georgia's first Alzheimer's-specific long-term care community, opened in 1995. The goals for this social model of care include specific training for staff in

Alzheimer's care with an emphasis on the use of positive interactions with residents, programs that incorporate the life experiences of the residents into their daily routines, and an environment within the center that maximizes each resident's well-being and dignity. "Our experience as an Alzheimer care provider has been and continues to be a learning experience. We believe in delivering service with a warm heart, a gentle touch, and a friendly smile," according to Kay Lloyd, staff educator.

Friendship Adult Day Care Center, Santa Barbara, California
Friendship Adult Day Care Center was founded in 1976 with a mission to preserve and enrich the quality of life of frail older adults and to provide respite and support for their caregivers. The program is a social model and serves more than 225 older adults in the community. An active horticultural therapy program called Elderflowers has become a small business. The "eldergardeners" create and sell crafts created from their garden. The center is working on a collaborative intergenerational program, GOLD, which is an acronym for "Growing OLD." GOLD members from the center visit children in public schools to foster intergenerational relationships.

Haven Nursing Center, Columbia, Louisiana
Haven Nursing Center is a third-generation family-owned and -operated long-term care facility. It was designed to meet the needs of a rural community by providing home health, hospice, assisted living, skilled care, intermediate care, a dementia unit, and a children's day care center for the employees in a single complex. The dementia unit serves 20 residents and is a social model that emphasizes intergenerational, horticultural, and pet therapy programs. The Best Friends approach seems to be put aside once a month when the residents and the children from the day care center in the same building vie for a bowling trophy. They may cheer on one another, but it is really the "best man or woman" and the "best boy or girl" who wins.

Helping Hand Day Center, Lexington/Bluegrass Chapter of the Alzheimer's Association, Lexington, Kentucky
The Helping Hand Day Center was opened in 1984 and was one of the first dementia-specific day centers in the United States. It soon became a laboratory for learning about high-quality care for *persons* with declining memory. The social model program involves some 150 volunteers, many of whom have the same training as the paid staff. The Best Friends approach to Alzheimer's care was born here as the volunteers realized that not only had they become friends with their participant but they had also become "Best Friends." A unique feature of the program is that visitors often ask the question, "Who is the participant and who is the volunteer?" and sometimes it is difficult to determine.

Heritage Court, The Samarkand Retirement Community, Santa Barbara, California
Heritage Court is a 17-room residential home that is part of The Samarkand Retirement Community in Santa Barbara. It is affiliated with Covenant Retirement Communities of Chicago. The goal of Heritage Court is to provide optimal care in a home environment. Staff and volunteers at the facility are proud to enjoy a close affiliation with the Santa Barbara chapter of the Alzheimer's Association; Heritage Court houses the chapter's Teaching/Learning Center. Through the center, professionals and students from the central coast of California receive training to enhance their skills in dementia care.

The Homestead, Hennis Care Centre of Bolivar, Bolivar, Ohio
The Homestead, a dementia-specific unit of Hennis Care Centre, opened in 2000 and has 18 private rooms. Their philosophy of care is to provide a homelike environment to the residents. For example, the nontraditional nursing station consists of a kitchen table and chairs, where residents are encouraged to sit and interact with staff. Bullet cards with a few important notes about each resident's interests, achievements, preferences, and family histories are available for all staff to read. These brief notes have been beneficial in the development of individually tailored activities, improving the quality of life for residents and increasing staff morale as the result of a positive environment.

Hotel Pawnee, A Retirement Residence, The Urban Group, North Platte, Nebraska
Hotel Pawnee is part of the Urban Group, a long-term care management and development company based in Santa Barbara, California. The administrators established an assisted living program to serve elderly people with mental and physical frailty and adults with cognitive impairment and chronic illness in 1988. Ten years later, an adult day health care program was added. Hotel Pawnee is committed to low-income and Medicaid waver-assistance residents. Residents with Alzheimer's disease are fully integrated into the community. The programs operate as a social model and serve 40 residents in the assisted living program and 6 older adults in the adult day health program. The community enjoys the benefits of housing a diverse population, with unexpected friendships and collaborations emerging when individuals with physical and mental limitations are teamed.

Karrington Cottages, a Sunrise Assisted Living Community, Rochester, Minnesota
Karrington Cottages was designed for five to seven residents to live in an apartment and share a kitchen, living room, and dining room. There are four apartments within a cottage, with common space that includes a porch and enclosed, secure courtyard. There are nine cottages connected by streets or lanes, which provides residents with a sense of living in an old-fashioned small town. Caregivers act as universal workers to assist the residents with doing laundry, preparing meals, and washing dishes, as well as providing meaningful activities and personal care as needed. This is a care-oriented rather than a task-oriented approach, and it provides an environment of friendship and family.

Laurel Heights Home for the Elderly, London, Kentucky
Laurel Heights Home for the Elderly was opened in 1966 to provide a home for London-area older adults who could not continue living at home. The facility provides all levels of care and serves 197 residents, many of whom have some form of dementia. Staff, residents, families, friends, and volunteers enjoy quiet visits and activities in the homelike lobbies, patios, and wheelchair-accessible garden, and appreciate the many plants in the solarium and breezeway. Each resident has a Best Friend who is a staff member from various disciplines such as laundry, the business office, or nursing. These special friendships have helped to transform the facility into a community.

Leena's Home (Leenankoti), Helsinki, Finland
Founded by the Alzheimer's Society of Finland in 1989, Leena's Home is a special care unit for 20 *persons* with dementia. The program's emphasis is to offer short-term stays of 2–4 weeks for *persons* who live with their families. The goal of this service is to maintain the func-

tional capacity of *persons* through good nursing care, provide case management, and improve the quality of life of the caregivers by providing respite. The primary nurses act as resources for the *person* as well as for the family members during ward and home visits. Leena's Home is the first of its kind in Finland and provides valuable data for research into high-quality care for *persons* with dementia.

Legacy St. Aidan's Place Daycare, Portland, Oregon
St. Aidan's Place is a nondenominational, nonprofit, social day center for older adults with memory loss or confusion resulting from Alzheimer's disease and related disorders. The center, staffed by a site coordinator, a program assistant, and a core of well-trained volunteers, is a cooperative effort among Legacy Health Systems, Caregiver Service, and St. Aidan's Episcopal Church with support from the Alzheimer's Association. Serving 12 participants each day, the center offers a wide range of activities to maximize abilities and build self-esteem, with an emphasis on using the arts (music, dance, exercise, poetry, drama, and visual arts) to foster self-expression.

Liberty Commons Assisted Living,
Liberty Healthcare Management Services, Inc., Wilmington, North Carolina
Liberty Commons Assisted Living is a residence that was created expressly for *persons* who do not require nursing facility care but who need more care than that offered by retirement communities. The concept of an assisted living residence was new to coastal North Carolina. Noted Cindy Stancil, director of operations: "It is a special place for individuals who have become insecure or lonely living at home or who have become confused due to a dementing illness. The home promotes a special relationship among staff, family, and residents. This relationship, called Partners in Caring, is a close working association that was designed to help residents live full, enriching, and dignified lives."

Margolic Psychogeriatric Center, Tel Aviv Medical Center, Tel Aviv, Israel
Margolic Psychogeriatric Center provides comprehensive psychogeriatric services to older adults in the Tel Aviv area via a multidisciplinary team. The center offers many programs, including a dementia day program with 55 daily participants. The purpose of the day center is to tap the remaining strengths and abilities of every member, especially the psychosocial abilities of interaction and communication, and to improve self-esteem and well-being. "We believe there is still room to grow and develop despite the many losses in dementia. This process takes place with the supportive therapeutic activities of expressive therapies, cognitive stimulation, and doing activities," stated Debi Lahav, coordinator of activities.

The Olive Branch Senior Care Center, Tallulah, Louisiana
The Olive Branch Senior Care Center has a special care unit that opened in 1998. This special care unit embodies an exciting and innovative concept in long-term care. Through the use of the Best Friends approach and an environment that includes children, plants, and animals, loneliness is replaced with companionship, helplessness with purpose, and boredom with anticipation. The unit serves 22 residents and is designed to promote each resident's remaining abilities. The rural setting allows residents to reminisce about life on the farm as they view the emu, cattle, and horses roaming in the pastures just beyond the enclosed outdoor space.

Omahanui Private Hospital, New Plymouth, New Zealand

Omahanui Private Hospital is a continuing care, extended-stay hospital providing total care for 30 *persons* in the province of Taranaki, New Zealand, on the shores of the Tasman Sea. Care goals at the facility include staff who are knowledgeable in Alzheimer's care and have positive interactions with residents, programs that incorporate the life experience of *persons* into the daily routine, and an environment within the facility that maximizes each resident's social well-being and dignity. "We believe in delivering service with a warm heart, a gentle touch, and a friendly smile. Omahanui is a very special place for very special people," said Patricia Wesley, administrator.

Pinegrove Special Care, Vista del Monte, Santa Barbara, California

Pinegrove, a 10-room special care unit at Vista del Monte retirement community, has invested in around-the-clock creative activities and individualized care. Vista del Monte comes under the umbrella of Internext Corporation, a national nonprofit corporation offering a variety of services across the continuum of care to older adults. Originally built for retired teachers, it is a beautiful campus near the Pacific Ocean with 240 residents in facilities ranging from independent living to skilled care. Special emphasis is placed on fitness; campus residents enjoy the fitness and aquatic center, completed in 1999.

Porterville Senior Day Care, Porterville, California

Porterville Senior Day Care is a "home away from home" for its participants. Staff members are Best Friends who assist one another in this homelike setting. The program works hard to separate the disease from the *person* and learn as much as possible about the *person* behind the disease. Staff remind one another constantly to "put themselves in the shoes of each participant." A unique feature of the program is the staff meetings. Caregivers, staff, volunteers, and members of the community are invited to share in updates on Alzheimer's disease and to learn tips on the "knack" of the Best Friends approach. Porterville is known as "your partner in caregiving."

Riverside Adult Day Program, Christiana Care Health Services, Wilmington, Delaware

Riverside Adult Day Program opened in 1994 and has a census of 19 daily participants with functional limitations, either physical or cognitive or a combination. All *persons* are fully integrated into the program and participate as they are able. The advantage of this small social model is participants' ability to develop close and intimate relationships. The staff and participants work and play together as a family. A participant expressed her love for the program, noting that every day at the program is special for her. Everyone goes out of his or her way to help one another.

St. Basil's Homes, New South Wales, Australia

St. Basil's Homes was incorporated in 1960. This charity endeavors to provide high-quality care to approximately 250 older adults in its nursing facility, hostels, and self-care units. St. Basil's Homes also operates a day center and provides 35 community eldercare packages that cater to older people still living at home. St. Basil's Homes are unique in that they offer care and services to people who are primarily of Greek origin and to elderly mainstream Australians, who are from a diverse range of cultural backgrounds. "We are a happy 'league of nations,' " said Judith Montano, director of care services.

Serenity Nursing Home, Johannesburg, South Africa
Serenity Nursing Home cares for people of all ages. The majority have various kinds of dementia. The residents share the facility on the same basis; there is no separation as a result of medical or other conditions or age. The unique feature is that everyone has a Best Friend, either a staff member or student. A nurse who was a Best Friend to a resident at Serenity commented, "I know my friend likes me. He always shares his chocolates with me. When he wins two at bingo, he gives me one."

Sunshine Terrace Adult Day Center, Logan, Utah
Sunshine Terrace Adult Day Center opened in 1984 and is now one of three programs (nursing facility, adult day center, and assisted living) operated by the Sunshine Terrace Foundation, a nonprofit community-sponsored organization. The average daily attendance is 32. The participants are encouraged to move beyond their impairments to discover or rediscover talents, skills, and interests. The program's design includes weekly themes and provides a continuing education model for frail older adults and adults with developmental disabilities. A major focus of the program is on music therapy. The participants have given concerts at six national conferences, and the bell choir has been featured in *The New York Times.*

Toca das Horttensias, Sao Paulo, Brazil
Associacao Toca das Horttensias was founded in 1995 and maintains a day center and respite care facility (Toca das Horttensias) for elderly *persons* with Alzheimer's disease and related disorders. The day center, a model program, serves 20 *persons,* and the respite program serves 16 *persons.* The day center is the first in Brazil to be dedicated to elderly *persons* with dementia. Many professionals have visited to learn new and innovative methods of care. A feature of both programs is the consistent use of the life story in the daily routine of each *person.*

Villa Alamar, Santa Barbara, California
Established in August 1996, Villa Alamar specializes in caring for *persons* with Alzheimer's disease and other dementias. Its mission is to create a secure, joyful environment for *persons* with Alzheimer's disease. Staff are committed to the dignity of the individual in an environment where their physical, mental, and spiritual needs are met, and their contributions to the lives of staff members are acknowledged every day. One highlight of life at Villa Alamar is the year-round wonderful weather, such that its 31 residents can wander in- and outside the building and in the secured courtyard. Another highlight is the nearby beach, a wonderful place to walk.

Villa Bella Residential Alzheimer's Care Center, Santa Barbara, California
Villa Bella was founded in 1993 as the first dementia-specific residence in Santa Barbara. It was designed specifically to provide a safe environment for its 36 residents. The program's goal is to provide a caring, homelike environment that focuses on residents' physical, social, and safety needs. The facility stresses individualized care plans and encourages its residents to enjoy the beautiful, sunny coastal California climate. Villa Bella has been featured in *People* magazine and mentioned on *Larry King Live* as an outstanding dementia care facility.

The Wealshire, Lincolnshire, Illinois
The Wealshire, located on 20 wooded acres in the Chicago suburb of Lincolnshire, is a unique, freestanding facility built specifically for the needs of *persons* with Alzheimer's disease. It provides a homelike atmosphere, activity-focused care based on individual ability,

and medical care through the facility's medical staff and its affiliation with the Northwestern University Alzheimer's Disease Center. "The home believes that its greatest challenge in dementia care is maintaining an individual's personhood through purposeful activities and socialization. The quality of life of each *person* can be enhanced. We have to fit into their world and not try to force them into ours," commented Carly R. Hellen, director of Alzheimer's care.

Wellington Parc of Owensboro, Owensboro, Kentucky
Wellington Parc opened in 1991. It is an 80-bed long-term care nursing facility designed exclusively for individuals with Alzheimer's disease or related cognitive impairment. Wellington Parc was the first dementia-specific long-term care community to open in Kentucky and has served as a model for many other facilities. Memory boxes located outside each resident's room, enclosed courtyards, and a specialized activity program are just a few of its unique features. Since its opening, Wellington Parc has expanded its services to include an adult day program.

West Park Long Term Care Center, Cody, Wyoming
West Park Long Term Care Center provides skilled and intermediate nursing care and opened a dementia care unit in 2000. All levels of care focus on the quality of life of its nearly 100 residents. The program is part of the West Park Hospital, a nonprofit organization founded in 1940. A beautiful contemporary-style facility built in 1984, West Park provides many rooms with a terrific view of the Rocky Mountains. Cody, a town of approximately 7,500 people, is the gateway to Yellowstone National Park, Grand Teton National Park, and many other sights, and residents take trips to these areas of interest during the summer.

Appendix B

Professionals Featured in *The Best Friends Staff*

Joyce Beedle, R.N., telephone (503) 760-5750
Joyce Beedle received a bachelor of science degree in nursing from the University of Arizona. She is the president of Alzheimer's Consulting Service. Her work regarding developing and/or remodeling Alzheimer's care units and caregiving issues takes her around the Pacific Northwest. Her book, *The Carebook: A Workbook for Caregiver Peace of Mind* (1990, Lady Bug Press, Portland, Oregon), is a resource of relevant information for people who are providing temporary care for *persons* with dementia to give respite to family caregivers.

Cynthia Belle, telephone (708) 771-6114
Cynthia Belle received her bachelor of arts degree from Loyola University in Chicago. A former teacher, she has spent 22 years working in long-term care; she has worked in dementia care since 1985. Cynthia teaches a 20-hour activity-focused care course for health professionals at all levels, with an emphasis on CNAs. She noted, "My love for training CNAs comes from what they have taught me." Belle also trains family, clergy, and other professionals in the basics of Alzheimer's care. She has developed professional curricula and has contributed to a number of publications in the field.

Susan D. Berry, M.S.
Susan Berry has degrees in therapeutic recreation and human development and gerontology. She has been a director of therapeutic recreation in numerous nursing facilities and psychiatric hospitals and was the director for Wesley Hall, one of the first Alzheimer's care units in the United States. Susan worked as the training coordinator for the Wisconsin Alzheimer's Information and Training Center and as a contracted trainer for the Alzheimer's Association of Southwest Michigan and Gerontology Network. She now provides private consultations and training and lives in Warsaw, Indiana.

Linda Blair, M.S.S.W., email Lblair@dcr.net
Linda Blair began her work in bereavement care at Hospice of the Bluegrass, Lexington, Kentucky, as a grief counselor and bereavement support group leader. She holds certification as a bereavement facilitator with specialized training in critical incident stress management and debriefing and prenatal loss grief care. Linda divides her time between individual and group

grief counseling and lecturing on grief issues. She teaches a biannual class entitled "When We Lose Our Friends" for volunteers and staff in the Helping Hand Day Center of the Lexington/ Bluegrass chapter of the Alzheimer's Association.

Elizabeth C. Brawley, A.S.I.D., I.I.D.A., email betsybrawley@attglobal.net
Betsy Brawley is president of Design Concepts Unlimited, an interior design firm specializing in long-term care and Alzheimer's special care. She is a past member of the National Board of Directors of the Alzheimer's Association and has been active in defining policy issues affecting older adults at state, national, and international levels. She is a frequent contributor to research and professional publications and is the author of the seminal book *Designing for Alzheimer's Disease: Strategies for Creating Better Care Environments* (1997, John Wiley & Sons, New York). Her web site is www.betsybrawley.com.

Carole A. Bromgard, M.A., email wcbromgard@msn.com
Carole Bromgard is a licensed professional counselor for the state of Colorado. She is the manager of a special care center for Alzheimer's residents at a Brighton Gardens Community in Lakewood, Colorado. Carole was formerly the owner of Family Elder Care Counseling, working with *persons* with Alzheimer's disease and their families. She is active as a part of the speaker's bureau and as a support group leader in the Rocky Mountain chapter of the Alzheimer's Association.

Dee Carlson, M.A., email carlbalm@comcast.net
Dee Carlson has specialized in the field of Alzheimer's disease and related dementias since 1990. She was formerly the director of Education and Family Services for the Mayo Clinic Alzheimer's Disease Center in Rochester, Minnesota. In 1996 she launched her own company, Alzheimer's Care: Consultation, Education & Training, Inc. (ACCET). ACCET offers assistance in developing, enhancing, or evaluating dementia care services, provides intensive training courses for caregivers, and gives numerous presentations at local, regional, and national conferences.

Leslie Congleton, telephone (503) 413-7032
Leslie Congleton holds a graduate certificate in gerontology and has 15 years of experience in the field of aging, with a particular interest in the design and development of creative and meaningful activities for *persons* with dementia. She is curator of "Kaleidoscope," a 23-piece traveling exhibit featuring the artwork of individuals with Alzheimer's disease. This exhibit inspires and educates audiences about the potential of *persons* with dementia. In addition to providing caregiver education programs, Leslie is program coordinator for Legacy Health Systems' Trinity Place Alzheimer's Day Respite Program in Portland, Oregon.

Barbara Susan Dicker, M.Ed., R.N., email Barbara.Dicker@cocwa.asn.au
Barbara Susan Dicker is a gerontological nurse practitioner employed in the residential aged sector in Perth, Western Australia, as a clinical nurse specialist/staff development consultant. She has actively promoted best practices in the area of case management, dementia care, and preventive care. Sue coordinated the Med-Smart Project, a medication-related education and counseling service for well seniors as well as the Dementia Care Communication Assistants course, both funded by the Commonwealth. Since 1997, she has acted as team facilitator of the Action Learning Project with goals to create a caring community and a high-quality lifestyle for staff and residents of a dementia-specific unit within a conventional nursing facility in Perth.

Deborah Dunn, M.F.T., email maryoakleyfndtnliaison@cox.net
Deborah Dunn is director of patient & family services for the Santa Barbara (California) chapter of the Alzheimer's Association. She counsels families and develops programs that support caregivers and *persons* with Alzheimer's disease. Before coming to the Alzheimer's Association, she was family counselor at the Friendship Adult Day Care Center, which is also spotlighted in this book. Her special interests include early-stage dementia and multicultural outreach. She heads a program called Juntos de la Mano, an outreach effort to Latino long-term care workers in Santa Barbara County.

Mynga Futrell, Ph.D., email instrnSys@aol.com
Mynga Futrell is a writer and curriculum developer. Her work includes coauthoring a college textbook for computer education (*Teachers, Computers, and Curriculum: Microcomputers in the Classroom,* 1999, Allyn & Bacon, Boston) and a manual for social studies teachers on nonconformist thinkers in history (*Different Drummers: Nonconforming Thinkers in History,* 1999, Tafford Publications, Victoria, British Columbia, Canada). Mynga began caring for her mother, who had Alzheimer's disease, in 1994. To help her friends and neighbors better understand the disease and continue their relationships with her mother, she developed a pamphlet, *What to Do When Your Friend or Neighbor Has Alzheimer's.* Mynga also developed booklets about her mother's life to help others reminisce with her.

Meredith Gresham, OT, email MDGresham@aol.com
Meredith Gresham coordinated and developed the internationally acclaimed Dementia Carers Training Programme with Professor Henry Brodaty at Prince Henry Hospital, Sydney, Australia, and has been active in the Alzheimer's Association of New South Wales (NSW). She has been responsible for the development and presentation of many dementia training sessions throughout Australia and overseas. Meredith has contributed to a number of publications in Australian and international journals and is a contributing author to numerous books. She is part of a team that is updating curricula in mental health and aging at NSW Institute of Psychiatry, Charles Sturt University. Meredith and her family moved to Avon, Connecticut, in 2000.

Lisa Gwyther, M.S.W., email lpg@geri.duke.edu
Lisa Gwyther is a widely known author, educator, researcher, and clinical social worker with 29 years of experience in aging and Alzheimer's services. She started and directs the Duke University Medical Center's Alzheimer's Family Support Program and also directs education for the Joseph and Kathleen Bryan Alzheimer's Disease Research Center, also at DUMC. She is revising her best-known book *Care of Alzheimer's Patients: A Manual for Nursing Home Staff* (see Appendix C). Lisa has received numerous awards for her outstanding work in dementia care.

Carly R. Hellen, OTR/L, email carlyhellen@yahoo.com
Carly Hellen is director of Alzheimer's care at The Wealshire in Lincolnshire, Illinois. She developed and is responsible for activity-based programming for residents in all stages of Alzheimer's disease. She is the author of *Alzheimer's Disease: Activity Focused Care* (second edition, 1998, Butterworth-Heinemann, Woburn, MA), a comprehensive manual providing practical and innovative strategies, interventions, and guidelines for professionals and family caregivers. Carly has authored numerous articles and book chapters and is a frequent presenter at Alzheimer's Association conferences.

Robin Hamon Kern, M.S.W., email robin.hamon@uky.edu
Robin Hamon Kern began working with *persons* with Alzheimer's disease as a student in 1989 and, after graduate school, became program manager of the Helping Hand Day Center program operated by the Lexington/Bluegrass chapter of the Alzheimer's Association. While working at the Alzheimer's Association, she developed a creative art training program, Hands and Hearts for Arts, designed to train staff and caregivers to use creative arts projects with *persons* with dementia. She is the family support coordinator for the Alzheimer's Disease Research Center at the University of Kentucky.

Kathy Laurenhue, M.A., email laurenhue@msn.com
Kathy Laurenhue, an international trainer and consultant and curriculum developer, is president of Better Directions, Inc., a multimedia training company that emphasizes a practical and lighthearted approach to Alzheimer's care. She was the author/editor for many years of *Wiser Now,* a monthly international newsletter for caregivers of people with Alzheimer's disease. She also was a producer and chief writer of *Best Practices in Assisted Living,* a 36-part video training series available from Primedia Workplace Learning.

Cindy Lynch, Ph.D.
Cindy Lynch built on her knowledge of adult development as she studied ways to help people deal with problems more effectively. She consulted with educators, researchers, and practitioners in a wide variety of professions. Her grandmother's struggles with dementia inspired her to apply her work to professional problem solving in dementia care. For example, she worked with Carolyn Read, a reading specialist, on an innovative Alzheimer's reading aloud project. In 2002, Cindy was killed in an automobile accident. She will be remembered for her excellent work.

Debbie McConnell, M.A., email kelco5@aol.com
Debbie McConnell is director of education for the Santa Barbara (California) chapter of the Alzheimer's Association and has worked in dementia care since 1990. She has worked in a variety of settings, including day services, university, and senior center programs. Her areas of interest include curriculum development, staff training, spirituality and aging, and program development. She heads a teaching/learning center that represents a collaboration between a nonprofit Alzheimer's Association chapter and a continuing care retirement community, The Samarkand.

Briana Melom, L.S.W., email Melom.Briana@mayo.edu
Briana Melom is a licensed social worker and director of education and family services at the Mayo Clinic Alzheimer's Disease Center, Rochester, Minnesota. She provides numerous educational opportunities for professional and family caregivers and facilitates support groups for *persons* with Alzheimer's disease and their families. Briana previously worked as a direct caregiver on the night shift at a dementia-specific assisted living facility where she later served as the admissions and education coordinator.

Alyce E. Parsons, telephone (805) 564-3341
As director of operations for Parsons House and The Urban Group (a provider of senior housing and assisted living services in three states), Alyce Parsons manages the marketing and day-to-day operations. She is an RCFE Licensed Administrator, a founding member of the Assisted Living Federation of America (ALFA), and holds a Bachelor of Arts degree from the

University of California, Berkeley. She is well studied in the field of therapeutic architectural design, and therefore understands the crucial role a project's design plays in creating a therapeutic environment. Her passion is the basis of the company's mission to serve older adults, offer unconditional love, nurture personal growth, and celebrate life to make a difference.

Robert E. Parsons, telephone (805) 564-3341
Robert Parsons is chairman and CEO of Parsons House and The Urban Group, a provider of senior housing and assisted living services in three states. He is a graduate of the University of California, Berkeley. In 1978, he became a founding partner of Armstrong Parsons Investment Real Estate. As the result of Armstrong Parsons's acquisition, The Urban Group was born in 1984. It provides affordable service-enhanced senior housing. Parsons House, LLC, was formed in 1997, adding market rate, service-oriented assisted living and Alzheimer's facilities to the services provided. The web site is www.parsonsgroupinc.com.

Susan Peters Rachal, M.Ed.
Susan Peters Rachal is a faculty member in gerontology education at the University of Louisiana at Monroe, Monroe, Louisiana. She has served on the Governor's Task Force on Alzheimer's Disease and Related Disorders and chaired the Special Needs Committee, which entailed conducting a statewide survey for caregivers that has been published and presented to Louisiana's governor and legislature. She also is a consultant for special care units in nursing facilities and assisted living environments and designed the programs at the Haven Nursing Center and The Olive Branch Senior Care Center.

Joanne Rader, R.N., M.N., FAAN, email joanne.rader@worldnet.att.net
Joanne Rader is an associate professor at Oregon Health Sciences University School of Nursing and is an independent consultant. She developed strategies to help nursing facilities reduce the use of physical restraints and inappropriate medications. She is involved in a research study to reduce the aggressive behaviors during bathing of *persons* with dementia under a grant from the National Institute for Nursing Research. She worked as a nurse in nursing facilities for more than 25 years. She coauthored the book *Individualized Dementia Care: Creative, Compassionate Approaches* (1995, Springer Publishing, New York).

Carolyn Read, Ph.D., email Cread3425@aol.com
Carolyn Read is a reading specialist, published poet, writer, and retired educator. She is the grant recipient for an innovative research project called Reading Aloud with Alzheimer's-Like Dementia Women. Working with Cindy Lynch, she designed the project to help dispel the insidious perception that elderly people, especially those with dementia, are voiceless and disposable. This project has the potential to provide a meaningful activity for *persons* with dementia. A graduate of the University of Denver, Carolyn lives and works in Colorado.

Lynn Ritter, Ph.D., email www.alzheimersNWO@msn.com
Lynn Ritter was employed for 11 years in a long-term care facility where she held the positions of activities coordinator and director of the facility's Alzheimer's special care unit, the first such unit in northwest Ohio. She also has been an adjunct faculty member at Bowling Green State University, Lourdes College, and Owens College, where she taught classes in the gerontology departments. Lynn has given presentations at local, state, regional, and national conferences. She is the professional education coordinator for the Alzheimer's Association, Northwest Ohio chapter.

Beverly Sanborn, L.C.S.W., email bwsanborn@cox.net
Beverly Sanborn is director of Alzheimer's field services for the Marriott Corporation Senior Living Services, Washington, D.C. She has more than 10 years of experience in the design and implementation of programs for *persons* with dementia, with a specialization in activity-based behavior management. Her work spans the continuum of care: adult day services, assisted living, skilled nursing, in-home companion, and other community-based services. She gives lectures and workshops throughout the United States and has authored and coauthored books and papers on dementia.

Vicki L. Schmall, Ph.D., email vschmall@comcast.net
Vicki Schmall is gerontology and training specialist/executive director of Aging Concerns, West Linn, Oregon, and professor emeritus at Oregon State University. She is widely known for her development of many aging- and caregiver-related educational materials and training programs for professionals, families, and older adults. Vicki has been active on the board of directors of the Oregon Trails chapter of the Alzheimer's Association from its inception. She coauthored the book *Taking Care of You: Powerful Tools for Caregiving* (2000, Legacy Health Care, Portland, Oregon).

Dorothy Seman, R.N., M.S., N.H.A., email dorothy.seaman@va.gov
Dorothy Seman has worked in health care in a variety of roles and settings for more than 30 years. She has served as clinical coordinator of the Alzheimer's Family Care Center in Chicago since 1986, which is affiliated with Rush-Presbyterian's Alzheimer's Disease Center. Dorothy also works for the VA Chicago Health Care System West Side Division, a medical center of the Department of Veterans Affairs. She gives numerous presentations every year and was the coauthor (with Sam Fazio and Jane Stansell) of *Rethinking Alzheimer's Care* (1999, Health Professions Press, Baltimore).

Marie B. Smart, L.S.W., telephone (859) 323-6729
Marie B. Smart began her work in the field of aging in 1982 at a state-funded home care program funded by the Area Agency on Aging in Kentucky. In 1988, she became family counselor at the Alzheimer's Disease Research Center, University of Kentucky, and is the Alzheimer's care specialist at The Breckinridge, a freestanding dementia personal care community. Marie has a special interest in support and education for family caregivers. She volunteers for the Lexington/Bluegrass chapter of the Alzheimer's Association as part of its Patient and Family Services Committee.

Beth Spencer, M.A., M.S.W., email spencer@smtp.munet.edu
Beth Spencer is assistant professor of gerontology at Madonna University, Livonia, Michigan, where she developed an undergraduate certificate in dementia care. She is the coauthor of *Understanding Difficult Behavior* (1996, Eastern Michigan University Press, Ypsilanti) and author of several articles on family caregiving. After many years of training and consulting in long-term care settings, Beth is coauthoring a training manual on dementia care for residential care staff (see Appendix C). She is a frequent presenter in regional and national conferences on many aspects of Alzheimer's disease care.

Virginia M. Sponsler, L.C.S.W.
Virginia M. Sponsler began her social work career in hospitals, where she was introduced to the world of Alzheimer's disease. She taught at California State University at Sacramento and

Portland State University. She is a counselor in private practice in Portland, Oregon, specializing in relationship, life stage, and family life issues, and is a teacher, consultant, and trainer. She also has taught courses for long-term staff working in dementia care in Oregon.

Tonya M. Tincher, M.S.W., email tonya.cox@alz.org
Tonya Tincher became the coordinator of the Helping Hand Day Center, Lexington/Bluegrass chapter of the Alzheimer's Association, in 1995. Later she was the program manager of the Helping Hand respite program, which includes the day center and in-home care. She is chapter programs director for the Lexington/Bluegrass chapter of the Alzheimer's Association. Tonya is active in many chapter activities, including serving on the Patient and Family Services Committee of the Alzheimer's Board. She leads workshops on Alzheimer's care locally and nationally.

Jitka M. Zgola, OT, email giverny@ns.sympatico.ca
Jitka Zgola is an occupational therapist with 20 years of experience in dementia care with clients, professionals, and family caregivers in direct service and administration. She provides teaching and consultation in dementia to agencies and professional groups throughout Canada, the United States, and Europe. She is the author of two books from The Johns Hopkins University Press: *Doing Things: A Guide to Programming Activities for Persons with Alzheimer's Disease and Related Disorders* (1987) and *Care That Works: A Relational Approach to Persons with Dementia* (1999), and is the author of *Bon Appetit! The Joy of Dining in Long-Term Care* (Health Professions Press).

Appendix C

Suggested Resources for Trainers

Books and Manuals

Alzheimer's Association. (1995). *Activity programming for persons with dementia: A sourcebook.* Chicago: Author.

Alzheimer's Association. (1995). *Terms and tips: An Alzheimer's care handbook* (Publication No. PF303 Z). Chicago: Author.

Alzheimer's Association. (1997). *Key elements of dementia care.* Chicago: Author.

Alzheimer's Association. (1999). *Family guide for Alzheimer's care in residential settings.* Chicago: Author.

Anderson, M., Beaver, K., & Culliton, K. (Eds.). (1996). *The long-term care nursing assistant training manual* (2nd ed.). Baltimore: Health Professions Press.

Andresen, G. (1995). *Caring for people with Alzheimer's disease: A training manual for direct care providers.* Baltimore: Health Professions Press.

Arizona Long-Term Care Gerontology Center. 1990. *Alzheimer's disease: Pieces of the puzzle. A training program for direct service staff.* Tucson: Author.

Assisted Living University. (1997). *Assisted living training system: Alzheimer's care for assisted living.* Oakton, VA: Author. (10206 Oakton Station Court, Oakton, VA 22124, telephone 800-258-7030.)

Avadian, B. (1999). *Where's my shoes? My father's walk through Alzheimer's.* Lancaster, CA: Northstar Books.

Beedle, J. (1990). *The carebook: A workbook for caregiver peace of mind.* Portland, OR: Lady Bug Press.

Bell, V., & Troxel, D. (1997). *The best friends approach to Alzheimer's care.* Baltimore: Health Professions Press.

Berman, K. (Ed.). (1996). *Friendship.* Kansas City: Ariel Books/Andrews & McMeel.

Brawley, E. (1997). *Designing for Alzheimer's disease: Strategies for creating better care environments.* New York: John Wiley & Sons.

Bridges, B. (1995). *Therapeutic caregiving: A practical guide for caregivers of persons with Alzheimer's and other dementia causing diseases.* Mill Creek, WA: BJB Publishing.

Castleman, M., Gallagher-Thompson, D., & Naythons, M. (1999). *There's still a person in there: The complete guide to treating and coping with Alzheimer's.* New York: Putnam.

Cohen, U., & Weisman, G. (1991). *Holding on to home: Designing environments for people with dementia.* Baltimore: The Johns Hopkins University Press.

Davies, H.D., & Jensen, M.P. (1998). *Alzheimer's: The answers you need.* Forest Knolls, CA: Elder Books.

Davis, R. (1989). *My journey into Alzheimer's disease.* Wheaton, IL: Tyndale House.

Fagan, M.F., William, C.W., & Burger, S.G. (1997). Meeting of Pioneers in Nursing Home Culture Change. (Available from Lifespan of Greater Rochester, Rochester, NY. Telephone 716-454-3224, extension 115.)

Fazio, S., Seman, D., & Stansell, J. (1999). *Rethinking Alzheimer's care.* Baltimore: Health Professions Press.

Gwyther, L. (1985). *Care of Alzheimer's patients: A manual for nursing home staff.* Chicago: American Health Care Association and Alzheimer's Association.

Gwyther, L. (1995). *You are one of us: Successful clergy/church connections.* Durham, NC: Duke University Center for Aging's Alzheimer's Family Support Program, Duke University Medical Center.

Hellen, C.R. (1998). *Alzheimer's disease: Activity-focused care* (2nd ed.). Woburn, MA: Butterworth-Heinemann.

Keating, K. (1983). *The hug therapy book.* Rochester, MN: Hazelden Educational Materials.

Kitwood, T. (1997). *Dementia reconsidered.* Birmingham, U.K.: Open University Press.

Kitwood, T., & Bredin, K. (1992). *Person to person: A guide to the care of those with failing mental powers.* Loughton, U.K.: Gale Centre Publications.

Kuhn, D., & Bennett, D. (1999). *Alzheimer's early stages: First steps in caring and treatment.* Alameda, CA: Hunter House.

Lustbader, W. (1992). *Counting on kindness: The dilemmas of dependency.* New York: The Free Press.

Lustbader W., & Hooyman, N.R. (1994). *Taking care of aging family members: A practical guide.* New York: The Free Press.

Mace, N.L., & Rabins, P.V. (1999). *The 36-hour day: A family guide to caring for persons with Alzheimer's disease, related dementing illnesses, and memory loss in later life* (3rd ed.). Baltimore: The Johns Hopkins University Press.

Meyer, M., & Derr, P. (1998). *The comfort of home: An illustrated step-by-step guide for caregivers.* Portland, OR: CareTrust Publications.

Montgomery, R., Karner, T., Schaefer, J., et al. (1999). *Resources for serving caregivers in culturally diverse communities.* Lawrence, KS: Health Resources & Services Administration.

Murphy, B. (1995). *He used to be somebody: A journey into Alzheimer's disease through the eyes of a caregiver.* Boulder, CO: Gibbs Associates.

Newstrom, J., & Scannell, E. (1989). *Games trainers play.* New York: McGraw-Hill.

Nilson, C. (1993). *Team games for trainers.* New York: McGraw-Hill.

Post, S. (2000). *The moral challenge of Alzheimer's disease: Ethical issues from diagnosis to dying* (2nd ed.). Baltimore: The Johns Hopkins University Press.

Rader, J. (1995). *Individualized dementia care: Creative, compassionate approaches.* New York: Springer Publishing.

Robinson, A., Spencer, B., & White, L. (1996). *Understanding difficult behaviors.* Ypsilanti: Eastern Michigan University.

Roche, L. (1996). *Coping and caring: Daily reflections for Alzheimer's caregivers.* Forest Knolls, CA: Elder Books.

Rose, L. (1996). *Show me the way to go home.* Forest Knolls, CA: Elder Books.

Schmall, V. (2000). *Taking care of you: Powerful tools for caregiving.* Portland, OR: Legacy Health Care.

Smith, B., Knudson, L., & Bennett, M. (1995). *A song to set me free: A model for music therapy and music-related activities for frail elderly and disabled adults.* Logan, UT: Sunshine Terrace Adult Day Center.

Snyder, L. (2000). *Speaking our minds: Personal reflections from individuals with Alzheimer's.* New York: W.H. Freeman.

Spencer, B., & Robinson, A. (2001). *Developing meaningful connection with people with dementia: A training manual.* Ypsilanti: Eastern Michigan University.

Stehman, J. (Ed.). (1996). *Handbook of dementia care.* Baltimore: The Johns Hopkins University Press.

Tideiksaar, R. (1998). *Falls in older persons: Prevention & management* (2nd ed.). Baltimore: Health Professions Press.

Valle, R. (1998). *Caregiving across cultures: Working with dementing illness and ethnically diverse populations.* Bristol, PA: Taylor & Francis.

Yale, R. (1995). *Developing support groups for individuals with early-stage Alzheimer's disease: Planning, implementation, and evaluation.* Baltimore: Health Professions Press.

Zgola, J. (1999). *Care that works: A relationship approach to persons with dementia.* Baltimore: The Johns Hopkins University Press.

Videos

Alzheimer's Association. (1995). *Alzheimer's disease: Inside looking. Twenty-two points, plus triple-word-score, plus fifty points for using all my letters. Game's over. I'm outta here.* Cleveland: Author.

Alzheimer's disease: At the time of diagnosis. (1996). (Available from Time-Life Medical Video, 800-950-7887.)

The Arizona Long-Term Care Gerontology Center. 1990. *Alzheimer's disease: Pieces of the puzzle.* Tucson.

A thousand tomorrows: Intimacy, sexuality and Alzheimer's. (1995). (Distributed by Terra Nova Films, 9848 S.Winchester Avenue, Chicago, IL 60643.)

Dress him while he walks: Behavior management in caring for residents with Alzheimer's disease. (Distributed by Terra Nova Films, 9848 S. Winchester Avenue, Chicago, IL 60643.)

Educational Media Services, Duke University. (1998). *From here to hope: The stages of Alzheimer's disease final, middle, and early.* (Available at 919-684-3748.)

Glaxo Wellcome. (1996). *Alzheimer's disease: Let's talk about it.* (Available at 800-824-2869.)

Helping Hand Day Center. (1991). *Best friends.* Baltimore: Health Professions Press.

Hoffman, D. (1996). *Complaints of a dutiful daughter.* (Available from Women Make Movies, Inc., 462 Broadway, Suite 500, New York, NY 10013. Telephone 212-925-0606 or email orders@wmm.com.)

Joseph & Kathleen Bryan Alzheimer's Disease Research Center. (1992). *Early onset memory loss: A conversation with Letty Tennis.* Durham, NC: Duke University.

Philogenesis Productions & Friendship Center. (1996). *My challenge with Alzheimer's disease.* (Distributed by Terra Nova Films, 9848 S. Winchester Avenue, Chicago, IL 60643.)

Primedia Workplace Learning. (1999). *Best practices in assisted living.* (Available at www.assistedliving.pwpl.com.)

Associations and Other Resources

Alzheimer's Association
919 North Michigan Avenue, Suite 1100
Chicago, IL 60611-1676
Telephone: (800) 272-3900
Website: www.alz.org

All Best Friends programs should establish a relationship with the local chapter of the Alzheimer's Association. Chapter services include newsletters (national and local), support groups, education and training, and advocacy. The national association has excellent publications and sponsors an annual national conference with a strong emphasis on long-term care. The association's Greenfield Library is highly regarded and can be accessed through the website.

Alzheimer's Disease Education & Referral Center (ADEAR)
Telephone: (800) 438-4380
Website: www.alzheimers.org

ADEAR is a clearinghouse sponsored by the National Institute on Aging with a quarterly newsletter, *Connections,* and other helpful publications.

Alzheimer's Disease International (ADI)
Website: www.alz.co.uk/

Alzheimer's Disease International is charged with supporting services for patients and families throughout the world; it sponsors excellent conferences that are held in a different country each year.

Alzheimer's Society Canada
Website: www.alzheimer.ca

Alzheimer's Society Canada is a nonprofit organization that works with regional associations to provide family support, education, advocacy and support for research.

American Association of Homes and Services for the Aging (AAHSA)
Telephone: (202) 783-2242
Website: www.aahsa.org

AAHSA represents the nonprofit long-term care communities in the United States.

American Society on Aging (ASA)
833 Market Street, Suite 511
San Francisco, CA 94103
Website: www.asaging.org
ASA is a national membership organization with excellent training programs and publications.

Assisted Living Federation of America (ALFA)
Telephone: (703) 691-8100
Website: www.alfa.org

ALFA represents the growing numbers of assisted living facilities in the United States.

National Association of Professional Geriatric Care Managers
Telephone: (520) 881-8008
Website: www.caremanager.org

Represents the social workers, nurses, and others who provide professional consultation to caregivers and people needing assistance with long-term care issues and financial management.

Pioneer Network
79 Clinton Avenue
Rochester, NY 14604
Telephone: (716) 464-3224 (extension 115)
Website: www.pioneernetwork.net

(From their website) "The Pioneer Network is a grassroots social movement to change the culture of aging for the 21st century. It is shaped and sustained by the work, interest, and support of a broad community of stakeholders in long-term care. We are an inclusive movement, gathering and sharing the best work in the field."

Journals and Newsletters

American Journal of Alzheimer's Disease and Other Dementias—bimonthly publication with academic articles on research, treatment, and practice; view online at www.alzheimersjournal.com

Early Alzheimer's: A Forum for Early-Stage Dementia Care—a quarterly newsletter concerning early-stage issues published by the Santa Barbara (California) chapter of the Alzheimer's Association, 2024 De la Vina Street, Santa Barbara, 93105. Subscription $55/year, (805) 563-0020

Perspectives: A Newsletter for Individuals Diagnosed with Alzheimer's Disease—a quarterly newsletter written for *persons* with early-stage dementia, published by Lisa Snyder, University of California–San Diego Alzheimer's Research Center, 9800 Gilman Drive, La Jolla, 92093. Subscription $24/year, (619) 622-5800

Web site

www.bestfriendsapproach.com

Index

Page numbers followed by "f" indicate figures.

Virginia Bell, M.S.W., enjoys an international reputation for her unique sensitivity to people with Alzheimer's disease. She has challenged many people to rethink their approaches to dementia care, most directly through her development of the Helping Hand Adult Day Center, sponsored by the Lexington/Bluegrass chapter of the Alzheimer's Association in Lexington, Kentucky. The Center was one of the first dementia-specific adult day programs established in the United States and remains one of the best. Ms. Bell was co-funded with David Troxel in the establishment of the Center by the Robert Wood Johnson Foundation's "Dementia Care and Respite Services" program, the first major initiative to evaluate and encourage the expansion of adult day services in the United States. Ms. Bell served for many years as organizer for the Center's volunteer training program and continues today as a program consultant. She also serves on the advisory board for the Lexington/Bluegrass chapter of the Alzheimer's Association.

Ms. Bell received her Master's in Social Work in 1982 at age 60. While pursuing her degree, she worked as a practicum student at the Sanders-Brown Center on Aging at the University of Kentucky and emerged with an interest in Alzheimer's disease, and specifically in how to help people with Alzheimer's disease and their caregivers. She worked as a family counselor at the Center on Aging, and in 1984 founded the Helping Hand Adult Day Center in her hometown of Lexington. She received the National Council on Aging's prestigious Ruth Von Behren Award for program excellence in 1994 for her work at Helping Hand.

Virginia Bell played a leading role in establishing a network of aging services throughout Kentucky. She has served on two Kentucky Governor's Task Forces studying Alzheimer's care and service delivery, and she was honored for this work with the University of Kentucky's Leadership Award in 1996. Her programs established at the Lexington/Bluegrass Alzheimer's Association for people with Alzheimer's disease and their families won four consecutive first-place awards from the national Alzheimer's Association in the late 1980s. In 1999, her ongoing efforts to improve the lives of older adults were recognized by the American Society on Aging with their Senior Award, presented to a member who exemplifies the abilities of people ages 65 and older and the contributions they can make to society.

A frequent and popular speaker in the field of aging, Ms. Bell's influence extends globally as she has been either a speaker or has served on the planning committee for the annual conference of Alzheimer's Disease International for more than a decade. Her writings have received widespread acclaim for their positive approach to caregiving and staff training. Her philosophy, as expressed in her books, her worldwide lectures, and the Alzheimer's Disease Bill of Rights (co-authored with David Troxel, which since its publication in 1995 has been extensively reprinted and translated into a dozen languages), serves as a touchstone for Alzheimer's care programs around the world.

Ms. Bell can be reached by email: BestFriendsVBell@aol.com.

David Troxel, M.P.H., is a recognized expert on the subject of best practices in Alzheimer's care and is a popular keynote speaker at conferences on Alzheimer's disease or aging services. He began his work in Alzheimer's disease in 1986 at the University of Kentucky Sanders-Brown Center on Aging, then one of only 10 federally funded Alzheimer's disease research centers. Along with Virginia Bell and others, he established a statewide network of support groups and services for Kentuckians with Alzheimer's disease and their caregivers. He was the first executive director of the Lexington/Bluegrass chapter of the Alzheimer's Association and, together with Virginia Bell, won an unprecedented four Excellence in Program Awards for patient and family services, the annual award given to local Alzheimer's Association chapters by the national association.

In 1990, Mr. Troxel became Executive Director of the senior service organization Alzheimer's Disease Care of San Luis Obispo, which ran adult day services programs, support groups, and a resource center for caregivers and people with Alzheimer's disease. From 1994 to 2004, he was Executive Director of the Santa Barbara chapter of the Alzheimer's Association. He is currently a long-term care consultant and writer.

After receiving his Master's in Public Health in 1986 from the University of Medicine and Dentistry of New Jersey (formerly Rutgers Medical School), Mr. Troxel became an active member of the American Public Health Association. He has served as a leader on the APHA action board since 1994, and in 1998 he received the APHA's Sarah Mazelis Award for outstanding practice in health education. He also serves on the Ethics Advisory panel of the national Alzheimer's Association.

Mr. Troxel has written and lectured nationally and internationally about Alzheimer's disease and Alzheimer's care. He is Associate Editor for *Early Alzheimer's,* an international newsletter sponsored by the Santa Barbara chapter of the Alzheimer's Association. Through his books and lectures, Mr. Troxel has inspired professionals around the world to start making sorely needed changes in the culture of care for the millions of people living with Alzheimer's disease.

Mr. Troxel can be reached by email: BestFriendsDavid@aol.com.

Build Your Best Friends™ Program with This Valuable Collection of Resources

Yes! Please send me the following:

(prices are subject to change without notice and may be higher outside the U.S.)

___ copies of **The Best Friends Approach to Alzheimer's Care** at $29.95 each $______

___ copies of **The Best Friends Staff** at $41.95 each $______

___ copies of **The Best Friends Book of Alzheimer's Activities, Volume One** at $36.95 each $______

___ copies of **The Best Friends Book of Alzheimer's Activities, Volume Two** at $36.95 each $______

___ copies of **Los Mejores Amigos en el Cuidado de Alzheimer** at $29.95 each $______

___ copies of **Best Friends** DVD at $54.95 each $______

Shipping & Handling:

For pretax total of	Add
$0.00 to $55.00	$6.49
$55.01 and over	12% of product total

For purchases outside of the continental U.S., call 410-337-9585 for shipping rates.

Subtotal $______

MD residents, add 6% sales tax $______

Shipping & Handling (see chart at left) $______

Total (in US $) $______

☐ Check or money order enclosed (payable to Health Professions Press)

☐ Mastercard ☐ Visa ☐ American Express ☐ Discover

Card No. ______________ Exp. Date ______________

Signature ______________

Name ______________ Daytime Ph. ______________

Title ______________

Organization ______________

Street Address ______________

(Orders cannot be shipped to P.O. Boxes) Check one: ☐ residential address ☐ commercial address

City/State/ZIP ______________

Email Address ______________

(Your email address will not be shared with any other party.)

☐ I want to receive e-mail notice of new products and special offers.

☐ Please send me a copy of your current catalog.

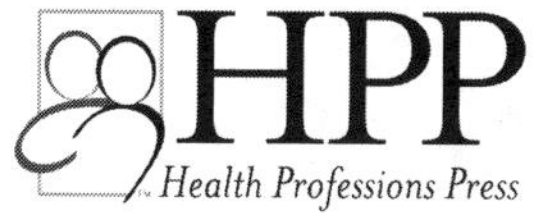

Health Professions Press
P.O. Box 10624, Baltimore, MD 21285-0624
Toll-Free: (888) 337-8808 • Fax: (410) 337-8539
www.healthpropress.com

List Code: ZBFS2